A SYNOPSIS OF REGIONAL ANATOMY

Johnston's Synopsis of
REGIONAL ANATOMY
A Revision Textbook

Tenth Edition

Revised and Edited by

ROGER WARWICK

B.Sc., Ph.D., M.D.

Professor of Anatomy, University of London,
(Director of the Department of Anatomy, Guy's Hospital Medical School)
Examiner in Anatomy to the Universities of London,
Manchester, Oxford, and Hong Kong, to the Royal
College of Surgeons of England and to the
Society of Apothecaries

WITH 28 PLATES AND 13 TEXT-FIGURES

J. & A. CHURCHILL LTD.

104 GLOUCESTER PLACE, LONDON

1968

First Edition		1921
Second ,,		1928
Third ,,		1934
,, ,,	*Reprinted*	1936
Fourth ,,		1939
Fifth ,,		1943
,, ,,	*Reprinted*	1945
Sixth ,,		1948
Seventh ,,		1951
,, ,,	*Reprinted*	1955
Eighth ,,		1957
Ninth ,,	(*R.W.*)	1963
Tenth ,,	,,	1968

Standard Book Number
7000 1381 4

Printed in Great Britain at the Pitman Press, Bath and published in London by J. & A. Churchill Ltd.

PREFACE TO THE TENTH EDITION

ATTITUDES to the content of courses in human anatomy are changing in most medical schools, and unfortunately to extremely varying extent. Suitable texts are hence difficult to provide. During the period of argument and experiment which will doubtless elapse before a new, and presumably appropriate uniformity of teaching emerges, a glut of transient and locally orientated texts is to be expected; this has, indeed, begun. The continuance of a stylized volume such as this is hence justifiable, for the present. Nevertheless, some modernization of the text has been effected in view of the tempo of today.

This has involved complete revision, with widespread abbreviation of language and the excision of many small and less relevant details. Continuing the policy of recent editions functional data and explanations of significance have been interpolated as far as possible in a text which must remain, in essence, a topographical description of the body, apparently preferred by many students.

A new introduction to the upper limb has been added and the section on the reticular system expanded. Apart from these a large number of smaller additions and amendments have been made to keep the text up-to-date. Despite this the volume has been shortened by a few pages. Nevertheless—and despite the removal of many "minutiae"—the book has never contained as much information as does this edition.

Two new plates, an arteriogram and a lymphogram, have been added; and the majority of the figures have been transferred to art paper and treated as plates. These have been distributed as appropriately through the text as the exigencies of production permit. The list of plates has been omitted, page references in the text being considered more useful. The index has been entirely revised and considerably amplified. Doubtless a few errors may persist here and elsewhere; for these apologies are offered.

London, 1968 ROGER WARWICK

CONTENTS

Section I.—THE UPPER LIMB

Section II.—THE LOWER LIMB

Section III.—THE THORAX

Section IV.—THE ABDOMEN

Section V.—THE HEAD AND NECK

Section VI.—THE CENTRAL NERVOUS SYSTEM AND ORGANS OF SPECIAL SENSE

Section VII.—OSTEOLOGY

NOMENCLATURE

The following lists include all common terms used in this text together with their new equivalents wherever these exist.

B.N.A. (*Birmingham Revision*)	*I.A.N.C.* (*New York* 1961)
Anterior nasal aperture	Piriform aperture
Anterior primary division (ramus)	Ventral ramus
Anterior tibial nerve	Deep peroneal nerve
Appendix	Vermiform appendix
Atrioventricular groove	Coronary groove
Auditory nerve	Vestibulocochlear nerve
Auditory striae	Striae medullares
Calcaneum (os calcaneum)	Calcaneus
Canal of Schlemm	Scleral venous sinus
Capsular ligament	Articular capsule
Capsule of Tenon	Bulbar fascia (Fascia bulbi)
Cricovocal membrane	Conus elasticus
Circumflex nerve	Axillary nerve
Circumvallate papilla	Vallate papilla
Coeliac artery	Coeliac trunk
Costocervical artery	Costocervical trunk
Extensor digitorum communis	Extensor digitorum
Extensor indicis proprius	Extensor indicis
Frenum of tongue	Frenulum linguæ
Flexor digitorum sublimis	Flexor digitorum superficialis
Fissure of Rolando	Central sulcus
Fissure of Sylvius	Lateral sulcus
Gasserian ganglion	Trigeminal ganglion
Genial tubercles	Mental spines
Hypogastric plexus	Superior hypogastric plexus
Ileocolic valve	Ileocæcal valve
Inferior dental nerve	Inferior alveolar nerve
Innominate (artery, etc.)	Brachiocephalic (artery, etc.)
Internal laryngeal artery	Superior laryngeal artery
Internal mammary artery	Internal thoracic artery
Lumbar fascia	Thoracolumbar fascia
Lateral ligament of elbow-joint	Radial collateral ligament
Lateral ligament of knee-joint	Fibular collateral ligament
Lateral popliteal nerve	Common peroneal nerve
Lateral sinus	Transverse sinus
Lymph glands	Lymph nodes
Medial ligament of elbow-joint	Ulnar collateral ligament
Medial ligament of knee-joint	Tibial collateral ligament

Medial popliteal nerve	Tibial nerve (includes posterior tibial nerve)
Median basilic vein	Median cubital vein
Spinal cord	Medulla spinalis
Nasopharyngeal tonsil	Pharyngeal tonsil
Nerve to latissimus dorsi	Thoracodorsal nerve
Nerve to rhomboids	Dorsal scapular nerve
Nerve to serratus anterior	Long thoracic nerve
Organ of Corti	Spiral organ
Oropharyngeal isthmus	Isthmus of the fauces
Palmar fascia	Palmar aponeurosis
Pelvic plexus	Inferior hypogastric plexus
Pharyngotympanic (Eustachian) tube	Auditive (auditory) tube
Pineal gland	Pineal body
Pituitary gland	Hypophysis cerebri
Plantar fascia	Plantar aponeurosis
Poupart's ligament	Inguinal ligament
Pinna	Auricle
Pouch of Douglas	Recto-uterine pouch or recess
Posterior primary division (ramus)	Dorsal ramus
Perineal membrane	Urogenital diaphragm
Posterior nasal aperture	Choana
Quadrigeminal body	Colliculus
Semilunar bone (wrist)	Lunate bone
Semilunar cartilage	Meniscus
Septum lucidum	Septum pellucidum
Stenson's duct	Parotid duct
Sternocostalis	Transversus thoracis
Subsartorial (Hunter's) canal	Adductor canal
Superior dental nerves	Superior alveolar nerves
Thyrocervical artery	Thyrocervical trunk
Transverse fissure of lung	Horizontal fissure of lung
Valves of Houston	Transverse rectal folds
Wharton's duct	Submandibular duct

FOREWORD TO THE READER

Before beginning to revise the facts of which you have gained information at first hand by dissecting the human body, you should first of all refresh your memory of the general principles which govern anatomical structure. You can do this very conveniently by reading again the introductions to the various sections (osteology, arthrology, myology, neurology, etc.) in your textbook of systematic anatomy, not once but several times, and you will find that it will be well worth while to do so, for you are now in a much better position to appreciate their content and to understand the examples which you will find cited. Further, if you stop occasionally to think, you will be able to recall many additional examples from your own observations. This may help you to correlate your knowledge and to get a better understanding of the meaning of anatomical structure and, after all, correlation and understanding are the best aids to memory.

In this edition you will find a number of X-ray Plates, and I hope that, when you examine them, you will not be content to concentrate only on the structures specifically indicated, for, if you try, you will be able to recognize many other important features. Do not forget that, when the field shown covers a large area, a certain amount of distortion is unavoidable in the peripheral parts.

I fear that you may underrate the value of this advice and that most of you will disregard it entirely, but even if only a few of you take it, I shall have been justified in devoting a whole page to this Foreword.

T. B. Johnston

Section I

THE UPPER LIMB

DETAILED revision of the upper limb should be preceded by some re-consideration of the limb as a whole in relation to the common functions to which it is so excellently adapted. Indeed, such considerations ought to be frequently in mind throughout the revision of any region. Without them the task of learning or revising anatomical details is not only tedious but misses its chief purpose. Functions occur only in structures, whether large, microscopic or biochemical. The study of function therefore inevitably demands structural details. On the contrary, structures can be studied *in vacuo* without reference to their significance in functional or any other terms. This is a highly sterile approach, and one especially prevalent in revision of macroscopic anatomy of the kind covered by this volume.

The arm as a whole works as a jointed lever, carrying a grasping tool, the hand. The hand can be carried to its work over a very wide range by movement at the shoulder joint. At the elbow the limb hinges to bring whatever is grasped to the mouth or into convenient range of the eyes. A kind of rotation around its long axis—supination or pronation (p. 45), enables the hand to face downwards to grasp and to be rotated upwards to turn an object into free view (or transfer it to the mouth). Because the central nervous system, which constantly controls the hand, has the outstanding capability of learning and perfecting an endless variety of new and highly skilled activities, the human hand is an exquisitely adaptable tool in itself, the essential partner, with the human brain, in creating the astonishing array of tools and techniques which have transformed human life. This outstanding ability of man's mind and hand to manipulate his environment has led to such a complex way of life, that he commonly considers himself as separated absolutely from all other forms of life, despite obvious evidence to the contrary.

Every detail of the upper limb, as is equally true of the whole body, can be correlated intimately with its customary activities. Not only in the nature of its different joints, but naturally in the muscles which move them, there is a constant parallel between structural arrangement and use. Some general principles in regard to muscles are therefore appropriate to mention here.

Muscles may act as *prime movers*, as do the flexors of the fingers in grasping. Prime movers can only produce actual movement if muscles arranged to give opposite effects simultaneously relax and lengthen. Such *opponent* muscles, or antagonists, may also act, as prime movers, or *protagonists*, when the direction of movement is reversed. This direction, in fact, depends upon the distribution of tensions in opposing groups of muscles. Provided that the central nervous control of such groups is adequate, the direction, range, and speed of movements can be varied with great nicety. This is especially so in the case of the hand, where a particularly high level of accuracy and skill can be developed.

When opposing groups of muscles act equally the actual movement is nil, and this effect is sometimes necessary in fixing a joint, such as the shoulder, to ensure a stable basis for the skilful actions of wrist, hand and fingers. A little observation of human activities will prove how often muscles are in fact thus used as *fixators*.

Muscles may collaborate in a third manner. Where prime movers pass over and can therefore act on more than one joint, e.g. the flexors of the finger, disadvantageous movements can be prevented by the synergic action of other groups. In clenching the fists the extensors of the wrist joint also contract, so that the flexors exert all their effect on the fingers, and not upon the wrist. In fact, the flexors and extensors fix the wrist in extension, while the finger flexors contract. In many muscular activities it is easy to discover that the obvious prime movers are assisted by such synergic muscles, often upon a very wide scale.

Finally, in all muscle activity the influence of gravity must not be overlooked. When an object is lowered by straightening out the elbow, this extension is not caused by contraction of extensor muscles, but by controlled relaxation of flexors, such as biceps. Similarly, bending or sitting down are not flexor activities, despite the generalized flexion of joints; gravity flexes them, as far as is permitted by deliberate lengthening of extensor muscles.

THE PECTORAL REGION AND THE AXILLA

These regions can be revised satisfactorily only from a subject in process of dissection in which the arm has not yet been removed from the trunk. In addition, the student should have by him, and should constantly refer to, a clavicle, a scapula and a humerus, belonging to the same side of the body as the axilla of the subject he is examining.

Cutaneous Nerves. The skin over the upper part of the deltoid and from the clavicle down to the second rib is supplied by descending branches from the cervical plexus (C. 3 and 4). Below the second rib the skin is supplied by the anterior and the lateral cutaneous branches of the second to the sixth intercostal nerves. The intercostobrachial nerve, which is the lateral cutaneous branch of the second intercostal nerve, supplies the skin of the axilla.

Mammary Gland. The gland lies in the subcutaneous fat and possesses no true capsule in a young adult female. It is hemispherical in shape, but tongue-like processes extend upwards to the second rib and downwards to the sixth, medially to the edge of the sternum and laterally to the mid-axillary line. One of these processes, termed the "axillary tail," curls round the lower border of the pectoralis major and comes into close relationship with the axillary vessels.

The deep surface of the gland rests on the connective tissue covering the pectoralis major and serratus anterior.

The gland is ectodermal in origin and arises as a number (fifteen to twenty) of solid epithelial ingrowths. Their deeper portions divide, subdivide and proliferate to form the lobules of the gland, while the original stem ingrowths become canalized to form the lactiferous ducts which open on the nipple. The gland is small in the child. The enlargement which occurs in the young female at puberty affects only the glandular tissue, and this also proliferates when the gland increases in size during the first pregnancy. The maximum size is reached during lactation after which retrogression ensues.

The *nipple* is traversed by the ducts of the gland and forms a small conical projection; though usually level with the fourth intercostal space, it is often lower in position. Its base is surrounded by a circular area of pigmented skin, termed the *areola*. Pinkish in the virgin, the areola darkens during the first pregnancy and never fully regains its former tint. It contains sebaceous (*areolar*) glands. At first a surface depression, the nipple becomes evaginated late in fœtal life.

Ducts. About fifteen ducts open independently of one another on the surface of the nipple. Each possesses a dilated ampulla just prior to its termination.

Lymphatics. The lymphatic vessels, which may act as channels for the spread of malignant disease from the breast to the associated lymph nodes, are of the greatest importance to the surgeon. (*a*) A *superficial plexus* of lymph vessels lies under the skin superficial to the gland. It receives afferents from the gland and sends its efferents, some to the pectoral lymph nodes, some to the infraclavicular lymph nodes, and others to (*b*) the *deep, or mammary plexus* of lymph vessels, which is closely related to the deep fascia on which the mammary gland rests. In addition the deep plexus receives, directly, most of the lymph vessels of the gland. The efferents from the deep plexus pass: (1) To the pectoral lymph nodes (p. 10); (2) to the subscapular lymph nodes (p. 11) (from both these groups efferent vessels pass to the lateral axillary and apical lymph nodes); (3) to the infraclavicular lymph nodes, and thence, *via* the apical lymph nodes, to the postero-inferior group of the deep cervical lymph nodes; (4) to the lymph nodes along the internal thoracic vessels, and thence to the mediastinal lymph nodes; (5) to the subdiaphragmatic plexus, crossing the costal margin and piercing the abdominal wall; and (6) to communicate with the deep plexus of the opposite side. Recent work has emphasised the importance of the internal thoracic nodes and also those associated with the posterior intercostal vessels. It has also shown that drainage across the midline is insignificant.

The *Blood Supply* is derived from perforating branches of the internal thoracic and intercostal arteries and from the external mammary branches of the lateral thoracic artery.

The **Axilla** is the region between the upper part of the arm and the side of the chest. It contains numerous lymph nodes and all the principal vessels and nerves of the limb. These enter the axilla from the neck through the narrow *apex*, bounded in front by the clavicle (middle third), behind by the upper border of the scapula and medially by the outer border of the first rib.

The size of the axilla is very much exaggerated after dissection because the fascial floor, which is normally drawn upwards by its connexion with the clavipectoral fascia and so produces the natural hollow of the arm-pit, has been removed together with a quantity of fat. In addition, the subscapularis has been freely separated from the serratus anterior, with which it is normally in direct apposition over its lower and medial two-thirds.

The *Anterior Wall of the Axilla* consists of two layers: (1) the pectoralis major; and (2) the subclavius, the clavipectoral fascia, the pectoralis minor and the suspensory ligament of the axilla.

The **Pectoralis Major** has (1) a clavicular part attached to the medial half of the clavicle, and (2) a sternocostal part fixed to the sternum and the upper six costal cartilages. The fibres converge on the upper part of the humerus, the lower fibres turning upwards behind the upper fibres so as to form a bilaminar tendon, attached to the lateral lip of the bicipital groove.

Actions. The pectoralis major adducts the arm and rotates it medially. The clavicular part, acting with the anterior fibres of the deltoid, flexes the arm to a right angle (p. 13), but the sternocostal part assists the latissimus dorsi to depress the flexed arm when the movement is carried out against resistance without the help of gravity. When the arms are fixed above the head, the sternocostal head draws the trunk upwards, as in climbing.

Nerve Supply. It receives branches from the lateral and medial pectoral nerves, which arise from the corresponding cords of the brachial plexus (C.5 to T1 for the clavicular part, C.7, 8, and T.1 for the sternocostal).

The **Subclavius** arises from the first costal cartilage and is inserted into the groove on the inferior surface of the clavicle.

It probably steadies the clavicle in its movements, and is supplied by a supraclavicular branch of the brachial plexus (C. 5 and 6).

The **Clavipectoral Fascia** is a thickened sheet of connective tissue which fills up the gap in the deep layer of the anterior wall between the subclavius and the pectoralis minor. It is continuous with the fascial covering of both muscles, and so, when traced laterally, is found to blend with the coracoclavicular ligament and the suspensory ligament of the axilla (*v. infra*). At its medial end it reaches the first and second costal cartilages and anterior intercostal membranes.

The fascia is covered medially by the clavicular part of the pectoralis major, but laterally it is related to the infraclavicular fossa. It is pierced by (1) the cephalic vein, *en route* to join the axillary vein; (2) the lateral pectoral nerve; (3) the acromiothoracic artery; and (4) the efferents from the infraclavicular lymph nodes.

The **Pectoralis Minor,** almost entirely covered by the pectoralis major, arises from the anterior ends of the third, fourth and fifth ribs, and narrows as it passes to be attached to the medial border of the coracoid process.

Actions. Under ordinary conditions it swings the shoulder forwards and downwards, but when the shoulder is fixed it may elevate its ribs of origin. Acting with the serratus anterior it draws the scapula forwards round the chest wall, as in pushing and stretching.

Its *Nerve Supply* is derived from the medial pectoral nerve, which also pierces it to reach the pectoralis major.

The so-called *suspensory ligament of the axilla* is merely dense connective tissue continuous with fascia around pectoralis minor and subjacent to the axillary skin, which is adherent to it.

The *Lateral Wall of the Axilla* is narrow, because the tendons of pectoralis major and latissimus dorsi come very close together at their humeral attachments. It is formed by a strip of the bicipital groove, hidden by the biceps and coracobrachialis muscles.

The great vessels and nerves are all closely related to the lateral wall, because, of course, they are entering the arm itself.

The *Posterior Wall of the Axilla* is formed, medially, by the subscapularis muscle and, laterally, by the latissimus dorsi and a very small part of the teres major.

The latissimus dorsi, as it passes to attachment to the floor of the bicipital groove, sweeps round the lower border of the teres major and covers nearly the whole of its anterior surface. Trace the latissimus dorsi and observe that, as a result of this sweep, its surfaces are reversed.

All the muscles on the posterior wall of the axilla are supplied by branches from the posterior cord of the brachial plexus (p. 9).

The *Medial Wall of the Axilla* is formed by the outer surface of the thoracic wall, covered by the serratus anterior muscle.

The **Serratus Anterior** arises from the upper eight ribs and passes backwards, closely applied to the chest wall, to be inserted into the ventral aspect of the medial border of the scapula; the lower four digitations are attached to its inferior angle.

Actions. The serratus anterior draws the scapula forwards round the chest wall, at the same time, by virtue of the greater pull exerted on the inferior angle, *rotating* it so that the inferior angle passes laterally and forwards. As a result the glenoid cavity is directed upwards. This rotation occurs when the arm is raised from the side, and reaches its maximum when the arm is elevated above the head. The serratus anterior and the trapezius co-operate to produce the movement. This rotation is often modified by other muscles, as in the commoner movement of stretching out the hand, in which the serratus anterior draws forwards the Scapula, and hence arm. When the shoulders are fixed, the muscle acts as an elevator of its ribs of origin.

It derives its *Nerve Supply* from the *long thoracic nerve* (*nerve to serratus anterior*) (C. 5, 6 and 7). The nerve descends along the medial wall of the axilla in the loose connective tissue on the muscle's surface. It enters the axilla through the apex, where it lies behind the great vessels and nerves.

The *Intercostobrachial Nerve*, which is the lateral cutaneous branch of the second intercostal nerve, pierces the medial wall of the axilla and crosses the region in the axillary fat. It supplies branches to the skin over the axillary floor, communicates with the medial cutaneous nerve of the arm (T. 1), and is distributed finally to skin over the dorsal aspect of the arm.

The **Axillary Artery** begins at the outer border of the first rib, as the continuation of the subclavian artery. It runs downwards and laterally (when the arm is by the side), and terminates at the lower border of the teres major, where it leaves the axilla and is now the brachial artery. Throughout its course it is closely associated with the cords of the brachial plexus and their branches to the arm, being enclosed with them in a dense sheath of connective tissue. When this axillary sheath is traced upwards through the apex of the axilla, it will be seen to be continuous with the prevertebral fascia.

The axillary artery is crossed superficially by the pectoralis minor, which serves to divide it, for descriptive purposes, into three parts.

The *First Part* of the axillary artery lies above the pectoralis minor and is related *anteriorly* to the clavipectoral fascia, the pectoralis major and the covering fasciæ and skin. It is crossed superficially by the lateral pectoral nerve and by the cephalic vein as it makes for the axillary vein. *Above, and to its lateral side*, lie the posterior and lateral cords of the plexus. *Posteriorly*, the medial cord of the plexus and the nerve to serratus anterior intervene between the artery and the first digitation of the serratus anterior. *Medially*, the axillary vein accompanies the artery and tends to overlap it anteriorly.

The *Second Part* of the axillary artery is covered *anteriorly* by the pectoralis minor and major muscles, fasciæ and skin. The three cords of the brachial plexus are related to the artery in the manner indicated by their names. *Posteriorly*, the artery and the posterior cord are separated from the subscapularis by a mass of fat. *Medially*, the medial cord intervenes between the artery and the axillary vein.

The *Acromiothoracic* and *Lateral Thoracic* arteries arise from the second part. The acromiothoracic pierces the clavipectoral fascia and sends two or more pectoral branches between the two pectoral muscles. The lateral thoracic artery runs along the lower border of the pectoralis minor.

The *Third Part* of the axillary artery lies below the lower border of the pectoralis minor. As the posterior fold of the axilla extends to a lower level than the anterior fold (a fact readily confirmed on the living subject), it follows that the terminal part of the artery escapes from under cover of the pectoralis major and is covered anteriorly only by the skin, fasciæ and certain nerves, although it is overlapped by the coracobrachialis muscle. The neurovascular bundle can therefore be palpated in this situation and the pulsations of the artery can be felt in the living subject. Higher up the artery is covered also by the pectoralis major.

The branches of the brachial plexus retain, for some distance, the relationships which their parent cords bear to the second part of the artery. Thus, the radial and circumflex nerves lie behind the artery, the musculocutaneous and the lateral root of the median lie to its lateral side, the ulnar and the medial cutaneous nerve of the arm lie to its medial side. The medial root of the median nerve, however, crosses in front of the artery to reach the lateral root, and the medial cutaneous nerve of the forearm gets displaced on to the anterior surface of the vessel.

In addition, the axillary vein lies to the medial side, the subscapularis, the latissimus dorsi and the teres major lie behind the artery, and the coracobrachialis, which overlaps the vessel anteriorly, and the humerus lie to its lateral side.

Branches. The **Subscapular Artery** arises at the lower border of the subscapularis and follows it down to the chest wall. Near its origin it is crossed by the ulnar nerve and the axillary vein. It gives off a *circumflex scapular* branch, which winds round the lateral border of the scapula, deep to the teres minor, and reaches the infraspinous fossa (for scapular anastomosis, see p. 16).

The **Circumflex Humeral Arteries** arise just below the subscapular. The *anterior* passes laterally in front of the surgical neck of the humerus, while the *posterior* passes backwards through the quadrilateral space (p. 16) in company with the circumflex nerve, and then winds round the posterior aspect of the surgical neck. These two arteries form an anastomosing circle round the surgical neck, from branches ascending to the shoulder joint and epiphysis. The posterior is much the larger, as it is the main artery to the deltoid. It sends a branch downwards to anastomose with the profunda artery, thus *linking up the third part of the axillary with the upper part of the brachial artery*.

The **Brachial Plexus** is formed by the ventral rami of the fifth, sixth, seventh and eighth cervical and the first thoracic spinal nerves, together with small communications from the fourth cervical and the second thoracic nerves. The union, separation, and reunion of these nerves in a definite manner constitute the plexus. It commences in the neck (p. 221) and is continued into the axilla.

In the neck, C. 5 and C. 6 unite to form the upper trunk; C. 7 forms the middle trunk; C. 8 and T. 1 form the lower trunk. Each trunk divides into anterior and posterior divisions, but these divisions are not always of equal size, and in the case of the lower trunk the posterior division is relatively small. The three posterior divisions unite to form the posterior cord; the anterior divisions of the upper and middle trunks constitute the lateral cord, and the anterior division of the lower trunk is continued on as the medial cord.

The separation of each trunk into an anterior and a posterior division is an indication of the subdivision of the musculature of the primitive limb into a ventral, or flexor, and a dorsal, or extensor, group.

The supraclavicular branches of the plexus arise before the stage of cords is reached. They are four in number:—

1. The *Dorsal Scapular Nerve* (*to the Rhomboids*) arises from the ventral ramus of C. 5 and pierces scalenus medius. Then it runs down the anterior border and surface of the levator scapulæ to reach the rhomboids.

2. The *Suprascapular Nerve* arises from the upper trunk (C. 5 and C. 6). When the brachial plexus is approached in the neck from its supero-lateral aspect, the suprascapular is the first branch that is encountered. It runs downwards and laterally, disappears behind the clavicle, and passes through the suprascapular notch to reach and supply the supra- and infra-spinatus muscles.

3. The *Long Thoracic Nerve* (*to Serratus Anterior*) is from the ventral rami of C. 5, C. 6 and C. 7 soon after they emerge from the intervertebral foramina. Its upper two roots pierce the scalenus medius and then descend on the surface of that muscle, meeting the lower root, which does not pierce the muscle, and ultimately joining with it. *Both the long thoracic nerve and the dorsal scapular nerve lie behind the prevertebral fascia in the neck* (p. 222). The nerve passes through the apex of the axilla behind the axillary vessels and the plexus, and runs downwards on the surface of serratus anterior, which it supplies.

4. The *Nerve to the Subclavius* arises directly from the anterior rami of C. 5 and C. 6 and descends in front of the plexus and the subclavian artery to reach the subclavius muscle.

In the Axilla, the cords of the plexus are closely related to the second part of the axillary artery. The medial cord crosses behind the artery to its medial side, the posterior cord runs down behind it, and the lateral cord lies along its lateral side. This relationship is also largely maintained by the branches of the cords.

The **Lateral Cord** gives off: (1) The *lateral pectoral nerve*, which runs forwards lateral to the axillary artery, pierces the clavipectoral fascia, and supplies the pectoralis major muscle. (2) The *musculo-cutaneous nerve* descends lateral to the artery, gradually deviating from it. It supplies coracobrachialis and then *pierces it*. (3) The *lateral root of the median nerve* is the direct continuation of the lateral cord along the lateral side of the artery. It is joined by the medial root, which crosses in front of the vessel.

The **Posterior Cord** supplies the posterior wall of the axilla. (1) The *upper subscapular nerve* arises high in the space and supplies the subscapularis. (2) The *thoracodorsal nerve* (*to latissimus dorsi*) runs downwards on the subscapularis to reach the subscapular vessels and lymph nodes, with which it is subsequently in close relationship. It supplies the latissimus dorsi. (3) The *lower subscapular nerve* runs laterally and slightly downwards across the subscapularis to reach the teres major. It gives branches to both muscles and crosses behind the subscapular vessels. (4) The *radial nerve* is the direct continuation of the posterior cord, and consequently intervenes between the axillary artery and the muscles on which it lies. It is the largest branch of the plexus and, before it leaves the axilla, it gives off branches to the long and the medial heads of the triceps and the posterior cutaneous nerve of the arm. (5) The *axillary nerve* runs laterally parallel to and just above the radial, with which it parts company at the lower border of the subscapularis. At this point it turns backwards through the quadrilateral space (pp. 8 and 16).

The **Medial Cord** of the plexus gives off: (1) The *medial pectoral*, which passes forwards medial to the artery, supplies and pierces the pectoralis minor and ends in the pectoralis major muscle. (2) The *medial cutaneous nerve of the arm* (T. 1) communicates with the intercostobrachial nerve (T. 2), runs downwards along the axillary vein, and supplies the skin over the medial surface of the arm. (3) The *ulnar nerve* runs downwards medial to the axillary artery, intervening between it and the axillary vein; it is smaller than the median nerve, but much larger than (4) the *medial cutaneous nerve of the forearm*, which descends in front of the artery. (5) The *medial root of the median nerve* crosses the artery obliquely in order to join the lateral root. Neither the median nor the ulnar nerve gives off any branches until just above the elbow joint.

The **Axillary Vein** begins at the lower border of the teres major, where it is continuous with the basilic vein. As it ascends through the axilla, it lies to the medial side of the axillary artery and tends to overlap it anteriorly. It receives tributaries which correspond to the branches of the artery and, in addition, it is joined by the venæ comitantes of the brachial artery, near its start, and by the cephalic vein, near its termination. Throughout its course it is intimately related to a chain of lymph nodes, of which the upper members lie in the apex of the axilla. Its relation to the medial cord, the ulnar nerve and the medial cutaneous nerve of the arm have already been pointed out. At the outer border of the first rib, the axillary vein becomes the subclavian vein.

The **Lymph Nodes of the Axilla** are arranged in four principal groups: (1) The *pectoral lymph nodes* lie along the lower border of the pectoralis major, and some may extend into the interval between it and the pectoralis minor. They receive *afferents* from the abdominal wall above the umbilicus and from the lateral portion of the mammary gland. Their *efferents* join the apical lymph nodes. (2) The *subscapular lymph nodes* are closely related to the subscapular vessels. They receive *afferents* from the tissues of the back, from the cervical region down to the iliac crests, and from the lateral portion of the mammary gland. Their *efferents* join the apical lymph nodes. (3) The *lateral lymph nodes* lie along the axillary vein, and receive most of the lymph vessels of the upper limb. The upper members of this group lie in the apex of the axilla, and are termed the *apical lymph nodes*. They receive *afferents* from the pectoral, subscapular, infraclavicular and lateral axillary groups, and their *efferents* pass to the lower groups of the deep cervical nodes or direct to the subclavian lymph trunk. (4) The *central lymph nodes* lie in the axillary fat near the base of the axilla. They have no direct area of drainage, but they receive *afferents* from the pectoral, subscapular and lateral lymph nodes and send their *efferents* to the apical lymph nodes.

Thus, All to apical nodes → Lower grps deep C nodes / Subclavian lymph trunk *

THE BACK

The *Cutaneous Nerves* which supply the skin of the dorsum of the trunk are all derived from the posterior primary rami of the spinal nerves, and their terminal branches do not extend further forwards than the posterior axillary line. The posterior primary rami of the first and eighth cervical nerves do not give off any cutaneous branches, and the seventh cervical frequently fails to do so. Further, the posterior primary rami of the upper three lumbar nerves turn downwards to supply the skin over the buttock, while those of the lower two lumbar nerves do not innervate skin.

The **Trapezius Muscle** arises from the external occipital protuberance, the ligamentum nuchæ and all the vertebral spines down to the twelfth thoracic spine. The fibres converge as they pass laterally, the upper being inserted into the lateral third of the clavicle, the middle into the medial border of the acromion process, and the lower into the upper border of the crest of the spine of the scapula. The muscle thus forms a large triangular sheet connecting the upper limb girdle to the axial skeleton.

Its *nerve supply* is derived from the accessory nerve (motor) and from C. 3 and C. 4 (proprioceptor).

Actions. In association with the other muscles attached to the scapula, the trapezius exercises a controlling influence over the position and movements of the shoulder girdle during active use of the arm and in *maintaining the level and poise of the shoulder*.

In elevation of the arm above the head (p. 13) the combined actions of the trapezius and the serratus anterior contribute substantially by bringing about a forward rotation of the scapula and consequently an upward inclination of the glenoid cavity.

The trapezius and rhomboids of both sides combine in the bracing back of the shoulders and approximation of the scapulæ. The rotary action of the trapezius on the scapula is counteracted by the rotary action of the rhomboids in the opposite direction. Elevation of the point of the shoulder results from the combined actions of the trapezius and the levator scapulæ. In this case also the rotary effects of the two muscles on the scapula are in opposite directions and therefore counteract each other.

The trapezius conceals the insertion of the levator scapulæ, both rhomboid muscles, and the upper part of the origin of the latissimus dorsi.

The **Latissimus Dorsi** arises from the lower six thoracic spines, under the trapezius, and from the lumbar fascia (p. 224). (It also receives fleshy fibres from the iliac crest, the lower three or four ribs and, sometimes, from the inferior angle of the scapula.) As it passes upwards and laterally to its insertion into the bicipital groove of the humerus, it is wrapped round the lower border of the teres major in such a way that its surfaces and borders become reversed.

The *thoracodorsal nerve* is derived from the posterior cord (C. 6, 7 and 8).

Actions. The latissimus dorsi is a powerful adductor of the arm; it can also extend it at the shoulder and rotate it medially. It assists in violent expiratory efforts, such as coughing, when its contractions can easily be felt in the posterior fold of the axilla. When both arms are fixed above the head, it helps the pectoralis major to draw the trunk upwards as in climbing.

The **Levator Scapulæ** arises from the upper four cervical transverse processes and is inserted into the upper part of the medial border of the scapula.

The **Rhomboids,** minor and major, extend from the lower cervical and upper thoracic spines downwards and laterally to the medial border of the scapula. Most of the fibres of the rhomboid major are inserted into the region of the inferior angle.

The *nerve supply* of the levator scapulæ is derived from C. 3 and C. 4, and often from the dorsal scapular nerve (C. 5), which descends in front of these muscles close to their insertion.

Actions. The rhomboids and levator scapulæ are antagonists of trapezius and serratus anterior as rotators of the scapula, being capable of restoring the bone to its normal position after the arm

PLATE I.—SURFACE LANDMARKS OF THE UPPER LIMB.

A

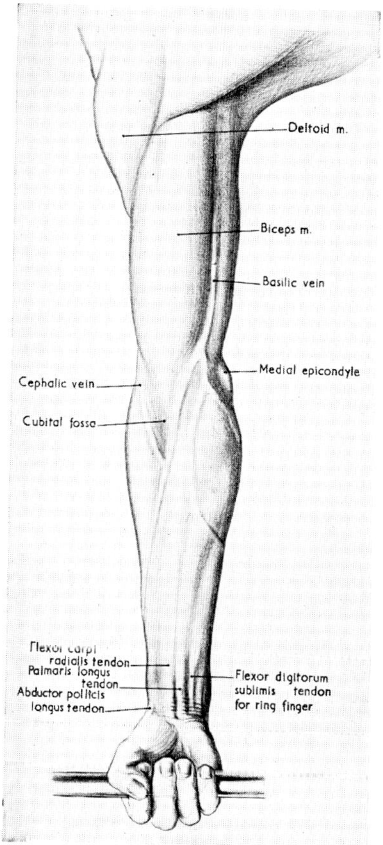

B

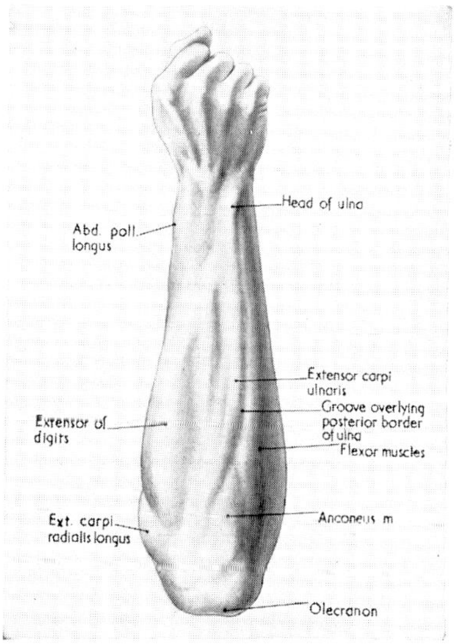

A.—The front of the upper limb, showing the visible surface landmarks in a muscular subject.

B.—The back of the forearm.

To face p. 12

PLATE II. SURFACE LANDMARKS OF THE ANTERIOR ABDOMINAL WALL.

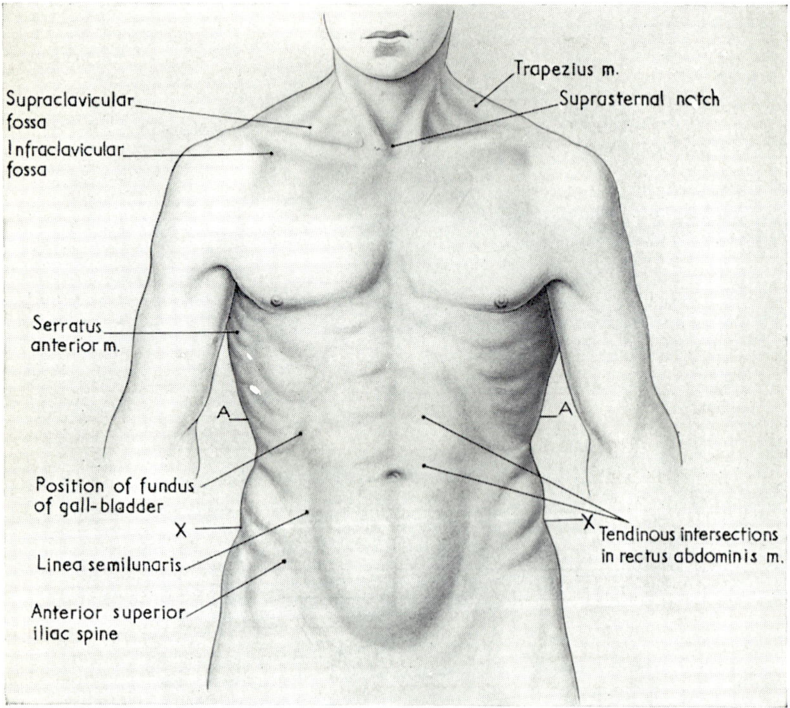

Note.—The line A—A represents the position of the transpyloric plane, and the line X—X the position of the intertubercular plane. The sternal heads of the sterno-mastoid muscle stand out clearly on either side of the suprasternal notch.

PLATE III. SURFACE LANDMARKS OF THE DORSAL ASPECT OF THE TRUNK.

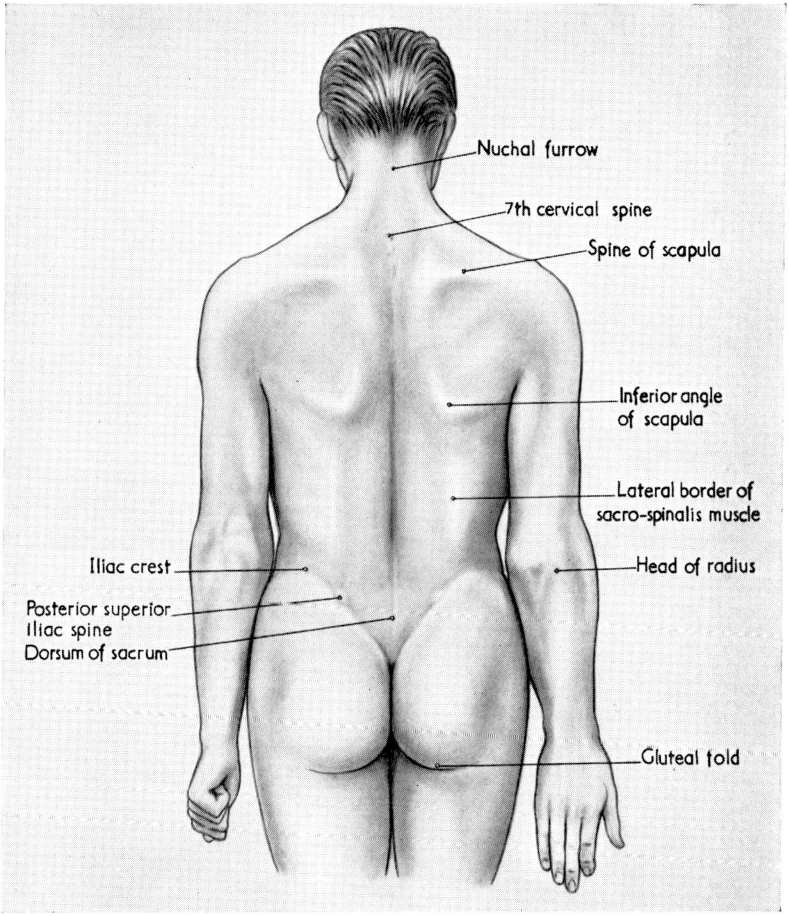

Plate IV. Surface Landmarks of the Left Lower Limb.

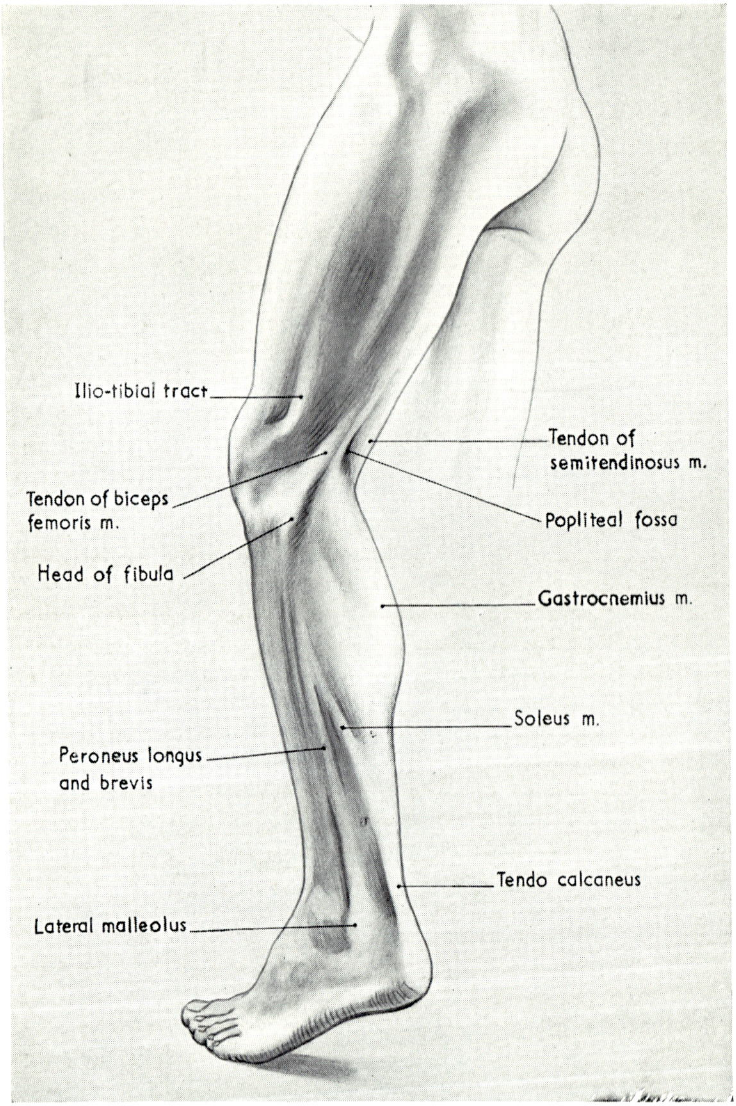

has been raised. In addition, with the trapezius, the rhomboids approximate the two scapulæ.

THE SCAPULAR REGION

For the satisfactory revision of this region the student must provide himself with a dissected and detached upper limb, the clavicle, scapula and humerus of the same side and, if possible, a dissected limb in which only the joints and ligaments have been preserved.

The skin over the upper part of the deltoid is supplied by the descending branches of the cervical plexus (C. 3 and 4), over the lower part of the muscle by the upper lateral cutaneous nerve of the arm, from the circumflex nerve (C. 5 and 6).

The **Deltoid** muscle is attached to the lateral third of the clavicle, the acromion (lateral border), and from the crest of the spine of the scapula (lower border). The fibres converge on the deltoid tuberosity of the humerus (p. 404). The anterior and posterior fibres are parallel, but the acromial fibres are multipennate—a clear indication that these fibres have heavier work to do. The reflection of the muscle exposes the insertions of the scapular muscles, the tuberosities of the humerus (p. 403), and the adjoining part of its shaft.

The *nerve supply* of the deltoid comes from the axillary nerve (C. 5 and 6).

Actions. The deltoid is a powerful abductor of the arm, moving it through an angle of about 90°, forward and lateral in the plane of the body of the scapula. The work of raising the limb against gravity is performed by the multipennate acromial fibres, sidesway of the unstable humeral head being prevented by the balanced tension of the anterior and posterior fibres.

When the arm is raised above the head, the deltoid and the supraspinatus, which abduct the humerus on the scapula, co-operate with the serratus anterior and the trapezius, which rotate the scapula. *These two groups of muscles work synchronously, and not at different stages, when the arm is elevated.*

Owing to the mobility of the scapula, abduction of the upper limb is more complicated than might appear at first sight. As the arm is raised above the head, the scapula swings forwards round the chest wall, and only when the humerus is kept in the same plane as the body of the scapula can the arm be fully raised. When the arm is above the head, the costal surface of the scapula faces medially. When the arm is by the side, it faces medially and forwards, as does the anterior surface of the humerus, a fact which can readily be confirmed in the living subject, since, when the arm is at rest by the side, *the lateral epicondyle is found on a more anterior plane than the medial epicondyle*. (The deltoid, acting as a whole, moves the humerus in the plane of the scapula and *not* in the coronal plane, and this must be borne in mind when it is desired to relax the paralysed muscle.)

The anterior and posterior fibres are capable of acting independently of the rest of the muscle. The former combine with the pectoralis major to draw the arm forwards and medially, the latter with the latissimus dorsi and teres major to draw it backwards.

The *Subacromial Bursa* extends medially below the coracoacromial ligament and the acromion, and laterally under cover of the middle fibres of the deltoid. Below, it is related to the supraspinatus tendon and the greater tuberosity. It does not usually communicate with the cavity of the shoulder joint.

The *Coracoacromial Ligament* extends from the lateral border of the coracoid process to the acromion immediately in front of the acromioclavicular joint. It is covered by the deltoid and, together with the coracoid process and acromion—the coracoacromial arch—it is said to give protection and support to the superior aspect of the shoulder joint. (This ligament is possibly no more than a vestige.)

The *Acromioclavicular Joint* is a small synovial joint between the acromion and the lateral extremity of the clavicle. The line of the joint, as seen from above, is antero-posterior, but the articular surfaces slope downwards and medially, so that the clavicle tends to override the acromion. The joint possesses a capsule with superior and inferior thickenings; from the superior a small, wedge-shaped articular disc passes into the joint. It is never complete, and frequently is insignificant in size.

The **Coracoclavicular Ligament** is a strong and functionally very important, *helping to suspend the scapula and upper limb from the clavicle*. It consists of two parts, usually separated by a bursa: (*a*) The *conoid part* is attached below to the angular bend of the coracoid process and above to the conoid tubercle of the clavicle. (*b*) The *trapezoid part* lies anterolateral to the conoid and passes upwards from the upper surface of the coracoid process to the trapezoid line on the clavicle.

Through this ligament the weight of the upper limb is partially transmitted to the clavicle, and thence medially along it to the axial skeleton. Under normal circumstances, however, the trapezius, the levator scapulæ and the rhomboids support the weight of the limb. (Should the clavicle be fractured medial to the coracoclavicular ligament, the transmission of the weight of the limb is interfered with. The muscles, deprived of their mechanical prop, are at a disadvantage, and the shoulder drops to a lower level, giving the characteristic deformity of a broken collar-bone.)

The **Supraspinatus** muscle arises from the medial two-thirds of the supraspinous fossa. It converges laterally into a tendon, which passes below the acromion and above the articular capsule of the shoulder joint, to the highest impression on the greater tuberosity of the humerus. *This tendon is directly related to the capsular ligament*, to which it is partly attached.

The **Infraspinatus** arises from the medial four-fifths of the infraspinous fossa. It converges into a tendon, passing laterally behind the articular capsule of the shoulder joint, to a facet immediately below the supraspinatus on the greater tuberosity. *The Tendon is* partially inserted into the capsule.

Nerve Supply. Both the foregoing muscles are supplied by the suprascapular nerve (C. 5 and 6), which enters the supraspinous fossa by passing backwards through the suprascapular notch, below the suprascapular ligament.

The **Teres Minor** arises from the upper two-thirds of the dorsal aspect of the scapula close to its lateral border. The fibres pass laterally into a tendon attached to the lowest facet on the greater tuberosity, and the upper part of this is, like the tendon of the infraspinatus, *intimately associated with the capsular ligament of the shoulder joint.*

Its *nerve supply* is derived from the axillary nerve (C. 5 and 6).

The **Subscapularis** muscle arises from the medial three-fourths of the subscapular fossa and from the grooved surface near the lateral border of the scapula. Its fibres converge on the lesser tuberosity of the humerus, where they are inserted. As it approaches its insertion, *its tendon is partially blended with the anterior aspect of the capsular ligament of the shoulder joint.* Medial to this connexion with the capsule the synovial membrane of the joint is protruded through a gap in the front of the capsule to form a "bursa" under the subscapularis tendon.

Its *nerve supply* is derived from the upper and lower subscapular nerves (p. 9).

Actions. The short scapular muscles are all attached to the humerus close to the shoulder joint and they are all partly blended with its capsular ligament. They are regarded as primarily synergic muscles to steady the head of the humerus during movements of the arm and to prevent it from slipping, or skidding, out of the glenoid cavity.

Although the subscapularis can act as a medial rotator, and the infraspinatus and teres minor as lateral rotators, when the arm is by the side, these actions are not necessarily of greatest importance.

At the start of abduction the downward pull of the infraspinatus, teres minor and subscapularis prevents the humeral head from slipping upwards on the glenoid cavity under the traction exerted by the deltoid muscle. These opponents with the help accorded by the supraspinatus, allow controlled movement to be initiated, and thereafter the mechanical advantage of the deltoid steadily increases.

The **Axillary Nerve** (C. 5 and 6) has already been seen in the axilla (p. 10), arising from the posterior cord of the brachial plexus and passing downwards on the subscapularis muscle, above the radial nerve and behind the axillary artery. On reaching the lower border of the subscapularis the nerve passes backwards across the border, above the teres major tendon, lateral to the long head of the triceps, and medial to the surgical neck of the humerus (*i.e.*, through a quadrilateral space). *After crossing the border of the subscapularis, the axillary nerve comes into close proximity with the inferior aspect of the capsular ligament of the shoulder joint, and this relationship is highly important* (p. 18).

As it turns backwards it gives off an articular twig to the joint and then divides into anterior and posterior branches: (*a*) The anterior branch keeps close to the humerus, running laterally behind it and then winding forwards across its lateral aspect to sink into the deltoid. After supplying the muscle, the terminal twigs emerge on its surface to supply the skin. (*b*) The posterior branch gives off the *nerve to the teres minor* (identified by a small swelling upon it), a few twigs to the deltoid, and then winds round the posterior border of the muscle to supply the skin over it. Here it is termed the *upper lateral cutaneous nerve of the arm.*

The *posterior circumflex humeral vessels* (p. 8) accompany the nerve after it leaves the axilla.

The **Teres Major** arises from a flattened oval area on the dorsal aspect of the inferior angle of the scapula below the area occupied by the teres minor. It is a short strap-like muscle which runs parallel to, but just below, the teres minor, and is inserted into the medial lip of the bicipital groove of the humerus. Near its insertion, it becomes tendinous and crosses in front of the long head of the triceps.

Its *nerve supply* is obtained from the lower subscapular nerve (p. 10).

Action. The teres major assists in the movements of adduction and medial rotation of the humerus.

The **Scapular Anastomosis.** In the neighbourhood of each of the large joints of the limbs there occurs a free arterial anastomosis, which is always situated close to the bones forming the articulation. In the case of the shoulder joint the circumflex humeral arteries form an anastomosing circle around the upper end of the humerus, and a free anastomosis occurs both on the costal and on the dorsal surface of the scapula.

The following arteries take part in the scapular anastomosis: (1) The suprascapular artery, which is distributed to both supra- and infra-spinous fossæ, (2) the deep branch of the transverse cervical, which runs down the medial border of the scapula in company with the nerve to the rhomboids, (3) the subscapular artery, which runs down the lateral border of the scapula, and (4) the circumflex scapular artery, which arises from the subscapular and is distributed to the infraspinous fossa.

The essential fact to be borne in mind is that, since (1) and (2) are derived from the first part of the subclavian artery, and (3) and (4) come from the third part of the axillary artery, *the scapular anastomosis represents an anastomotic connexion between these two important and widely separated vessels.* This connexion may sometimes be useful, but the primary function of these anastomosing arteries is to supply epiphyses.

The **Shoulder Joint** is a synovial joint of the "ball and socket" variety. It is characterised by the wide range of movement which its structure permits (Plate V, p. 32).

The articular head of the humerus is large compared with the glenoid cavity, which forms a very shallow receiving surface even in the living state, when it is deepened by the presence of the glenoid labrum, a fibrocartilaginous rim attached round its margin. *The bony constituents of the joint, therefore, are arranged to give a marked range of movement.*

The *Capsular Ligament* is very loose, a condition necessarily associated with free movement. Its humeral attachment runs round the anatomical neck, but on the medial side, it descends for about half-an-inch and includes a U-shaped portion of the shaft within the capsule. (N.B. This attachment crosses the junction between epiphysis and diaphysis.) On the scapula it is attached above the supraglenoid tubercle, so that the long head of the biceps lies within the capsule. Elsewhere it is attached to the glenoid labrum.

The *Transverse Ligament* bridges the gap between the two tuberosities. Its upper border blends with the capsular ligament, while its lower border is free, and in this way a deficiency is left to allow for the exit of the long head of the biceps.

The *Coracohumeral Ligament*, an accessory ligament of the shoulder joint, extends from the coracoid process to blend with the capsular ligament and the transverse ligament.

The *Synovial Membrane* lines the capsular ligament, covers the glenoid labrum, surrounds the long tendon of the biceps, and covers such bone as is intracapsular and non-articular. It protrudes from under the transverse ligament, forming a sheath round the extracapsular part of the long tendon of the biceps, and also through a gap in front of the capsule, to form a bursa under subscapularis.

The anterior, superior and posterior aspects of the capsular ligament are greatly strengthened by the subscapularis, the supraspinatus, and the infraspinatus and teres minor respectively (p. 15). Below, the capsule forms a dependent pocket when the arm is by the side, but, when the arm is abducted, it is stretched tightly below the lower, part of the head of the humerus. In the latter position it is supported by the long head of the triceps, but this support is not so efficient as the support given to the other portions of the capsule by their associated muscles. *Below*, the capsular ligament is comparatively *weakest*, and in dislocations of the shoulder joint it is this part which is torn. As the dislocated head passes downwards through the tear it comes into close relation with the axillary nerve and the posterior circumflex humeral vessels (p. 16). These structures usually escape injury, but every now and then dislocation of the shoulder is complicated by injury to the circumflex nerve or laceration of the vessels.

It will be clear from the foregoing that the shoulder joint depends as much on the support of the surrounding muscles as on bony or ligamentous arrangements.

In addition to the structures already mentioned, the joint is related, *above*, to the subacromial bursa, the coracoacromial arch and the deltoid; *in front*, to the anterior part of the deltoid, the coracobrachialis and the short head of biceps; and, *behind*, to the posterior part of the deltoid.

At this stage in his revision the student is in a position to work out the muscle groups which are concerned in the various movements that occur at the shoulder; this is by far the best way of appreciating and remembering them.

THE UPPER ARM

For the satisfactory revision of this and subsequent regions of the upper limb the student must provide himself with a dissected upper limb, with the necessary bones and, if possible, with a specimen dissected to show the joints.

The *Nerve Supply* to the skin of the shoulder region has already been considered. The lateral aspect of the upper arm below the deltoid is supplied by the lower lateral cutaneous nerve of the arm (radial nerve, C. 5 and 6). Branches from the medial cutaneous nerve of the forearm (C. 8 and T. 1) supply the skin over the biceps muscle. The skin of the medial and posterior aspects is supplied by (1) the medial cutaneous nerve of the arm (T. 1); (2) the intercostobrachial nerve (T. 2); and (3) the posterior cutaneous nerve of the arm (C. 8).

Two large *veins* ascend in the superficial fascia of the upper arm: (1) The *cephalic vein*, joined in the lower part of the upper arm by the radial veins (p. 24), ascends in the groove on the lateral side of the biceps until it reaches the insertion of the deltoid. It then follows the anterior border of that muscle, lying between it and the pectoralis major until it reaches the infraclavicular fossa, where it pierces the clavipectoral fascia to join the axillary vein.

(2) The *basilic vein*, joined in the lower part of the upper arm by the ulnar veins (p. 24), ascends in the groove on the medial side of the biceps. Half-way up the arm it pierces the deep fascia and is medial to the brachial artery. *At the lower border of the teres major it enters the axilla and becomes the axillary vein.* *

DORSAL ASPECT OF THE UPPER ARM

This region contains the triceps muscle, the radial nerve and profunda brachii artery.

The **Triceps Muscle** arises by three distinct heads of origin:—

(*a*) The *long head* springs from the infraglenoid tubercle at the upper end of the lateral border of the scapula, and is superficial throughout.

(*b*) The *lateral head* arises from a linear ridge on the posterior surface of the humerus above the spiral groove, and also from the fibrous arch which spans the groove. This head is covered at its upper end by the posterior fibres of the deltoid, but in the greater part of its extent it is superficial.

(*c*) The *medial head* arises from the posterior surface of the humerus below the spiral groove. It is covered by the other two heads except in the lower part of the upper arm, where it becomes superficial.

The common tendon of the triceps is attached to the upper surface of the olecranon, and the posterior limit of its attachment is usually raised into a prominent ridge. It is separated from the posterior ligament of the elbow joint by a small synovial bursa.

The *nerve supply* of each head is a separate branch from the radial nerve (C. 7 and 8).

Action. The triceps is a powerful extensor of the elbow.

The **Radial Nerve** starts from the posterior cord of the brachial plexus in the axilla. It runs downwards and laterally on the posterior wall of the axilla, lying behind the artery and below the axillary nerve. In the upper part of the arm it passes backwards, downwards and laterally between the long and medial heads of triceps to gain the spiral groove of the humerus, accompanied by the profunda vessels. In the groove the nerve runs downwards and laterally between the lateral and medial heads of the triceps, and *in contact with the bone.* At the lower end of the groove it runs forwards through the lateral intermuscular septum, and then downwards in front of that structure and between the brachialis on the medial side, and the brachioradialis and the extensor carpi radialis longus on the lateral side. Just above the elbow it gives off the posterior interosseous nerve (p. 39).

Branches. (*a*) *Muscular* branches are given off: (1) to the long and medial heads of triceps, before the nerve enters the spiral groove; (2) to the lateral and medial heads of triceps and to the anconeus, as the nerve lies in the groove; (3) to the brachioradialis, the extensor carpi radialis longus and the brachialis, after the nerve has entered the anterior compartment of the arm.

(*b*) (1) The *posterior cutaneous nerve of the arm* arises before the nerve enters the groove and supplies the skin on the back of the arm.

(2) The *lower lateral cutaneous nerve of the arm* arises just before the nerve pierces the lateral intermuscular septum and supplies the skin over the lateral and anterior aspects of the lower part of the arm.

(3) The *posterior cutaneous nerve of the forearm* arises in common with the preceding nerve and runs down the middle of the back of the forearm. At the wrist, it communicates with the lateral cutaneous nerve and the terminal branch of the radial. It supplies a strip of skin from the elbow to the wrist, and may take part in the cutaneous supply of the dorsum of the hand.

(*c*) A few *articular* twigs are given to the elbow joint.

The **Profunda Brachii Artery** arises from the brachial artery high up in the arm, and accompanies the radial nerve along the spiral groove. In addition to supplying the triceps muscle, it gives off an ascending branch to anastomose with the posterior circumflex humeral artery, and its terminal branches take part in the anastomosis round the elbow joint (p. 23).

THE FRONT OF THE UPPER ARM

The *Deep Fascia* which ensheaths the upper arm sends two extensions inwards to the bone, incidentally separating the upper arm into two osteo-fascial compartments and, more realistically, increasing the area of surface available for muscular attachments. (*a*) The lateral intermuscular septum is attached to the lateral epicondyle and supracondylar ridge of the humerus as high up as the insertion of the deltoid. *At the junction of its upper and middle thirds it is traversed by the radial nerve.* (*b*) The medial intermuscular septum has a corresponding attachment on the medial side of the humerus and is traversed by the ulnar nerve. It is a much denser and stronger structure.

The **Biceps Muscle** has two heads of origin: (*a*) The *long head* arises from the supraglenoid tubercle on the scapula, and passes through the shoulder joint ensheathed by synovial membrane. It emerges from under cover of the transverse ligament and occupies the bicipital groove, at the lower end of which the tendon gives place to a fleshy belly. This is joined, in the lower third of the upper arm, by the belly of (*b*) the *short head*, which arises from the tip of the coracoid process in company with the coracobrachialis. The tendon of the biceps is inserted into the posterior part of the tuberosity of the radius, a small bursa intervening between it and the anterior part of the tuberosity.

An aponeurotic band, termed the *bicipital aponeurosis*, passes from the medial side of the biceps tendon to the deep fascia covering the pronator teres. It lies in front of the brachial artery and the median nerve, and is crossed, superficially, by the basilic vein and the medial cutaneous nerve of the forearm. Its medial edge can be palpated without difficulty in the living subject, when the biceps is in action.

Each belly receives a branch from the musculocutaneous nerve (C. 5 and 6).

Action. The biceps is a powerful supinator of the radius and flexor of the elbow joint.

The **Coracobrachialis** arises from the tip of the coracoid process and is inserted about half-way down the medial side of the humerus. It is usually traversed by the musculocutaneous nerve, from which it obtains its nerve supply (C. 7).

Action. The coracobrachialis assists in the movements of flexion and adduction at the shoulder joint.

The **Brachialis** muscle arises from the front of the lower half of the humerus. It crosses in front of the elbow joint to be inserted into the anterior surface of the coronoid process of the ulna.

Its *nerve supply* is derived from the musculocutaneous nerve, but the lateral head of the muscle, which ascends behind the deltoid tuberosity, receives a small branch from the radial nerve.

Action. The brachialis is a powerful flexor of the elbow joint.

The **Musculocutaneous Nerve** arises from the lateral cord of the brachial plexus and passes downwards and laterally through the coracobrachialis and then is continued downwards behind the biceps and in front of the brachialis. Just above the elbow it emerges at the lateral side of the biceps tendon and pierces the deep fascia. Thereafter it is termed the *lateral cutaneous nerve of the forearm*, and its branches supply the skin of the lateral aspect of this region. In the neighbourhood of the wrist these nerves communicate with the terminal branch of the radial nerve and the posterior cutaneous nerve of the forearm.

Branches. (*a*) *Muscular*, to coracobrachialis, both heads of biceps and brachialis.

(*b*) *Cutaneous*, to skin of forearm.

(*c*) *Articular*, to elbow joint.

The **Brachial Artery** is the direct continuation of the axillary artery. It commences at the lower border of the teres major, *where it is medial to the humerus*, and terminates half-an-inch below the elbow joint, in the middle line of the limb.

Relations. Anterior. Under the deep fascia the artery is partly overlapped from its lateral side by the coracobrachialis and the biceps, but otherwise it is superficial throughout its course and its pulsations can readily be felt. In the upper part of its course the medial cutaneous nerve of the forearm lies in front of the artery; about the middle of its course the artery is crossed anteriorly by the median nerve; in the lower part of its course it is crossed by the *bicipital aponeurosis*, by which it is separated from the basilic vein. The median nerve crosses the artery very obliquely, and not infrequently it may cross behind it.

Lateral. The median nerve, the coracobrachialis, and the biceps lie to its lateral side above, while the tendon of the biceps is closely related to its lateral side below.

Posterior. The artery lies on the triceps, the insertion of the coracobrachialis and also, in the lower half of its course, on the brachialis. The radial nerve passes between the artery and the triceps immediately below the teres major.

Medial. The ulnar nerve is closely applied to the artery and separates it from the basilic vein in the upper part of the arm. In the lower part of the arm, the ulnar nerve passes away from the artery, and the basilic vein is separated from it by the deep fascia. Below the insertion of the coracobrachialis, the median nerve is closely associated with the medial side of the artery.

Branches. As well as (1) un-named *muscular branches*, the artery has (2) a *profunda branch* (p. 20), which accompanies the radial nerve and arises high up in the arm; (3) an *ulnar collateral branch*, which accompanies the ulnar nerve and takes part in the anastomosis round the elbow joint; (4) a *supratrochlear branch*, which arises near the termination of the artery and takes part in the anastomosis round the elbow joint.

The **Median Nerve** is closely related to the brachial artery throughout the whole of its course in the arm. At first to the lateral side, it gradually crosses in front of the vessel and then runs down to the elbow along its medial side. The nerve is, therefore, very superficial in the arm, but just at the elbow it is crossed by the bicipital aponeurosis.

The **Ulnar Nerve** runs downwards on the medial side of the artery, lying between it and the basilic vein. At the insertion of the coracobrachialis, the nerve gradually inclines backwards and medially away from the artery, and, accompanied by the ulnar collateral vessels, traverses the medial intermuscular septum, behind which it descends, covered posteriorly by the medial head of the triceps. At the elbow it lies behind the medial epicondyle, and here it is prone to injury. In this situation the nerve can be compressed against the bone in the living subject, and tingling sensations can be aroused in the area of distribution of its cutaneous branches.

The **Cubital Fossa** is an intermuscular region lying in front of the elbow and extending downwards for a short distance into the forearm (Plate IA, p. 16). It is bounded on the lateral side by the brachioradialis muscle and on the medial side by the pronator teres. Above, it is limited by an imaginary line joining the two epicondyles of the humerus.

The fossa contains the median nerve, the termination of the brachial and the origins of the radial and ulnar arteries, the tendon of the biceps, and the radial nerve with the commencement of its posterior interosseous branch. (These structures are enumerated from the medial to the lateral side.) In addition, the *supratrochlear lymph nodes* lie above its upper and medial part. These lymph nodes receive afferents from the medial two or three digits, and the corresponding areas of the palm and forearm. Their efferents join the lateral axillary lymph nodes (p. 11).

Behind, the fossa is limited by the supinator on the lateral side, and the brachialis on the medial side.

The **Anastomosis around the Elbow Joint** constitutes a free communication between the brachial artery on the one hand and the upper ends of the radial and ulnar arteries on the other. The profunda from the upper part of the brachial, the ulnar collateral usually from the intermediate part, and the supratrochlear from the lower part, link up with branches which arise from the radial, ulnar and posterior interosseous arteries, close to their points of origin. The anastomosis, like all periarticular anastomoses, lies close to the bones and supplies them.

THE FRONT OF THE FOREARM

The *Nerves* which supply the skin of the front of the forearm are derived from the anterior branches of (1) the medial cutaneous nerve of the forearm (C. 8 and T. 1), and (2) the lateral cutaneous nerve of the forearm (C. 5 and 6). The former is distributed along the ulnar, and the latter along the radial, side of the forearm, and the two areas overlap only to a slight extent, as the spinal cord segments concerned are not consecutive, *C. 7 having no area of supply on the front of the forearm.*

Superficial Veins. The *cephalic vein* arises from the radial side of the dorsal venous arch of the hand, and, winding round the radial border of the forearm, ascends to the apex of the cubital fossa. There it receives a tributary from the deep structures of the forearm, and gives off the median cubital vein. It then ascends in the groove on the lateral side of the biceps. In its course it receives a variable number of radial veins from the dorsal aspect of the forearm.

The *basilic vein* arises from the ulnar side of the dorsal venous arch and gradually winds round the ulnar border of the forearm as it ascends to the arm, where it lies in the groove on the medial side of the biceps. In its course it receives one or two ulnar veins from the dorsal aspect of the forearm (Plate IA, p. 16).

The *median cubital vein* leaves the cephalic at or near the apex of the cubital fossa and runs upwards and medially to join the basilic vein. It crosses in front of the brachial artery and the median nerve, but is separated from both structures by the bicipital aponeurosis.

The upward flow in the veins of the limbs is aided by a number of different factors. (1) The outflow from the capillary bed provides a certain degree of "vis a tergo." (2) Muscular contractions exert a squeezing effect, especially on the deep veins. Although this tends to drive the blood in both directions, the presence of competent venous valves ensures that there will be very little backward flow. At the same time blood is driven into the superficial veins and onwards towards the heart. (3) Alterations in the posture of the limbs, *e.g.*, elevation of the arms, obviously exercise a favourable influence. (4) Negative intrathoracic pressure tends to suck blood into the right atrium from the great veins of the thorax and so assists the onward flow in the veins of the limbs.

The **Superficial Group of Flexor Muscles** comprises the pronator teres, the flexor carpi radialis, the palmaris longus, the flexor digitorum superficialis and the flexor carpi ulnaris. These muscles possess a common tendinous origin, which makes a strong impression on the anterior and medial aspects of the medial epicondyle. In addition, each is attached to the covering deep fascia and the fascial partitions which exist between them.

The **Pronator Teres** also possesses a small *deep head of origin*, which springs from the medial border of the coronoid process of the ulna. It is the most laterally placed member of the group, and runs downwards and laterally to be inserted into a roughened area about halfway down the lateral aspect of the radius. At its insertion the radial artery and the radial nerve cross in front of it, while the median nerve passes downwards between its two heads of origin, and the ulnar artery runs deep to both heads.

Actions. The chief action of the muscle is pronation, but it also helps in flexion of the elbow.

The **Flexor Carpi Radialis** runs downwards, with a gradual inclination laterally, to the wrist. It pierces the lateral attachment of the flexor retinaculum, occupies the groove on the front of the trapezium, and so reaches the palmar surfaces of the bases of the second and third metacarpal bones, into which it is inserted. At the wrist the tendon of the flexor carpi radialis lies lateral to the median nerve and medial to the radial artery.

The **Palmaris Longus,** which is not always present, passes downwards with a slight inclination laterally and, crossing in front of the flexor retinaculum, gains insertion into the palmar aponeurosis. At the wrist it lies in front of the median nerve, which tends to project to its lateral side.

Actions. Both the flexor carpi radialis and the palmaris longus act as flexors of the wrist joint. In addition, the former, acting in combination with the radial extensors of the wrist, abducts the hand. When they are thrown into contraction against resistance, the tendons of both muscles show up clearly under the skin above the front of the wrist, the flexor carpi radialis tendon being the more lateral (Plate IA, p. 16).

The **Flexor Digitorum Superficialis (Sublimis)** has an extensive origin along an oblique line, which is interrupted opposite the interval between the radius and the ulna. Commencing at the common flexor origin on the medial epicondyle, the origin extends along the medial ligament of the elbow joint to the medial border of the coronoid process. The radial head from an oblique line on the front of the radius, is in line with the preceding fibres, and through the gap left between the two heads the median nerve and the ulnar artery pass downwards. The radial head is covered over by the pronator teres, the flexor carpi radialis and the palmaris longus, but the rest of the muscle is superficial.

In the lower part of the forearm four tendons are developed, and these enter the palm behind the flexor retinaculum, where the tendons for the middle and ring fingers lie in front of those for the index and little fingers.

Eventually the tendons are inserted into the *borders* of the middle phalanges (p. 32).

Action. The flexor digitorum superficialis flexes the fingers, primarily at the proximal interphalangeal joints, and secondarily at the metacarpophalangeal joints. It also assists in flexing the wrist joint, but it can only do so at the expense of its digital action, and hence, when a tight grip is required, the carpal extensors, functioning as synergic muscles, oppose any tendency to flexion.

Nerve Supply. The four preceding muscles are all innervated by the median nerve.

The **Median Nerve** leaves the cubital fossa by passing downwards between the two heads of the pronator teres reaches to the deep surface of the flexor digitorum superficialis, which separates it from flexor carpi radialis and palmaris longus. At the wrist, it emerges from the lateral border of the muscle and lies behind the palmaris longus tendon. Finally, it enters the palm by passing behind the flexor retinaculum. In the upper part of its course it crosses in front of the ulnar artery, from which it is separated by the deep head of the pronator teres. Throughout the rest of its course in the forearm the nerve lies on the anterior surface of the flexor digitorum profundus, but when this muscle is separated from the flexor superficialis by blunt dissection, the nerve usually remains adherent to the deep surface of the latter.

Branches. As it lies in the cubital fossa, the median nerve gives off (1) articular twigs to the elbow joint, and (2) branches to supply the pronator teres, the flexor carpi radialis, the palmaris longus and the flexor digitorum superficialis. In the upper part of the forearm it gives off additional branches to the last-named muscle, and (3) the *anterior interosseous nerve.*

In the lower part of the forearm it gives off a cutaneous branch to supply a small area of skin over the central part of the palm.

The **Flexor Carpi Ulnaris** possesses a second head of origin, which arises from the medial side of the olecranon process and is continuous below with an aponeurosis which binds the muscle to the posterior border of the ulna. It passes vertically down the medial side of the forearm, and its tendon is inserted primarily into the pisiform bone and via this into the hamate and fifth metacarpal bones, which provide its true insertion. At the wrist it overlies the ulnar nerve and has the ulnar artery immediately to its lateral side, intervening between it and the tendons of the flexor digitorum superficialis. In this situation it can be palpated in the living subject very readily, especially when the forearm is pronated.

Its *Nerve Supply* comes off from the ulnar nerve as it lies behind the medial epicondyle.

Action. The flexor carpi ulnaris is a flexor of the wrist joint. Acting in combination with the extensor carpi ulnaris it adducts the hand, or, conversely, it prevents abduction of the hand, *e.g.*, when the thumb is fully extended. (Confirm this by palpation.)

The **Ulnar Nerve** runs downwards from its position behind the medial epicondyle, crosses the medial ligament of the elbow joint and passes between the two heads of the flexor carpi ulnaris. It is then continued downwards to the wrist under cover of that muscle, and on the surface of the flexor digitorum profundus. In the lower two-thirds of the forearm the ulnar artery lies close to its lateral side.

Branches. 1. *Articular*, to the elbow joint.

2. *Muscular*, to the flexor carpi ulnaris and to the medial half of the flexor digitorum profundus.

3. *Cutaneous*, palmar and dorsal. The palmar cutaneous is a small nerve which arises in the middle of the forearm and ultimately supplies the skin over the hypothenar eminence.

The *dorsal branch* arises about three inches above the wrist and winds round the ulnar border of the forearm under cover of the tendon of the flexor carpi ulnaris. It is ultimately distributed on the dorsum of the hand (p. 36).

The **Ulnar Artery** arises in the cubital fossa, half-an-inch below the elbow joint, and passes downwards and medially deep to the pronator teres, the flexor carpi radialis, the palmaris longus and the flexor digitorum superficialis. It then passes under cover of the flexor carpi ulnaris, and, coming into relationship with the ulnar nerve, it runs straight downwards to the wrist lateral to the muscle and the nerve. In the upper part of its course it crosses behind the median nerve, from which it is separated by the deep head of the pronator teres.

Posteriorly, the artery lies at first on the brachialis, but in nearly the whole of its course through the forearm it has the flexor digitorum profundus behind it.

Consideration of the anterior relations of the vessel will show that, *in the upper part of its course, it is deeply situated. Near the wrist, however, it becomes comparatively superficial*, for it emerges from under cover of the flexor carpi ulnaris and lies between that tendon and the tendons of the flexor digitorum superficialis.

Branches. In addition to giving branches to the neighbouring muscles, the ulnar artery gives off recurrent branches from its upper end to the anastomosis round the elbow joint, and small branches from its lower end to the anastomosis round the wrist joint.

Its largest branch is the *Common Interosseous Artery*, which arises in the cubital fossa and, after a short course downwards and backwards, ends by dividing into the anterior and the posterior interosseous arteries (pp. 29 and 40).

The **Radial Artery** is comparatively superficial throughout its whole course, but particularly in its lower half. It arises from the brachial in the cubital fossa and runs downwards, curving laterally, to the wrist. In the upper part of its course it is overlapped by the brachioradialis, but *in the lower half of its extent it is covered only by the skin, the superficial and the deep fascia.*

In its *upper third*, the artery crosses the tendon of the biceps and the insertion of the supinator. The radial nerve lies to its lateral side, but is not an immediate relation. In its *middle third*, the artery crosses the pronator teres and the radial head of the flexor digitorum superficialis. The nerve is closely applied to its lateral side. In its *lower third* the artery lies on the flexor pollicis longus, the pronator quadratus and, finally, on the radius, where its pulsations can readily be felt in the living subject. It is no longer in relation to the nerve, which leaves it by winding round the radial border of the forearm deep to the brachioradialis tendon.

Branches. In addition to branches to the neighbouring muscles, a recurrent branch to the anastomosis round the elbow and a branch to the anastomosis round the wrist joint, the radial artery gives off a *superficial palmar branch*, which arises just above the wrist and runs down into the hand, either through or superficial to the muscles of the thenar eminence (p. 33) which it supplies. It frequently completes the superficial palmar arch.

The **Deep Group of Flexor Muscles** comprises the flexor pollicis longus, the flexor digitorum profundus and the pronator quadratus.

The **Flexor Pollicis Longus** arises from the anterior surface of the radius, between the oblique line and the upper border of the pronator quadratus, and also from the adjoining part of the interosseous membrane. Its tendon passes downwards behind the flexor

PLATE V. ANTERO-POSTERIOR RADIOGRAPH OF RIGHT SHOULDER REGION IN A YOUNG ADULT.

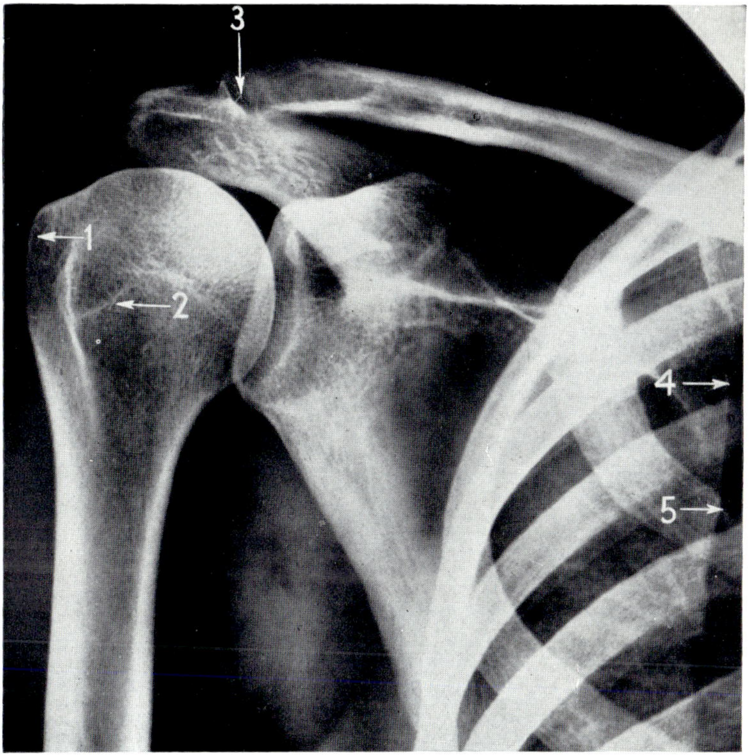

1. Greater tuberosity
2. Upper epiphyseal line indicated by a thin strip of dense bone.
3. Acromioclavicular joint.
4. Medial border of scapula.
5. Second rib.

Observe that the greater tuberosity of the humerus is the most lateral bony point in the shoulder region, and note the density of the shadow produced by the lateral border of the scapula.

To face p. 28

PLATE VI. ANTERO-POSTERIOR RADIOGRAPH OF THE SHOULDER REGION OF A BOY OF 12 YEARS OF AGE.

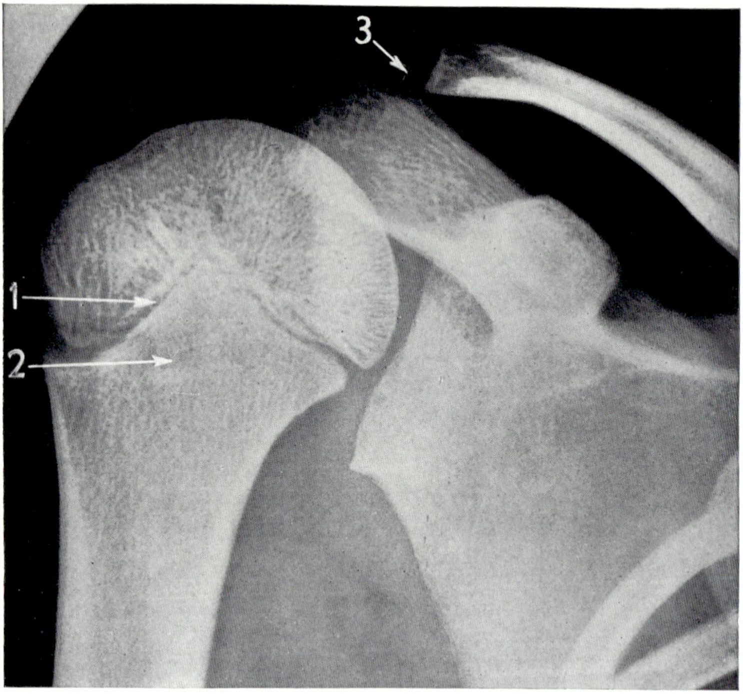

1. Upper epiphyseal cartilage of humerus.
2. Upper end of diaphysis. Note its wedge-like appearance.
3. Gap between clavicle and acromion, occupied by the cartilaginous lateral end of the clavicle and by the cartilage of the acromion and the acromio-clavicular joint.

Note that the increased density in the area medial to the upper part of the glenoid is due to the presence of the coracoid process, which is foreshortened in this view.

PLATE VII. ANTERO-POSTERIOR RADIOGRAPH OF THE ELBOW REGION IN A YOUNG ADULT.

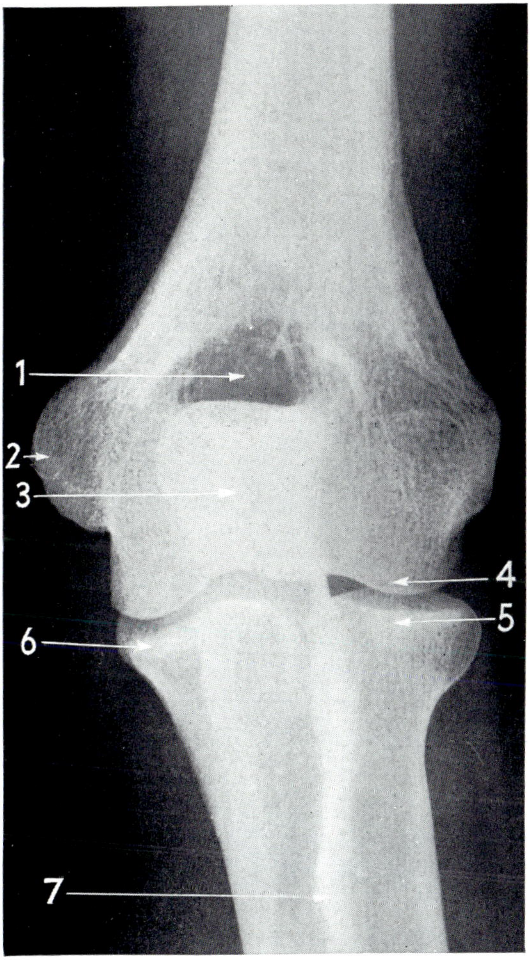

1. Olecranon fossa.
2. Medial epicondyle.
3. Olecranon overlying shadow of trochlea.
4. Capitulum.
5. Head of radius.
6. Edge of coronoid process.
7. Tuberosity of radius.

Note the downward projection of the medial edge of the trochlea, and the "carrying angle."

Plate VIII. The Left Hand of a Girl of 15 Years in Full Abduction (left) and Full Adduction (right).

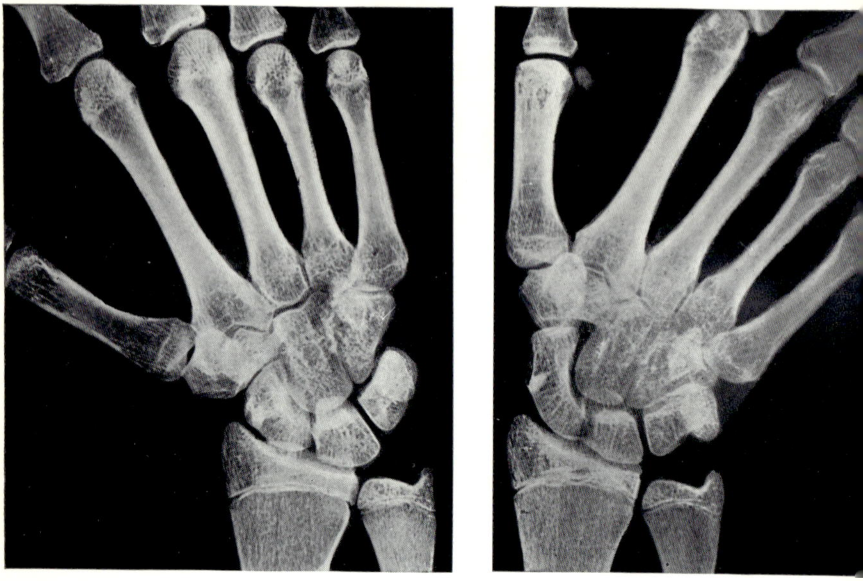

Note that the scaphoid is much foreshortened owing to rotation round its transverse axis in abduction and compare with its appearance in full adduction.

Note too, that the lunate articulates only with the radius in full adduction and that, whereas in full abduction the medial edge of the capitate is in line with the medial edge of the lunate, in adduction these margins become angulated on each other, showing that movement has occurred also at the transverse carpal joint.

In confirmation of the latter statement, compare the positions of the hamate and triquetral bones relative to each other, and observe that in adduction the pisiform becomes approximated to the ulnar styloid process.

Owing to the sex and age of the subject, the epiphyses of all the metacarpal bones and proximal phalanges shown have united with the corresponding diaphyses.

retinaculum to reach the thumb, and is inserted into the palmar surface of the base of the distal phalanx.

The *Action* of the muscle is indicated by its name.

The **Pronator Quadratus** arises from the front of the ulna in its lower fourth, and is inserted into the corresponding part of the radius.

Actions. It is a pronator of the forearm and hand.

Nerve Supply. Both the preceding muscles are supplied by the anterior interosseous nerve.

The **Flexor Digitorum Profundus** arises from the upper three-fourths of the medial and anterior surfaces of the ulna, and from the corresponding part of the interosseous membrane. It is covered anteriorly by the flexor digitorum superficialis and by the flexor carpi ulnaris, while the median nerve and the ulnar artery and nerve run down on its anterior surface.

Above the wrist it gives rise to four tendons, which enter the palm by passing behind those of the flexor digitorum superficialis and the flexor retinaculum. They are inserted into the bases of the distal phalanges (p. 32).

Its *Nerve Supply* is derived from the ulnar and the anterior interosseous nerves.

Action. Primarily, the flexor digitorum profundus flexes the distal phalanges of the fingers; secondarily, it flexes the proximal interphalangeal and the metacarpophalangeal joints. In the ordinary action of closing the hand, flexion of the metacarpophalangeal joints precedes flexion of the proximal interphalangeal joints, and both these movements have been almost completed before the terminal phalanges become flexed (p. 36).

The **Anterior Interosseous Nerve** arises from the median nerve at the upper end of the forearm and runs downwards, in front of the interosseous membrane, between the flexor pollicis longus and the flexor digitorum profundus, accompanied by the artery of the same name. It supplies branches to both these muscles, and ends by supplying the pronator quadratus.

The **Anterior Interosseous Artery** arises from the common interosseous and runs downwards, with the anterior interosseous nerve, to the upper border of the pronator quadratus. *There it pierces the interosseous membrane,* behind which it descends to take part in the anastomosis around the wrist joint.

Branches. In addition to muscular branches, nutrient branches to the bones of the forearm and a communicating branch to the anastomosis round the wrist joint, the anterior interosseous artery gives off the *median artery,* which runs with the median nerve. The anterior interosseous artery is part of the primitive stem artery of the limb and is the first of the forearm arteries to develop. (Its median branch is relatively large at first and breaks up into a superficial palmar network which later becomes resolved into the superficial palmar arch. Occasionally the median artery is found persisting as a comparatively large vessel and in these cases it takes part in the formation of the superficial palmar arch.)

THE PALMAR ASPECT OF THE WRIST AND HAND

The *Superficial Fascia* of the palm of the hand is intersected by numerous fibrous bands which extend between the skin and the deep fascia, in consequence, it lacks mobility.

Cutaneous Nerves. Palmar cutaneous branches arise from the ulnar, median, and radial nerves, but the branch from the latter may be replaced, in part or completely, by a branch from the lateral cutaneous nerve of the forearm.

The digital nerves will be described later (p. 33).

The *Deep Fascia* of the palmar aspect of the wrist is specially thickened to form the *flexor retinaculum*, which forms a bridge across the carpus so as to complete an osteo-fascial tunnel restraining the flexor tendons of the thumb and fingers.

On the medial side it is attached to the pisiform and the hook of the hamate (p. 408); on the lateral side it is attached to the tubercle of the scaphoid and to the trapezium. At a point which corresponds to the *distal* flexion skin crease of the wrist it is continuous with the deep fascia of the front of the forearm, and below it blends with the palmar aponeurosis.

Anterior to the retinaculum, the palmaris longus and the ulnar artery and nerve pass into the palm. *Behind* the retinaculum lie the tendons of the flexor pollicis longus and the flexor digitorum superficialis and profundus, with their synovial sheaths, and the median nerve. The lateral attachment of the retinaculum is pierced by the flexor carpi radialis tendon.

The *deep fascia of the palm* consists of weak lateral and medial parts, covering the small muscles of the thumb and little finger respectively, and a strong central part, better named the *palmar aponeurosis*, which covers the flexor tendons. Above the aponeurosis blends with the flexor retinaculum, and distally it splits into four slips opposite the heads of the metacarpal bones. Each slip is continuous below with the fibrous sheath of the finger and, at the sides, is connected to the deep transverse ligaments. From the edges of the palmar aponeurosis, weak septa pass backwards into the palm to subdivide it into medial, intermediate and lateral compartments which may impede spread of infection.

Each finger is provided with an arched *fibrous sheath* continuous above with the palmar aponeurosis and attached to the sides of the phalanges and across the base of the distal phalanx. This fibrous sheath, together with the phalanges and the palmar ligaments of the interphalangeal joints, forms a blind osteo-fascial tunnel, in which lie the flexor tendons of the finger. It is specially strong opposite the phalanges, but is thin opposite the joints to permit of free flexion.

These three structures, the flexor retinaculum, the palmar aponeurosis, and the fibrous flexor sheaths constitute a continuous structure. which holds the tendons in position and so increases the efficiency of the grip. It is at least equally important to note that the palmar skin is tethered to the deep fascia (p. 30) and through the latter to bone. By this mechanism great forces can be transmitted from the hand to the rest of the body.

The palmar aponeurosis gives no slip to the thumb, in contradistinction to the arrangement in the foot. *The wide range of movement of the thumb, which is in part due to this fact, is an important feature of the primate hand.*

The **Superficial Palmar Arch** is the direct continuation of the ulnar artery into the palm. After crossing in front of the flexor retinaculum, the artery runs laterally across the palm immediately behind the palmar aponeurosis. On the lateral side of the palm it is sometimes completed by the superficial palmar branch of the radial artery but frequently the communication with the radial artery is made through the *arteria radialis indicis* (p. 42) or the arteries of the thumb. In its course the arch forms a curve convex downwards the lowest part lying on a level with the extended thumb.

As it crosses the palm the arch lies on the flexor digiti minimi, the flexor tendons of the fingers and the lumbricals, and the digital branches of the median nerve.

Four *digital branches* pass to the fingers. Of these the most medial runs down the ulnar side of the little finger, and the others pass to the medial three clefts, dividing into two for the supply of the adjoining borders of two fingers. Each finger therefore receives two arteries on its palmar surface, each derived from a different digital branch.

As they leave the arch the digital arteries lie in front of the digital nerves, but they cross one another before reaching the fingers, where the arteries lie posterior to the nerves.

The *deep branch of the ulnar artery* arises in front of the flexor retinaculum and plunges between the flexor and the abductor digiti minimi to join and complete the deep palmar arch.

The **Flexor Tendons of the Fingers and their Synovial Sheaths.** The flexor tendons are crowded together in the carpal tunnel behind the flexor retinaculum, but they diverge in the central compartment of the palm, where the tendons of the flexor digitorum superficialis lie superficial to those of the deep flexor. Entering the fibrous sheath of its own finger, each superficialis tendon splits opposite to the proximal phalanx and allows the profundus tendon to perforate it. The tendon then re-unites behind the profundus, undergoes a partial decussation of fibres, and again splits to be attached to the *borders* of the middle phalanx. The deep tendon is continued onwards to be inserted into the palmar surface of the base of the distal phalanx.

As they lie behind the flexor retinaculum the flexor tendons of the fingers are enclosed in a *common synovial sheath*, which possesses a parietal layer, lining the walls of the carpal tunnel, and a "visceral" layer, closely applied to the tendons. The arrangement is precisely as if the tendons had been invaginated into an elongated bursal sac from its lateral side. The common synovial sheath extends upwards for 2 or 3 inches into the forearm and downwards into the palm. *Here its medial extremity is carried down, without interruption, on the tendons of the little finger to line its fibrous sheath. Elsewhere in the palm the common sheath ends blindly, opposite to the middle of the shafts of the metacarpal bones.*

Digital Synovial Sheaths, closed at both ends, line the fibrous sheaths of the ring, middle and index fingers and invest their tendons from the base of the distal phalanx to the head of the metacarpal bone.

The *Vincula Longa and Brevia*, which connect the tendons to the phalanges, are synovial folds, similar to a mesentery.

The **Flexor Pollicis Longus** tendon passes behind the flexor retinaculum and then runs downwards among the muscles of the thenar eminence, on the palmar surface of the metacarpal bone of the thumb. On the proximal phalanx it enters a fibrous sheath, similar to those already described for the fingers, and is inserted into the palmar surface of the base of the distal phalanx. It possesses a synovial sheath, which extends upwards on the tendon for 2 or 3 inches into the forearm and downwards to its insertion. This sheath may communicate with the common sheath, as they lie in close contact behind the flexor retinaculum.

The four **Lumbrical Muscles** arise from the tendons of the flexor digitorum profundus in the palm. Each is inserted into the radial side of the dorsal digital expansion of its own finger (p. 39).

The *Nerve Supply* of the lateral two lumbricals is from the median nerve, while the medial two are supplied by the ulnar nerve.

Actions. The lumbricals flex the fingers at the metacarpophalangeal joints. If they contract when the digital flexors are passive, the pull of the lumbricals tends to relax the flexor profundus tendons and so permits the extensor digitorum to extend the interphalangeal joints, as in the upstroke in writing.

The **Median Nerve** enters the central compartment of the palm by passing behind the flexor retinaculum, where it is in contact with the common synovial sheath but is not invested by it. It at once breaks up into *lateral* and *medial divisions.*

The *Lateral Division* gives off, usually by a common trunk, the nerves of supply to the abductor brevis, the flexor brevis and the opponens pollicis muscles. It then gives off digital branches to both sides of the palmar aspect of the thumb and to the radial side of the index finger. The last-named supplies the first lumbrical muscle.

The *Medial Division* breaks up into two, and these pass downwards behind the superficial palmar arch to the clefts between the index and middle and the middle and ring fingers. There they divide to supply the adjoining sides of the fingers named.

These palmar digital nerves supply not only the whole palmar aspect, but also the distal half of the dorsal aspect of each digit, and a similar arrangement holds good for the digital branches of the ulnar nerve.

The *Small Muscles of the Thumb* form the thenar eminence.

The **Abductor Pollicis Brevis** arises from the scaphoid, the trapezium and the flexor retinaculum, and is inserted into the radial side of the base of the proximal phalanx of the thumb. It is subcutaneous and is supplied by the median nerve.

Action. Abduction of the thumb occurs in an antero-posterior plane, i.e., *at right angles to the plane of abduction of the fingers. The difference is due to the fact that the metacarpal bone of the thumb, as compared with the other metacarpals, is rotated so that its dorsal surface is directed laterally* (p. 408). The movement occurs both at the carpometacarpal and at the metacarpophalangeal joint, and, when the thumb is abducted fully, the digit and its metacarpal bone are no longer in the same straight line.

The **Flexor Pollicis Brevis** is also subcutaneous and lies along the ulnar side of the preceding muscle. It arises from the flexor retinaculum and is inserted in common with the abductor. (The so-called first palmar interosseous muscle is often considered a part of the flexor pollicis brevis, *v.*p. 35.)

Its *Nerve Supply* comes from the median nerve but it not infrequently receives an additional supply from the deep branch of the ulnar nerve and is often solely supplied by it. Its *Action* is indicated by its name.

The **Opponens Pollicis** muscle lies deep to the two preceding muscles. It arises from the flexor retinaculum, deep to the flexor brevis, and is inserted into the whole length of the radial (or anterior) border of the first metacarpal bone. Its *nerve supply* comes from the median nerve.

Action. Opposition is the movement which carries the tip of the thumb into contact with the tip of any of the fingers. In addition to flexion of the carpometacarpal and metacarpophalangeal joints, it involves a small degree of abduction and of medial rotation of the metacarpal bone of the thumb.

The **Adductor Pollicis** lies in the lateral part of the palm. Its *Tranverse Head* arises from the shaft of the third metacarpal bone behind the flexor tendons and lumbrical muscles. Its fibres converge to be inserted into the ulnar side of the base of the proximal phalanx of the thumb. Near its insertion the muscle is superficial in the web of the thumb.

The *Oblique Head* lies along the radial border of the transverse head. It arises from the bases of the second and third metacarpals and the adjoining carpal bones, and is inserted by a common tendon with the transverse head.

The *Nerve Supply* of both muscles is derived from the ulnar nerve.

Action. The adductors restore the abducted thumb to its normal position of rest, and, in association with the flexor pollicis longus and the opponens pollicis muscle, are chiefly responsible for the power of the grip, as far as the thumb is concerned.

The *Small Muscles of the Little Finger* form the hypothenar eminence.

The **Abductor Digiti Minimi** arises from the pisiform bone and is inserted into the ulnar side of the base of the proximal phalanx of the little finger. It is very superficial and lies along the ulnar border of the hand.

The **Flexor Digiti Minimi** lies along the radial side of the abductor and is also subcutaneous. It arises from the flexor retinaculum and is inserted in common with the abductor.

The **Opponens Digiti Minimi** lies deep to the two preceding muscles. It arises from the flexor retinaculum and is inserted into the ulnar border of the fifth metacarpal bone.

All the small muscles of the little finger receive their *Nerve Supply* from the ulnar nerve.

Their *Actions* are indicated by their names.

The **Ulnar Nerve** enters the palm close to the medial side of the superficial palmar arch. As it crosses the flexor retinaculum superficially it divides into a superficial and a deep terminal branch.

The *Superficial Terminal Branch* divides, almost at once, into a digital branch which runs downwards to supply the ulnar border of the little finger, and a branch which runs down behind the palmar aponeurosis to the cleft between the ring and the little fingers, where it divides into two branches to supply the adjoining sides of these two fingers.

Near their origin these two branches can be rolled against the hook of the hamate (p. 408).

The *Deep Terminal Branch* passes backwards between the abductor and the flexor digiti minimi, and then turns laterally across the palm in close relationship with the deep palmar arch and behind the flexor tendons. It supplies (1) the small muscles of the little finger; (2) the third and fourth lumbricals; (3) all the interossei; and (4) both heads of the adductor of the thumb, *i.e., all the muscles of the hand excepting the abductor brevis, opponens and flexor brevis pollicis and the first and second lumbricals, all supplied by the median nerve*. (Not infrequently it gives a branch to the flexor pollicis brevis.)

The **Deep Palmar Arch** crosses the upper part of the palm in contact posteriorly with the metacarpal bones and interosseous muscles, and related anteriorly to the flexor tendons. Throughout its course it is accompanied by the deep terminal branch of the ulnar nerve, the arch being completed on the medial side by union with the deep branch of the ulnar artery.

The radial artery enters the palm from behind by passing forwards between the heads of the first dorsal interosseous muscle at the proximal end of the space between the first and second metacarpal bones. It then turns medially, behind the oblique head of the adductor of the thumb and, opposite the third metacarpal bone, it emerges between that muscle and the transverse head.

The arch sends branches proximally to the anastomosis round the wrist, and downwards to join the digital branches of the superficial arch at the clefts of the fingers.

The **Interosseous Muscles** of the hand comprise four dorsal and four palmar muscles. (The first palmar is sometimes described as the medial part of the flexor pollicis brevis.) The former abduct the fingers from, and the latter adduct them to, the middle line of the hand.

The second, third and fourth *Palmar Interossei* arise from the palmar surfaces of the second, fourth and fifth metacarpal bones respectively. The second is inserted into the ulnar side of the base of the proximal phalanx of the index, and the remaining two into the radial side of the corresponding bones of the ring and little fingers, respectively. Each is also attached to the adjoining part of the dorsal digital expansion (*cf.* Lumbricals, p. 32). The first arises from the base of the first metacarpal bone and is inserted into the ulnar side of the base of the proximal phalanx of the thumb. *It is a flexor and adductor of the thumb at the metacarpo-phalangeal joint* (*v.* p. 33).

The *Dorsal Interossei* arise, each by two heads, from the adjoining sides of the two metacarpal bones between which they lie. The first is inserted into the radial side of the base of the proximal phalanx of the index; the second is inserted similarly on the proximal phalanx of the middle finger; the third, on the ulnar side of the same bone; and the fourth, on the ulnar side of the proximal phalanx of the ring finger. Each receives additional insertion into the dorsal digital expansion.

In addition, both the palmar and the dorsal interossei act with the lumbricals to flex the fingers at the metacarpophalangeal joints (see also p. 32).

The nerve supply of all the interossei is derived from the deep terminal branch of the ulnar nerve.

It is most important to remember that, according to clinical evidence, *all the muscles of the hand*, no matter whether they are supplied by the median or by the ulnar nerve, *receive their innervation ultimately from the first thoracic spinal segment.*

THE BACK OF THE FOREARM AND HAND

The skin of the back of the forearm is supplied by the posterior branch of the medial and the lateral cutaneous nerves of the forearm. A strip of skin down the middle of the surface is supplied by the posterior cutaneous nerve of the forearm.

The terminal part of the radial nerve and the dorsal branch of the ulnar nerve supply the skin of the back of the hand and fingers. The former, which winds round the radius deep to the brachioradialis tendon about 3 inches above the wrist, is continued downwards superficial to the extensor retinaculum and supplies the skin over the lateral two-thirds of the dorsum of the hand and gives dorsal digital branches to the thumb and index fingers, and to the radial side of the middle finger.

The dorsal branch of the ulnar nerve winds round the ulna about 3 inches above the wrist and descends superficial to the extensor retinaculum. It supplies the rest of the skin over the dorsum of the hand and the little and ring fingers and the ulnar side of the middle finger.

The dorsal digital nerves usually do not extend much beyond the

proximal interphalangeal joints, the rest of the dorsum of each finger receiving its nerve supply from the palmar digital nerves.

An irregular *dorsal venous arch* lies in the superficial fascia on the dorsum of the hand. It receives the *digital veins* and from its ulnar and radial extremities, respectively, the *basilic* and *cephalic veins* arise.

The *Deep Fascia* over the posterior aspect of the forearm is specially thickened in the region of the wrist, where it forms the *extensor retinaculum*, an *oblique* band, about half-an-inch deep, which is attached to the *anterior* border of the radius above its styloid process on the lateral side, and to the pisiform and triquetral bones on the medial side. Further, it is attached to certain longitudinal ridges on the posterior aspect of the lower end of the radius, and so completes a number of short osteo-fascial tunnels for the passage of the extensor tendons (p. 41).

The **Superficial Group of Muscles** have a common tendinous attachment to the lateral epicondyle of the humerus. In addition, each arises from the covering deep fascia and from the fascial septa which intervene between it and its neighbours. The brachioradialis and the extensor carpi radialis longus, which belong to this group, arise proximal to the common tendon.

The **Brachioradialis** muscle arises from the upper two-thirds of the lateral supracondylar ridge of the humerus and the adjoining part of the anterior surface of the lateral intermuscular septum. It overlaps the brachialis and descends in front of the lateral epicondyle, forming the lateral boundary of the cubital fossa (Plate IA, p. 16). About half-way down the forearm the muscular belly becomes a tendon, attached to the lower end of the radius, just above the styloid process.

Its *Nerve Supply* is from the radial nerve, which lies under cover of the muscle in the lower part of the upper arm.

Action. The brachioradialis is a flexor of the elbow joint and acts to best advantage when the forearm is in the mid-prone position. When the semi-prone forearm is flexed against resistance, the muscle becomes very conspicuous.

The **Extensor Carpi Radialis Longus** is closely associated with the preceding muscle. It arises from the lower third of the lateral supracondylar ridge and intermuscular septum, and descends over the lateral epicondyle deep to the brachioradialis. At first lateral to the radius, it gains the dorsal surface half-way down the forearm. It has a long tendon, which is continued downwards to the wrist, where it passes under cover of the extensor retinaculum and is inserted into the dorsum of the base of the second metacarpal bone.

It receives its *Nerve Supply*, near its origin, from the radial nerve.

The **Extensor Carpi Radialis Brevis** arises from the common origin and runs downwards, at first overlapped by, and later to the medial side of, the extensor carpi radialis longus. Its tendon commences at the middle of the forearm and passes under cover of the extensor retinaculum, through a compartment which it shares with the longus. It is inserted into the dorsum of the base of the third metacarpal bone.

Its *Nerve Supply* is derived from the posterior interosseous nerve.

Both the radial extensors of the wrist are crossed at the junction of the lower and middle thirds of the forearm by two of the deep muscles—the abductor pollicis longus and the extensor pollicis brevis—which here become superficial.

Actions. Both the radial extensors act as their names indicate, and, when co-operating with the flexor carpi radialis, they abduct the hand. They are, however, used more frequently as synergic muscles than as prime movers and are called into play to extend and fix the wrist in gripping.

The **Extensor Digitorum** arises from the common origin and runs downwards, medial to the extensor carpi radialis brevis. It divides into four tendons, which pass under the extensor retinaculum and then diverge to the fingers. On the dorsum of the hand the individual tendons are connected to one another and also, in the cases of the first and fourth, to the extensor indicis and the extensor digiti minimi. Partly on account of these connections, complete extension of an individual finger at the metacarpophalangeal joint is not possible so long as the other fingers are kept flexed, although, in the case of the index, the range of extension is almost complete. The connections can be seen by watching the play of the tendons on the dorsum of the hand when each finger, in turn, is flexed at the metacarpophalangeal joint, the other fingers being kept extended.

As each extensor tendon, incorporated in the dorsal digital expansion, crosses the metacarpophalangeal joint, it is separated from the thin capsular ligament by a bursa, and immediately distal to the joint some of its deeper fibres are inserted into the bone. Near the proximal interphalangeal joint the tendon splits into a central portion, which is inserted into the base of the middle phalanx, and two lateral portions which converge to be inserted into the base of the distal phalanx. The extensor digitorum extends the fingers at all the digital joints (p. 33).

The **Dorsal Digital Expansion** is a fibrous sheet lying on the dorsal surface of the proximal phalanx of each of the fingers. It has the shape of a truncated isosceles triangle, the base of which is proximal and covers the metacarpophalangeal joint in the position of extension. The extensor digitorum forms a thickened band down the middle of the expansion, the base of which connects it to the corresponding interosseous muscle on each side by numerous curved fibres. The edges of the expansion are oblique and are continuous with the tendon of the lumbrical muscle on the lateral side and the corresponding interosseous muscle on the medial side. In the intervals between its borders and the extensor tendon, the expansion consists of a thin but uninterrupted membranous sheet. It resembles a hood and is drawn distally when the metacarpophalangeal joint is flexed, providing good purchase for the lumbrical and interosseous muscles, which produce the movement, simultaneously extending the interphalangal joints.

The **Extensor Digiti Minimi** is medial to the extensor digitorum. It passes through a separate compartment of the extensor retinaculum and forms the dorsal extensor expansion for the little finger, being joined by the small fourth tendon of the extensor digitorum.

The **Extensor Carpi Ulnaris** is between the preceding muscle and the anconeus in the upper part of the forearm, but in the lower two-thirds of the forearm its medial border lies along the subcutaneous posterior border of the ulna (Plate IB, p. 16). It passes through the most medial compartment of the extensor retinaculum and is inserted into the base of the fifth metacarpal bone.

Action. The extensor carpi ulnaris extends the wrist and, with the corresponding flexor, adducts the hand. Like the radial extensors of the wrist, it is used more often as a synergic muscle (p. 38).

The *Nerve Supply* of the three preceding muscles is derived from the posterior interosseous nerve.

The **Anconeus** does not belong to the superficial group of extensor muscles but it can conveniently be considered at this stage. Its origin, from the posterior aspect of the lateral epicondyle, is narrow and tendinous, but the fibres diverge widely to be inserted into an elongated triangular area on the lateral aspect of the olecranon and the adjoining part of the posterior surface of the ulna. It covers the posterior part of the annular ligament of the radius.

Action. The anconeus assists the triceps to extend the elbow; it may be responsible for the movement of the ulna which occurs during pronation. It gets its *nerve supply* from the radial nerve.

The **Posterior Interosseous Nerve** is really the continuation of the radial nerve where it forks in the cubital fossae. Piercing the supinator, it winds round the lateral aspect of the radius in the substance of the muscle to reach the dorsum of the forearm. It emerges from the posterior surface of the supinator and so gains the fascial interval between the superficial and the deep muscles. It supplies the muscles of both groups and runs downwards to the upper border of the long extensor of the thumb. It passes deep to this muscle and reaches the interosseous membrane, on which it descends, in company with the terminal part of the anterior interosseous artery. On the back of the wrist joint it ends in a small flattened expansion, from which branches run to the carpal joints.

The posterior interosseous nerve supplies all the muscles in this region with the exception of the brachioradialis, the extensor carpi radialis longus and the anconeus, which are innervated by the radial nerve itself.

The **Posterior Interosseous Artery** arises from the common interosseous near the upper border of the interosseous membrane and passes backwards between the radius and the ulna above the membrane. It then passes between the supinator and the abductor pollicis longus, and reaches the interval between the superficial and the deep muscles. After giving off numerous muscular branches it ends by taking part in the anastomosis round the wrist joint. A *recurrent branch* runs upwards to take part in the anastomosis round the elbow joint.

THE DEEP MUSCLES OF THE BACK OF THE FOREARM

The **Supinator** arises from the supinator crest of the ulna and from the adjoining part of the small triangular area which lies immediately in front of it. Its fibres pass backwards and laterally round behind the upper quarter of the shaft of the radius and are inserted into the posterior, lateral and anterior aspects of that bone over an area limited below by the insertion of the pronator teres. Its *Nerve Supply* is derived from the posterior interosseous nerve and its *Action* is to assist in supination.

The **Abductor Pollicis Longus** arises from the posterior surface of the ulna just below the insertion of the anconeus, from the interosseous membrane, and from the posterior surface of the radius below the insertion of the supinator. Its upper border marches with the lower border of the supinator, and runs obliquely downwards and laterally, so that the radial origin is at a lower level than the ulnar origin. At the junction of the middle and lower thirds of the forearm its tendon emerges between the extensor digitorum and the extensor carpi radialis brevis. It then runs downwards, superficial to the tendons of the radial extensors of the wrist, and passes under cover of the extensor retinaculum, grooving the lateral aspect of the lower end of the radius. It is inserted into the radial side of the base of the metacarpal bone of the thumb.

The **Extensor Pollicis Brevis** arises from the radius and the interosseous membrane immediately below the preceding muscle, which it accompanies, on its medial side, to the wrist. It is inserted into the base of the proximal phalanx of the thumb.

The **Extensor Pollicis Longus** arises from the ulna and the interosseous membrane, below the origin of the abductor pollicis longus. Its tendon passes through an oblique compartment of the extensor retinaculum, grooving the medial side of the dorsal tubercle of the radius, and is continued downwards and laterally to be inserted into the base of the distal phalanx of the thumb.

When the thumb is actively extended, a surface depression, often termed the "anatomical snuff-box," is visible superficial to the base of the first metacarpal bone. It is bounded on the medial side by the prominent tendon of the extensor pollicis longus and on the lateral side by the less conspicuous tendons of the extensor pollicis brevis and the abductor pollicis longus.

The **Extensor Indicis** arises from the ulna and the interosseous membrane immediately below the preceding muscle and runs downwards and laterally to the extensor retinaculum, under which it runs in company with the tendons of the extensor digitorum. It terminates by joining the dorsal expansion of the index tendon of that muscle.

The four preceding muscles are all supplied by the *posterior interosseous nerve.*

Their *Actions* are indicated by their names, but the abductor pollicis longus assists also in extending the thumb and in abducting the hand. In addition, the extensor pollicis longus, in full action, adducts the extended thumb and rotates it laterally.

The **Extensor Retinaculum** bridges over six grooves, which contain tendons of extensor muscles. Each tunnel is provided with a synovial sheath which extends on the tendons in both directions beyond the retinaculum.

1. The most lateral groove lies on the *lateral aspect* of the lower end of the radius and contains the tendons of the abductor pollicis longus and extensor pollicis brevis.

2. On the most lateral part of the posterior aspect of the radius the tendons of the extensor carpi radialis longus and brevis share a groove.

3. To their medial side the tendon of the extensor pollicis longus passes obliquely through the retinaculum in a compartment of its own.

4. The medial part of the posterior surface of the radius shows a

wide, shallow groove, which is occupied by the extensor digitorum and the extensor indicis as they lie under cover of the retinaculum.

5. The extensor digiti minimi occupies a small groove situated over the inferior radio-ulnar joint.

6. The extensor carpi ulnaris grooves the posterior aspect of the head of the ulna and occupies the most medial compartment.

The **Radial Artery** winds round the lateral aspect of the wrist and reaches the dorsum of the hand. After leaving the radius (p. 28) the artery passes round on the lateral ligament of the wrist joint and under the abductor pollicis longus and extensor pollicis brevis tendons. Reaching the dorsum, it runs downwards *over the trapezium* and then turns forwards and medially between the two heads of the first dorsal interosseous muscle. Before it does so, the artery is comparatively superficial and its pulsation can easily be felt to the lateral side of the extensor pollicis longus tendon, at the base of the "anatomical snuff-box."

In its short course on the dorsum of the hand the radial artery gives off a communicating branch to the anastomosis round the wrist and small dorsal metacarpal branches, which, in turn, divide into dorsal digital arteries (of the thumb and index).

On entering the palm the radial artery at first lies deep to the oblique head of the adductor pollicis. In this position it gives off (1) the *arteria radialis indicis*, which run downwards, in front of the first dorsal interosseous muscle and behind the transverse head of the adductor, to the radial side of the index finger; and (2) the *arteria princeps pollicis*, which runs downwards and laterally on to the palmar surface of the first metacarpal bone, where, under cover of the long flexor tendon, it divides into two collateral branches for the thumb.

JOINTS OF THE UPPER LIMB

The acromioclavicular and shoulder joints have already been described (pp. 14 and 17).

The **Elbow Joint** is a synovial joint of the hinge variety. The capitulum and trochlea of the lower end of the humerus, the trochlear notch of the ulna, and the upper surface of the head of the radius all take part in the articulation. The transverse axis of the lower articular end of the humerus is not horizontal but slopes medially and downwards, making an angle of about 85° with the long axis of the shaft. A similar arrangement is found to a lesser extent affecting the radial and ulnar articular surfaces. Consequently, when the limb is extended at the elbow, the forearm being supine, the long axis of the humerus meets the long axis of the forearm at an angle, open laterally, of about 170°. This is termed the *carrying angle*. Owing to its presence, the forearm comes into line with the long axis of the arm in the mid-prone position, *and it is in this position that the hand is most frequently used.*

The **Articular Capsule (Capsular Ligament)** of the joint is attached (1) to the humerus, (2) to the ulna, and (3) to the annular ligament of the superior radio-ulnar joint.

The *humeral attachment* lies along the upper borders of the radial and coronoid fossæ in front, reaches the base of the epicondyle on each side—so as to exclude the common flexor and extensor origins from the joint—and, posteriorly, crosses the olecranon fossa near its upper border.

The *ulnar attachment* follows the margins of the trochlear notch except on the lateral side, where it is interrupted by the radial notch.

Below and to the lateral side the capsule blends with the annular ligament.

The *anterior* and *posterior ligaments* are strengthening bands in the capsule. The *radial collateral* (*lateral*) *ligament* is attached to the lower aspect of the lateral epicondyle. It forms a rounded band, which blends below with the annular ligament. The *ulnar collateral* (*medial*) *ligament*, triangular in outline, consists of (1) an anterior band, from the medial epicondyle to the upper end of the medial border of the coronoid process; (2) a transverse band, running from the medial border of the olecranon to the coronoid process; (3) a posterior band, from the base of the medial epicondyle to the medial side of the olecranon; (4) a thin, triangular sheet of fibres, attached above to the medial epicondyle and below to the transverse band.

The *Synovial Membrane* lines the interior of the capsular ligament, is reflected into the three humeral fossæ, and on the lateral side is continuous with the synovial membrane of the superior radio-ulnar joint.

Extrasynovial pads of fat are incorporated in the anterior and posterior aspects of the capsule, projecting into the coronoid fossa during extension and the olecranon fossa during flexion.

The *anterior relations* of the joint include the brachialis and, in front of that muscle, the median nerve, brachial artery and tendon of biceps. *Posteriorly*, the tendon of triceps is separated from the joint by a small bursa.

On the *medial side*, the ulnar nerve and its accompanying vessels lie in contact with the medial ligament.

The *active movements* at the elbow joint are limited to flexion and extension. Flexion is arrested by the meeting of the soft parts of forearm and upper arm, and extension by the tension of the anterior ligament and the brachialis. The coronoid and olecranon processes do not actually come into contact with the humerus during these movements.

All the movements which can be performed actively at any joint can be carried out passively when the surrounding muscles are kept relaxed, *e.g.*, under general anæsthesia. Under these conditions, however, additional movements, which cannot be performed actively, can be obtained, and these are termed "passive" or "accessory" movements. They indicate the occurrence of a certain amount of play in the joint and are of value when it is subjected to violent stresses.

The *passive* or *accessory movements* of the elbow joint are very limited in range. When the surrounding muscles are completely relaxed, the ulna can be abducted or adducted and the head of the radius can be moved forwards and backwards on the capitulum of the humerus, but the degree of movement is small in both cases.

The **Superior Radio-Ulnar Joint** is a synovial joint of the pivot type.

The **Annular Ligament** forms a collar for the head of the radius. It is attached to the anterior and posterior borders of the radial notch of the ulna, and superiorly it blends with the capsular ligament of the elbow joint. The lower border of the ligament is free in order to allow the head of the radius to rotate inside its collar during pronation and supination.

A thin layer of cartilage covers the surface of the annular ligament where it is in articular contact. Elsewhere the lining is synovial membrane, extending from that in the elbow joint, the two joints having a continuous cavity.

The **Interosseous Membrane** is attached to the opposed borders of the radius and ulna. Below, it extends as far as the inferior radio-ulnar joint, but above, it stops short below the tuberosity of the radius. Most of the constituent fibres pass downwards and medially from the radius to the ulna, and may help to transmit stresses from the former bone to the latter. It certainly provides attachment for flexor and extensor muscles.

In its lower part the membrane is pierced by the anterior interosseous vessels.

Anteriorly, the membrane is related to the deep flexor muscles of the forearm (p. 29) and to the anterior interosseous vessels and nerve.

Posteriorly, it is related to the deep extensor muscles and to the terminal parts of the posterior interosseous nerve and the anterior and posterior interosseous vessels.

The **Inferior Radio-Ulnar Joint** is a synovial joint of the pivot type. The ulnar notch of the radius articulates with the head of the ulna, and the joint is closed below and shut off from the radiocarpal joint by a triangular articular disc.

A weak articular capsule, possessing feeble anterior and posterior ligaments, invests the joint and is in continuity with the capsular ligament of the radiocarpal joint.

The *Synovial Membrane* lines the capsular ligament and projects upwards as a small cul-de-sac—often termed the *recessus sacciformis*—in front of the lower end of the interosseous membrane.

The triangular **Articular Disc** is attached by its apex to the depression at the base of the ulnar styloid process and by its base to the lower border of the ulnar notch of the radius. Its anterior and posterior margins blend with the corresponding ligaments of the radiocarpal joint. Usually complete, it may be perforated, and in these cases the joint cavities of the inferior radio-ulnar and radiocarpal joints communicate.

The **Movements of Pronation and Supination** are rotatory movements around a vertical axis. So far as the movements of the radius relative to the ulna are concerned, this axis passes through the centre of the head of the radius above, and through the ulnar attachment of the triangular articular disc below. In the movement the head of the radius rotates within the annular ligament, but the lower end of the bone moves bodily forwards in pronation, and backwards in supination, the radial styloid moving round the circumference of a circle whose radius is the breadth of the lower end of the radius plus the breadth of the triangular articular disc.

When the movements of the ulna are not hindered, pronation is complicated by the simultaneous movement of the lower end of the ulna in a lateral direction, and in this case the combined movements of the radius and ulna occur around a longitudinal axis which passes through the centre of the head of the radius above and through the area of contact of the opposed thumb and index fingers below. On this account instruments such as screwdrivers and corkscrews can be employed effectively without the complication of any side to side movement.

When the movements of the ulna are hindered, *e.g.*, if the dorsum of the hand is rested on a plane surface, the ulna remains stationary and the lower end of the radius, carrying the hand with it, rolls over to the medial side.

The student should satisfy himself on these points by investigating the movements of his own forearm and hand under these two conditions, remembering, however, that the latter condition is abnormal.

Passive Movements. Both the head of the radius and the head of the ulna can be moved passively in a forward and backward direction.

The **Radiocarpal or Wrist Joint** lies just proximal to the upper skin crease on the front of the wrist. It is a synovial joint of the condyloid variety. The radius and the triangular articular disc, above, articulate with the scaphoid, lunate and triquetral bones below. The articular surfaces of the former constitute an ellipsoid concave surface, which is adapted to the ellipsoid convex surface presented by the carpal bones concerned.

The **Articular Capsule** is of moderate strength and is attached above to the lower ends of the radius and ulna, and below to the proximal row of the carpus. The *anterior and posterior ligaments* strengthen their respective aspects of the capsule, but are not specially noteworthy.

The *Medial and Lateral Ligaments* extend, respectively, from the ulnar styloid to the triquetral bone and from the radial styloid to the scaphoid. They are rounded, cord-like bands, which are sufficiently lax to permit a fair range of movement in abduction and adduction. The lateral ligament is crossed by the radial artery as it passes backwards below the styloid process of the radius.

The *Synovial Membrane* lines the interior of the capsular ligament but *the joint cavity does not communicate with the joint cavities of the intercarpal joints, nor with the cavity of the inferior radio-ulnar joint, unless the disc is perforated.*

The *active movements* at the wrist involve both the radiocarpal and the transverse carpal joints since the muscles concerned in their production are inserted into the bases of the metacarpal bones. The movements comprise flexion, extension, abduction (or radial deviation), adduction (or ulnar deviation) and circumduction, which results from a combination of the preceding movements. In *extension* from the mid-position, most of the movement occurs at the radiocarpal joint, but in *flexion* the intercarpal joint takes the major part. In *adduction*, which, owing to the shortness of the ulnar styloid process, is much freer than abduction, nearly all the movement occurs at the radiocarpal joint, but in *abduction* from the mid-position the intercarpal joint is mainly concerned (Plate VIII, p. 33).

Axial rotation of the carpus and hand cannot be performed actively, but this does not imply any disadvantage owing to the movements imposed on the hand in pronation and supination of the forearm.

The *passive movements* include backward and forward movement of the carpus on the radius and ulna, and a surprising degree of rotation.

The **Intercarpal Joints.** The *Pisiform Joint* is a separate small synovial joint of the plane or gliding variety. It possesses a simple capsular ligament and synovial membrane. The insertion of the flexor carpi ulnaris provides strong ligaments (p. 27).

The *Transverse Intercarpal Joint* is synovial and is interposed between the bones of the proximal and distal rows of the carpus. It permits movement between the two rows, especially in flexion and in abduction at the radiocarpal joint (Plate VIII, p. 16). The carpal bones are connected to one another by palmar and dorsal ligaments, and at the radial and ulnar extremities of the joint by lateral and medial ligaments.

The joint cavity, lined by synovial membrane, extends not only between the two rows, but also upwards between the scaphoid and the lunate and between the lunate and the triquetral, and downwards between the bones of the distal row. As a general rule this joint cavity communicates freely with the joint cavity of the four medial carpometacarpal and intermetacarpal joints.

The non-articular opposed surfaces of the carpal bones are connected to one another by interosseous ligaments.

The **Carpometacarpal Joint of the Thumb** is a synovial joint of the saddle variety, and *does not communicate with the other joints in the neighbourhood.* The saddle-shaped base of the first metacarpal bone articulates with the trapezium, and a joint is formed which permits of a wide range of movement. The joint possesses a capsular ligament lined by synovial membrane.

Active movements of flexion and extension, abduction and adduction, and a certain amount of rotation occur at this joint and give the thumb its characteristic range of movement. The only *passive movement* obtainable is separation of the two bones, effected by traction.

The **Metacarpophalangeal Joints** are synovial joints of the condyloid variety. Each joint possesses a separate capsular ligament and synovial membrane, and palmar, medial and lateral ligaments.

The *Palmar Ligaments* are strong and usually contain some fibrocartilage. They are more firmly attached to the phalanx than to the metacarpal bone. Dorsally the capsular ligament is thin and is separated from the extensor tendon by a bursa.

The *collateral ligaments* are oblique cord-like bands placed at the sides of the joints. Each runs downwards and forwards from the head of the metacarpal bone to the base of the phalanx.

The *active movements* at these joints comprise flexion, extension, abduction, adduction and a limited degree of circumduction. The movement of abduction is free when the fingers are extended, but is negligible when they are flexed. This is *not* due to tension of the collateral ligaments, as often stated, for the flexed fingers can readily

FIG. 1. The segmental distribution of the nerves of the brachial plexus to the skin of the upper limb.

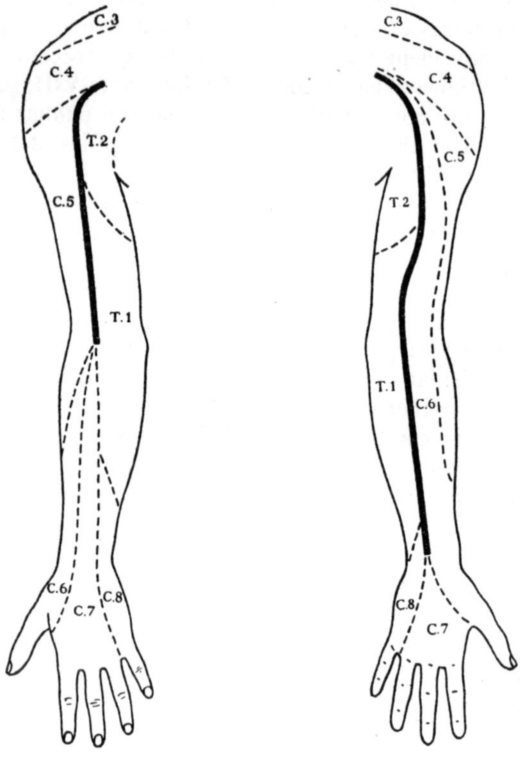

Note that the *axial line* (heavy black), across which overlap is minimal, extends more distally on the ventral than on the dorsal aspect. Overlap across the interrupted lines is considerable.

be abducted *passively*. Other *passive movements* are backward, forward and side to side movement of the phalanx on the head of the metacarpal bone, in addition to rotation.

The **Interphalangeal Joints** are very similar in structure to the metacarpophalangeal joints.

The palmar ligaments of the medial four metacarpophalangeal joints are connected to one another by the *deep transverse ligaments of the palm*, which serve to bind the heads of the medial four metacarpal bones firmly to each other. The tendons of the interossei pass behind the ligaments as they approach their insertion, while the tendons of the lumbricals lie in front of them.

THE SEGMENTAL INNERVATION OF THE UPPER LIMB

On its first appearance in the embryo, at about the end of the third week of intrauterine life, the upper limb possesses ventral and dorsal surfaces and rounded, pre-axial (or headward) and post-axial (or tailward) borders. It grows from the lateral surface of the trunk and is innervated by the anterior primary rami of fifth cervical to first thoracic segments, the former being distributed along the pre-axial border, and the latter along the post-axial border, and the intervening nerves supplying successive strips on both ventral and dorsal surfaces.

During development the ventral (or flexor) surface of the upper limb becomes approximated to the ventral surface of the trunk and undergoes a process of lateral rotation around its long axis, although the change is masked in the forearm and hand by the simultaneous occurrence of pronation. As a result of these changes the lateral aspect of the arm and the radial border of the forearm correspond, roughly, to the pre-axial border, while the medial aspect of the arm and the ulnar border of the forearm correspond to the post-axial border, the thumb being the pre-axial digit and the little finger the post-axial digit. It will be found, therefore, that the sensory nerves which innervate the lateral aspects of the arm and forearm are derived from the upper nerves of the plexus, while the lower nerves innervate the medial aspect of the limb (Fig. 1, p. 48).

Section II

THE LOWER LIMB

LIKE the upper limb the lower limb is a multi-jointed lever, having a relatively freely movable joint at its proximal end and provided with a specialised distal end, the foot, which functions as a stable support for the body-weight in the erect attitude, both at rest and in walking, running, etc. It should be noted that when the feet are under load, *i.e.*, bearing weight, many of the muscles of the leg act in reverse, *i.e.*, they tend to approximate their origins to their insertions instead of vice-versa. The best example of this reversal is provided by the glutei, medius and minimus, which prevent sagging or wobble at the hip when the body-weight is borne on one foot, as in walking. Under these circumstances the gluteal muscles of the weight-bearing side act on their origins, and by their pull on the ilium they prevent the sagging that would otherwise occur to the opposite side. Paralysis of these two muscles is readily diagnosed from the laboured, lurching gait, and is one of the most serious of all disabilities in the lower limb.

It should be remembered, too, that the small muscles of the foot are not able to act in the way their names suggest when the foot is under load. Their main function then is to brace the foot and assist in maintaining its arches.

THE FRONT OF THE THIGH

This region cannot be revised satisfactorily after the limb has been removed from the trunk, and revision should be done on disections in which it is still attached to the trunk, and with the help of an articulated pelvis and a femur of the same side of the body.

Superficial Nerves. The *Lateral Cutaneous Nerve of the Thigh* arises from the lumbar plexus (L. 2 and 3) and emerges behind the lateral end of the inguinal ligament. It divides into anterior and posterior branches, which supply the skin of the whole of the lateral aspect of the thigh as far down as the knee joint, where the terminal part of the anterior branch takes part in the patellar plexus. Some twigs from the posterior division supply the skin of the anterior part of the buttock.

The *Femoral Branch of the Genitofemoral Nerve* (L. 1 and 2) is also a derivative of the lumbar plexus. It is usually small and supplies a limited area of skin below the middle of the inguinal ligament.

The *Intermediate Cutaneous Nerve of the Thigh* arises from the femoral nerve and supplies the skin over the anterior aspect of the thigh through lateral and medial branches, which end in the patellar plexus.

The *Medial Cutaneous Nerve of the Thigh*, from the femoral nerve, assisted by a few branches from the obturator nerve, supplies the medial aspect of the thigh and joins the patellar plexus.

The *Patellar Plexus* lies in front of the patella and ligamentum patellæ. It is formed by the numerous communications between the terminal branches of the lateral, intermediate and medial cutaneous nerves of the thigh and the infrapatellar branch of the saphenous nerve (p. 55).

The **Long Saphenous Vein** begins at the medial side of the dorsal venous arch of the foot and ascends in front of the medial malleolus, and then to the medial side of the knee. As it runs up through the thigh it inclines forwards and laterally, and it passes through the deep fascia at the saphenous opening. Superficial veins from the thigh, the anterior abdominal wall and the external genitalia join the upper part of the vessel.

Numerous valves are found in the long saphenous vein, especially below the knee (p. 24). Two are situated at the upper end of the vessel, just below its junction with the femoral vein.

The **Superficial Inguinal Lymph Nodes** lie in the superficial fascia below and parallel to the inguinal ligament. The medial members of the group receive *afferents* from the adjoining part of the abdominal wall (below the umbilicus), and the superficial lymph vessels from the perineum. The lateral members of the group drain the adjoining part of the anterior abdominal wall and receive the superficial lymph vessels from the gluteal region.

The lower members of the group lie in the superficial fascia along the upper part of the long saphenous vein. They receive the superficial lymph vessels of the lower limb.

These superficial lymph nodes send their efferents through the deep fascia to join the *Deep Inguinal Nodes*, which lie in relation to the femoral vein—one of them occupying the femoral canal. In addition, the deep inguinal nodes receive afferents from the deeper tissues of the penis or clitoris and the deep lymph vessels of the lower limb, including the efferents from the popliteal lymph nodes. From the deep group the efferents pass to the lymph nodes which lie along the external iliac artery (Plate XII, p. 65).

The **Fascia Lata** of the thigh is remarkably developed on the lateral aspect, and in this region is known as the *Iliotibial Tract*. It is attached to the outer lip of the iliac crest above and to the lateral condyle of the tibia and the head of the fibula below. The tensor fasciæ latæ and most of the fibres of the gluteus maximus are inserted into the iliotibial tract (p. 61) and, acting through it, they keep the limb braced in the erect posture.

When, with the thigh flexed, the leg is extended against gravity, the iliotibial tract stands out and can be felt as a prominent band just above the knee joint on its antero-lateral aspect. It is separated from the lateral border of the vastus lateralis by a conspicuous depression.

The *Saphenous Opening* is a gap in the fascia lata which transmits the long saphenous vein and some small arteries. It lies about 1½ inches below the medial end of the inguinal ligament, and measures 1 inch long by ½-inch wide. The lower and lateral borders of the opening form the sharp and crescentic *falciform margin* and lie anterior to the femoral sheath. The medial border lies on a plane posterior to the lateral and inferior borders, and is little more than a ridge in the fascia covering the pectineus muscle. The margins of the opening are connected by loosely-knit connective tissue termed the *cribriform fascia.*

The opening acquires some importance from the fact that a femoral hernia, as it increases in size, passes through the deep fascia at this point and becomes subcutaneous.

At its upper limit the fascia lata is continuous with the lower aspect of the inguinal ligament and, when the thighs are extended, it exerts a downward pull on the aponeurosis of the external oblique muscle.

From the deep surface of the fascia lata three septa pass in to the linea aspera and divide the thigh into an anterior or extensor, a medial or adductor, and a posterior or flexor compartment. Of these septa the lateral, which separates the hamstrings from the extensors, is much the strongest.

The **Femoral Triangle** is situated in the upper part of the thigh and its position is indicated in the living subject by a depression, which lies below the fold of the groin and is accentuated when the thigh is flexed against gravity. It is bounded above by the inguinal ligament, on the lateral side by the sartorius, and on the medial side by the medial border of the adductor longus. Its floor is formed by the anterior surfaces of the adductor longus and pectineus muscles, and to a much smaller extent by the iliopsoas, which occupies the upper and lateral angle.

The contents of the triangle include the femoral nerve and its branches, the femoral sheath with its contained structures, the femoral artery and its branches, and the femoral vein and its tributaries.

The **Femoral Sheath** is a continuation into the thigh of the loose connective tissue of the abdomen. Its anterior wall is continuous with the fascia transversalis (p. 143), and its posterior wall with the fascia iliaca (p. 176). The femoral artery, as it enters the thigh, lies in the lateral part of the sheath, separated by connecting tissue from the femoral vein, which lies to its medial side. The medial part of the sheath is occupied by some extraperitoneal fat and one of the deep inguinal lymph nodes, and these are separated from the femoral vein by a partition. Inferiorly, the sheath blends with the adventitious coats of the femoral vessels.

N.B. It should be remembered that the walls of the sheath are firmly adherent to the walls of the vessels and that, despite the customary use of the word "compartments," no spaces of any kind exist within the femoral sheath.

The femoral sheath thus possesses three "compartments," of which the medial is the smallest. This is termed the **Femoral Canal,** and is closed inferiorly by the blending of its medial wall with the outer coat of the femoral vein. The upper end of the canal is widely open into the peritoneal cavity. It is at this *femoral ring* that a femoral hernia may become strangulated. In front is the inguinal ligament; behind the pubic bone; to its lateral side lies the femoral vein; medially is the sharp free border of the lacunar ligament (p. 140).

A femoral hernia passes through the femoral ring into the femoral canal, and then, pushing the anterior wall of the sheath in front of it, emerges through the saphenous opening, to lie immediately under the skin. The canal is alleged to permit expansion of the femoral vein, preventing contact with the edge of the lacunar ligament.

The **Femoral Artery** enters the thigh by passing behind the inguinal ligament at the mid-point of a line joining the pubic symphysis to the anterior superior iliac spine. It runs almost vertically downwards and slightly backwards and, about the junction of the middle and lower thirds of the thigh, it pierces the adductor magnus to gain the popliteal fossa. It can be mapped out on the surface by the upper two-thirds of a line drawn from its commencement to the adductor tubercle of the femur (Plate XI, p. 60).

In the femoral triangle the artery is superficial, being covered only by the skin and fasciæ. Anteriorly it is related to the anterior wall of the femoral sheath above, and to the medial cutaneous and saphenous nerves below.

Posteriorly the artery rests at first on the psoas, which separates it from the rounded head of the femur, then on the pectineus, and finally on the adductor longus muscle. As it descends, it lies to the medial side of the neck and shaft of the femur.

The femoral vein lies medial to the artery in the uppermost part of the thigh, but at a lower level it comes to lie behind it. The profunda femoris vessels pass behind the artery as it lies on the pectineus. The femoral nerve is lateral to the artery as it enters the thigh, and its branches are lateral and anterior to the vessel.

At the apex of the triangle the artery passes under the sartorius and enters the adductor (subsartorial) canal.

Branches. 1. Several superficial branches arise from the femoral, but the only one worthy of mention is the *Superficial External Pudendal*, which runs medially in front of the femoral vein across the spermatic cord to supply pudendal skin.

2. The *Deep External Pudendal* artery arises about 1½ inches below the inguinal ligament and runs medially behind or in front of the femoral vein and in front of the pectineus and adductor longus muscles. Piercing the fascia lata, it is distributed to the scrotum or labium majus, as the case may be.

3. The *Profunda Femoris* artery is a large vessel which arises from the postero-lateral aspect of the femoral artery in the upper part of the triangle. It runs downwards and then curves medially behind the femoral vessels, lying at first on the iliacus, and then on the pectineus and the adductor brevis. It passes behind the adductor longus, which separates it from the femoral vessels, and then lies on the adductor magnus, where it *ends as the fourth perforating artery*.

As it lies in the femoral triangle, the profunda gives off the lateral and medial femoral circumflex and the upper two perforating arteries. These will be considered later.

The **Femoral Vein** is the upward continuation of the popliteal vein (p. 68). It ascends through the adductor canal and the femoral triangle in close association with the femoral artery, having very similar relations (p. 53). Below, the vein lies to the lateral side of the artery, but in most of its course it lies posteriorly, except in the upper part of the thigh, where it lies to the medial side. It receives the long saphenous vein (p. 51) and tributaries corresponding to the branches of the artery. It is provided with a valve—usually bicuspid—near its upper end and also just above the point where it is joined by the profunda femoris vein.

The **Femoral Nerve** *is the nerve of the anterior or extensor compartment of the thigh.* Within the false pelvis, the nerve lies deeply in the groove between the psoas and the iliacus, behind the fascia iliaca. It enters the femoral triangle by passing behind the inguinal ligament in a continuation of the same intermuscular groove. Consequently the nerve lies behind the fascia lata, and it is placed lateral to the femoral artery and sheath. Having reached the thigh, the femoral nerve breaks up almost immediately into a leash of terminal branches. These are arranged in anterior and posterior groups.

From the anterior division there arise the intermediate (p. 50) and medial cutaneous nerves of the thigh and branches to the *pectineus* and the *sartorius*.

The *Medial Cutaneous* does not pierce the deep fascia until it reaches the lower third of the thigh. It supplies skin of the medial side of the thigh and ends in the patellar plexus, but some of its branches extend beyond the knee and supply the skin of the upper and medial part of the leg.

From the posterior division there arise the saphenous nerve and the branches to the extensor muscles in the thigh.

1. The *Saphenous Nerve* runs downwards and medially and gains the anterior aspect of the femoral artery, on which it is carried down into the adductor canal. At the lower end of the canal the nerve pierces the deep fascia on the medial side of the knee between the sartorius and the gracilis tendons. An *infrapatellar branch* joins the patellar plexus after piercing the sartorius muscle. In the leg the nerve, now accompanied by the long saphenous vein, runs down the medial aspect of the limb, supplying the overlying skin. It is continued downwards in front of the medial malleolus to the medial border of the foot, where it terminates at the base of the great toe.

2. The *Nerve to the Rectus Femoris* supplies the muscle and the hip joint.

3. The *Nerves to the Vasti* supply these muscles and also send twigs to the knee joint. The nerve to the vastus lateralis accompanies the descending branch of the lateral circumflex femoral artery.

The **Sartorius** arises from the anterior superior iliac spine and runs downwards across the front of the thigh to be inserted into the upper part of the medial surface of the tibia. It forms the lateral boundary of the femoral triangle and the roof of the adductor canal.

Its *Nerve Supply* is derived from the femoral nerve.

Action. The sartorius flexes both the hip and the knee joints, turning the knee outwards to bring the foot under inspection.

The **Pectineus** arises from the superior ramus of the pubis and runs downwards in front of the capsular ligament of the hip joint to the posterior aspect of the femur, lateral to the lesser trochanter.

Its *Nerve Supply* is derived from the femoral nerve.

Action. Although supplied by the femoral nerve, the pectineus is an adductor as well as a flexor of the hip. It probably assists the other short muscles round the hip (p. 62) to control and steady the head of the femur during movements of the hip joint.

The **Psoas Tendon** enters the thigh behind the femoral artery and *covers the capsular ligament of the hip joint* in the interval between the iliofemoral and the pubofemoral ligaments. A bursa intervenes between the tendon and the capsule, and may sometimes communicate with the joint. The tendon is attached to the lesser trochanter of the femur.

The **Iliacus** enters the thigh on the lateral side of the psoas tendon and is partly overlapped by the sartorius. Its medial fibres are inserted into the psoas tendon, while its lateral fibres are attached to the femur immediately below the lesser trochanter.

Actions. The ilio-psoas flexes the thigh on the body, at the same time rotating the femur medially. *When the thigh is fixed it flexes the trunk on the thigh.*

These muscles are described further on pp. 176 and 177.

The **Lateral Circumflex Femoral Artery** arises from the lateral aspect of the profunda femoris near its origin and runs laterally, amongst the terminal branches of the femoral nerve, and behind the sartorius and the rectus femoris. It breaks up into ascending, transverse and descending branches, each of which takes part in the formation of an important arterial anastomosis.

The *ascending branch* runs upward under tensor fasciæ latæ and, in the region of the anterior superior spine, anastomoses with branches of the *deep circumflex iliac* and *superior gluteal arteries* (p. 65).

The *transverse branch* winds round the posterior aspect of the upper part of the femur, where it joins the crucial anastomosis (p. 65).

The *descending branch* follows the anterior border of the vastus lateralis and the nerve to that muscle. In the lower part of the thigh it runs down on the femur and takes part in the anastomosis round the knee (p. 68).

The lateral circumflex artery varies considerably in its mode of origin. Frequently it arises directly from the femoral, or its descending branch may arise from the femoral and its other branches from the profunda, or *vice versâ.*

The **Quadriceps Femoris** consists of four distinct parts, viz., the rectus femoris, the vastus intermedius, the vastus medialis and the vastus lateralis, which have a *common tendon of insertion* into the patella and, via this large sesamoid bone, into the tibia.

The **Rectus Femoris** arises by a straight head from the upper part of the anterior inferior iliac spine and by a reflected head from the ilium, just above the acetabulum. The two heads unite in front of the hip joint, and the muscular belly runs down the front of the thigh to be inserted into the common extensor tendon. Deeply situated at its origin, it appears in the angular interval between the sartorius and the tensor fasciæ latæ, and descends superficial to the following three muscles.

The **Vastus Lateralis** arises from a broad linear strip which begins at the upper end of the trochanteric line, skirts the base of the greater trochanter, and follows the gluteal tuberosity and the lateral lip of the linea aspera half-way down the femur. It also arises from the lateral intermuscular septum, and it is inserted into the common tendon. From its lower margin a fibrous expansion is given off, which strengthens the capsule of the knee joint and gains attachment to the tibia.

The **Vastus Medialis** also arises from a linear strip of bone. Beginning at the lower part of the trochanteric line, the origin follows the spiral line and the medial lip of the linea aspera, while the lowest fibres arise from the tendon of the adductor magnus. The muscle covers the medial surface of the femur, and is partly blended with the vastus intermedius. It is inserted into the common tendon and into the medial border of the patella. Like the vastus lateralis, it gives off a fibrous expansion to the capsule of the knee joint. The lowest fibres of the muscle, which are almost horizontal in direction, form the fleshy mass which can be seen medial to the upper part of the patella in the living subject.

The **Vastus Intermedius** arises from the anterior and lateral aspects of the shaft of the femur. It is a large, fleshy muscle, closely related to the femur throughout its course, and inserted into the deep aspect of the common tendon.

All four heads of the muscle are innervated by the *femoral nerve*.

Action. The quadriceps acts as a powerful extensor of the knee joint, but, in addition, the rectus femoris is a flexor of the hip joint.

The **Adductor Canal** is an intermuscular canal situated on the medial aspect of the thigh in its middle third. It contains the femoral vessels and the saphenous nerve.

Its *roof*, or antero-medial wall, is formed by a fibrous expansion which lies deep to the sartorius muscle. Its *floor*, or posterior wall, is formed in its upper two-thirds by the adductor longus and in its lower third by the adductor magnus. The *antero-lateral wall* of the canal is formed by the vastus medialis.

The **Femoral Artery** enters the subsartorial canal at the apex of the femoral triangle. Within the canal the artery inclines downwards and backwards relative to the long axis of the femur, so that, as it leaves the canal by passing through the opening in the adductor magnus, it passes on to the popliteal surface of the bone. The saphenous nerve lies on the anterior aspect of the vessel and gradually crosses in front of it to its medial side. The femoral vein lies behind the artery above, but is on its lateral side in the lower part of the canal and posterior to it in the popliteal region.

Branches. Near the lower end of the canal the femoral artery gives off the *descending genicular artery.* This vessel gives off a superficial branch which accompanies the saphenous nerve, an articular branch which takes part in the anastomosis round the knee joint (p. 68), and also muscular branches.

THE MEDIAL SIDE OF THE THIGH

This region includes the adductor group of muscles, the obturator nerve and the medial circumflex femoral artery. It can only be revised satisfactorily from a limb in process of dissection and not yet detached from the trunk.

The **Adductor Longus** arises from the body of the pubis, in the angle between the crest and the symphysis. Narrow and tendinous at its origin, the muscle fans out as it runs downwards and laterally to be inserted into the medial lip of the linea aspera. Its anterior surface lies in the floor of the femoral triangle and also in the floor of the adductor canal, in intimate relationship with the femoral vessels.

The **Adductor Brevis** lies on a more posterior plane. It arises from the body of the pubis below the adductor longus, and runs downwards, backwards and laterally to be inserted into the posterior aspect of the femur from the lesser trochanter to the linea aspera. Anteriorly it is overlapped above by the pectineus and below by the adductor longus.

The **Adductor Magnus** is a large triangular muscle, which lies on a plane posterior to the adductor brevis. It arises from the pubic arch under cover of the adductor brevis, and from the anterior portion of the ischial tuberosity. The pubic fibres run laterally to the medial edge of the gluteal tuberosity, along which they are inserted. The succeeding fibres, becoming more nearly vertical, are inserted into the linea aspera and the upper part of the medial supracondylar line. *The fibres which arise from the ischial tuberosity run almost vertically downwards and end in a short tendon, which is inserted into the adductor tubercle on the medial condyle of the femur —the ischio-condylar part* (p. 414).

The posterior surface of the adductor magnus is related to the hamstring muscles and the sciatic nerve. Its anterior surface is covered above by the adductor brevis and below by the adductor longus except at its lowest part, which extends beyond the latter muscle and forms part of the posterior wall of the subsartorial canal. Opposite the middle third of the medial supracondylar line there is a gap in the insertion of the muscle, and this allows the femoral vessels to enter the popliteal fossa.

The **Gracilis** arises from the margin of the upper part of the pubic arch and the adjoining part of the body of the pubis, and runs downwards along the medial side of the thigh. It is subcutaneous throughout, and its deep surface is related to the medial borders of the other adductor muscles. In the lower third of the thigh the fleshy fibres end in a long tendon, which is inserted into the upper part of the medial surface of the tibia, under cover of the expanded tendon of the sartorius. No difficulty should be experienced in distinguishing the gracilis from the sartorius in the detached limb. The gracilis possesses a long tendon and its muscular belly gradually diminishes in width from its origin to its tendon of insertion, whereas the sartorius tendon is very short and the width of its muscular belly is unchanged from its origin to the level of the knee.

In the living subject, when the knee is flexed actively, and simultaneously abducted, against resistance, two tendons stand out prominently on its postero-medial aspect. The more medial is the tendon of the gracilis and the more lateral the tendon of the semitendinosus. The semimembranosus, which does not produce a surface elevation, lies deeply in the interval between the two.

Nerve Supply. All the adductor muscles are supplied by the obturator nerve. The adductor magnus, however, is a compound muscle. Its pubic, or adductor, portion is supplied by the obturator nerve, but its ischio-condylar portion is a derivative of the hamstring group and is supplied by the sciatic nerve (medial, flexor, division).

Actions. All of the above muscles are adductors of the thigh. In addition, the gracilis is a flexor of the knee joint, and the adductors brevis, longus and magnus (upper part) assist in flexion and lateral rotation of the thigh. The lower part of the magnus—like the hamstring muscles—extends the thigh.

The **Obturator Nerve** is derived from the lumbar plexus (L. 2, 3 and 4) and, after emerging from the medial border of the psoas (p. 191), runs forwards and downwards on the side wall of the pelvis to the upper part of the obturator foramen. Here it divides into anterior and posterior divisions. *It is the nerve of the medial (adductor) compartment of the thigh.*

The *anterior division* passes over the upper border of the obturator externus and runs downwards behind the pectineus and then behind the adductor longus, and in front of the adductor brevis. It supplies (1) the adductor brevis, (2) the adductor longus, and (3) the gracilis, and gives an articular branch to the hip joint.

The *posterior division* supplies (1) the obturator externus muscle and pierces its upper part. It then descends behind the adductor brevis, and in front of the adductor magnus. The terminal branches supply (2) the adductor magnus, and (3) an articular branch to the knee joint.

The **Medial Circumflex Femoral Artery** arises usually from the profunda femoris, but it frequently springs from the femoral artery. It at once passes backwards and slightly downwards between the tendon of the psoas and the lateral border of the pectineus. It then passes between the surface of the obturator externus muscle, which lies above it, and the upper border of the adductor brevis, which lies below it. Finally it reaches the interval between the quadratus femoris and the adductor magnus, and there gives off its terminal muscular branches.

Branches. In addition to unnamed *muscular branches* to the adductors and an *acetabular branch* to the hip joint, the medial circumflex femoral gives off (1) an ascending and (2) a transverse branch.

1. The *Ascending Branch* arises as the artery lies in contact with and supplies the obturator externus muscle, and follows the tendon of that muscle to the trochanteric fossa, where it anastomoses with branches from the superior and inferior gluteal arteries, which are derivatives of the internal iliac artery.

2. The *Transverse Branch* follows the upper border of the adductor magnus and joins the crucial anastomosis (p. 65).

The *Perforating Arteries* are derived from the profunda femoris and are usually four in number, the lowest being the terminal part of the parent trunk. They run laterally across the linea aspera, perforating the various muscular attachments, and terminate under cover of the vastus lateralis and intermedius. Each is connected with its neighbour: the first perforating is connected to the crucial and trochanteric anastomoses: and the fourth anastomoses with muscular branches of the popliteal artery. In this way a series of anastomoses is established on the back of the thigh, which links up the popliteal artery below, with the femoral at the origin of the profunda femoris, and with the superior and inferior gluteal arteries above. The perforating arteries mainly supply muscle.

The **Obturator Externus** muscle arises from the outer surface of the obturator membrane and from the bony margins of the foramen. Its fibres converge laterally into a strong tendon which passes below the hip joint and then across the posterior aspect of the neck of the femur to the trochanteric fossa, where it is inserted. The tendon, accompanied by the ascending branch of the medial circumflex femoral artery, lies deeply in the interval between the quadratus femoris and the upper border of the adductor magnus.

PLATE IX. ANTERO-POSTERIOR RADIOGRAPH OF THE REGION OF THE HIP-JOINT IN A YOUTH OF 15 YEARS OF AGE.

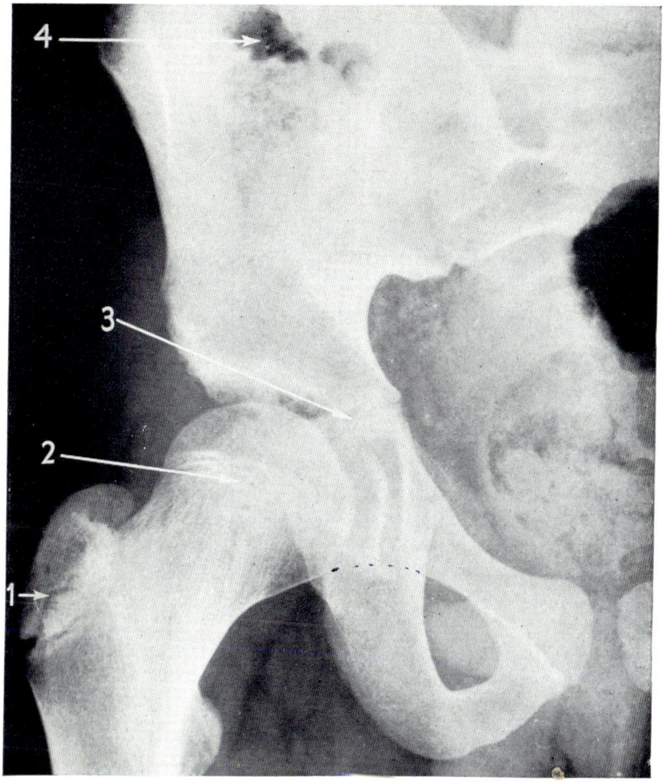

1. Epiphysis of greater trochanter.
2. Epiphyseal cartilage of head of femur.
3. Fusion of ilium with ischium and pubis not yet complete.
4. Bubble of gas in cæcum.

Note that the curve of the lower border of the neck of the femur is in line with the curve of the upper border of the obturator foramen.

To face p. 60

PLATE X. LATERAL RADIOGRAPH OF THE KNEE-JOINT IN A GIRL OF 15 IN THE POSITION OF SEMI-FLEXION.

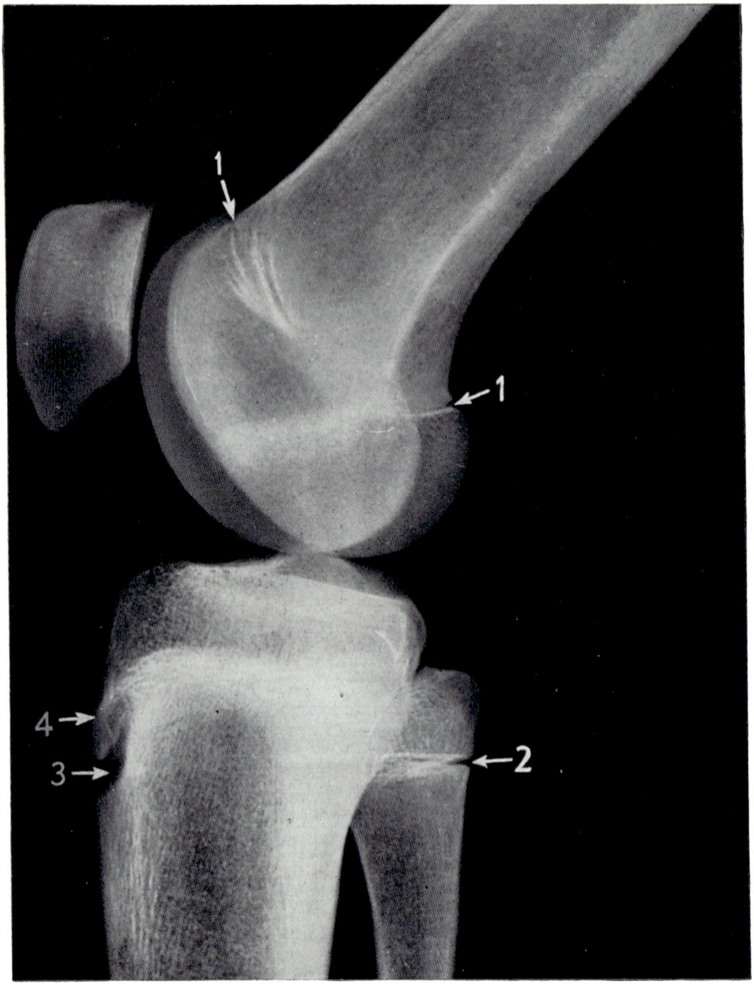

1. Lower femoral epiphyseal line.
2. Upper fibular epiphyseal line.
3. Upper tibial epiphyseal line.
4. Tibial tubercle.

Observe the position of the patella relative to the line of the knee-joint and note that the bone is fully ossified.

Plate XI. Antero-posterior Radiograph of the Knee in a Young Adult.

The interval between the femur and the tibia is occupied by the articular cartilage covering the bones and by the semilunar cartilages of the knee-joint.

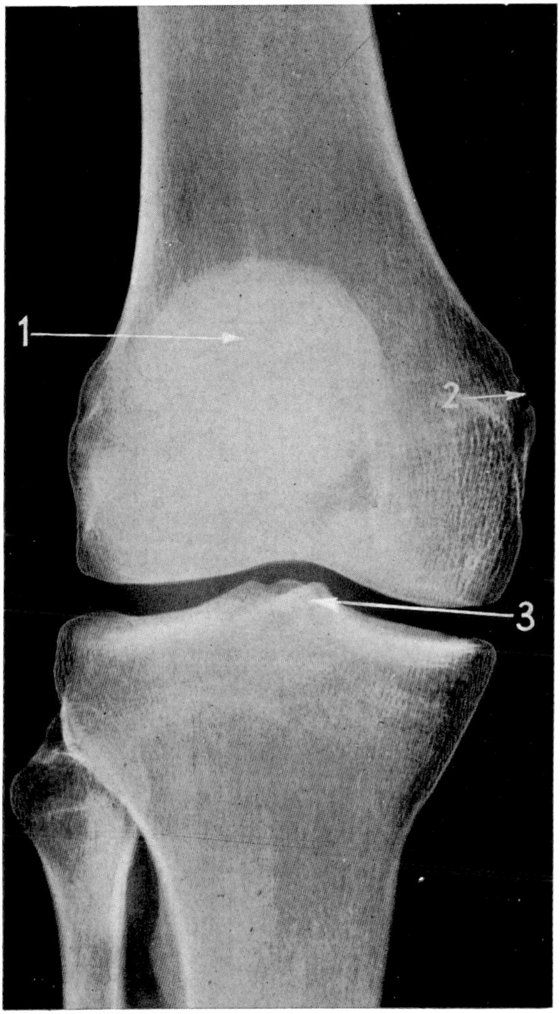

1. The patella. Note that its lower border lies above the level of the knee-joint. 2. The adductor tubercle. 3. The medial intercondylar tubercle.

PLATE XII. LYMPHOGRAM OF LOWER EXTREMITIES.

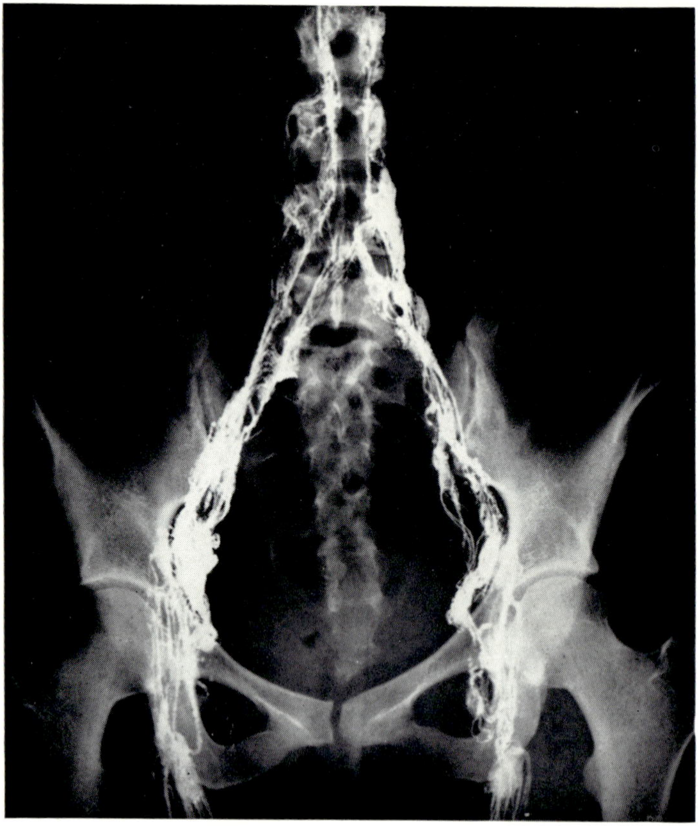

Radio-opaque material, introduced into the subcutaneous tissues of both legs, has arrived at the superficial inguinal lymph nodes and has passed on to the intra-abdominal lymphatics.

The *Nerve Supply* is derived from the posterior division of the obturator nerve.

Action. The obturator externus is a powerful lateral rotator of the thigh and helps the other short muscles round the hip joint to control the movements of the joint (p. 85). *

THE GLUTEAL REGION

For the satisfactory revision of this region, the student must have access to a limb in process of dissection. He should also provide himself with a bony pelvis and a femur of the corresponding side.

The *Superficial Nerves* which supply the skin of the gluteal region are derived partly from the posterior primary rami and partly from the anterior primary rami of the spinal nerves.

1. The terminal branches of the posterior primary rami of the first three lumbar nerves and derivatives of the posterior primary rami of the first three sacral nerves supply the skin of the upper and posterior part of the buttock.

2. The lateral branches of the ilio-hypogastric (L. 1) and of the last thoracic nerve (both from anterior primary rami) supply the skin of the upper and anterior part of the buttock.

3. Branches from the posterior division of the lateral cutaneous nerve of the thigh (L. 2 and 3, anterior primary rami) supply the skin of the lower and anterior part of the buttock.

4. Branches from the posterior cutaneous nerve of the thigh (S. 1, 2 and 3, anterior and posterior primary rami) curl round the lower border of the gluteus maximus to be distributed to the skin of the lower and posterior part of the buttock.

The *Superficial Lymph Vessels* of the gluteal region join the lateral lymph nodes of the superficial inguinal group.

The **Gluteus Maximus** is a large and powerful muscle, coarsely fasciculated. It arises continuously from the posterior part of the gluteal surface of the ilium, the dorsal aspects of sacrum and coccyx, and the posterior surface of the sacrotuberous ligament. The fibres run laterally and downwards to be inserted partly into the femur and partly into the fascia lata. The lower half of the deep fibres is attached to the gluteal tuberosity on the femur, while the rest of the muscle is inserted into a splitting of the fascia lata at the upper and posterior part of the iliotibial tract. Note that the fold of the buttock (Plate III, p. 16) does *not* correspond to the lower border of the muscle, which crosses it obliquely about its mid-point.

The *Nerve Supply* is derived from the inferior gluteal nerve (p. 63). *

Actions. The gluteus maximus acts as an extensor and lateral rotator of the thigh and plays an important part in walking and running. The great size of the muscle is not attributable to its constant use in these acts, but to the fact that, *when the body is bent at the hips, it is this muscle which restores it to the erect posture.* It is brought into action therefore every time one rises from a sitting, bending, or squatting to a standing position.

The deep surface of the muscle is related to a large number of muscles and to the vessels and nerves issuing from the greater sciatic foramen. The muscles include the posterior part of the gluteus medius, the piriformis, the obturator internus tendon and the two gemelli, the quadratus femoris, the upper part of the insertion of the adductor magnus and the origins of the hamstrings. Above the piriformis the superior gluteal vessels and nerve leave the upper part of the greater sciatic foramen. Below the piriformis the inferior gluteal and internal pudendal vessels, the sciatic nerve, the posterior cutaneous nerve of the thigh, the inferior gluteal and the pudendal nerves, and the nerves to the obturator internus and to the quadratus femoris, come into relationship with the deep surface of the gluteus maximus.

Two *bursæ*, which frequently communicate with each other, lie (*a*) between the tendon of the gluteus maximus and the greater trochanter, and (*b*) between the tendons of the gluteus maximus and the vastus lateralis.

The **Piriformis** arises from the front of the sacrum (p. 192) and, passing through the greater sciatic foramen, runs laterally and forwards to be inserted into the upper border of the greater trochanter.

Its *Nerve Supply* is derived from the anterior primary rami of S. 1 and S. 2. *

The **Obturator Internus** tendon emerges through the lesser sciatic foramen and runs forwards and laterally to be inserted into the upper border of the greater trochanter. The bony floor of the lesser sciatic notch is coated with cartilage to facilitate the play of the tendon, and a large bursa is interposed between the two.

The *Superior and Inferior Gemelli* are small muscles associated with the upper and lower borders of the tendon of the obturator internus, and the whole is sometimes referred to as the *tricipital tendon.*

The **Quadratus Femoris** arises from the lateral aspect of the ischial tuberosity and passes laterally to be inserted into a small rounded prominence on the intertrochanteric crest of the femur. Its upper border lies edge to edge with the inferior gemellus.

The *Nerve Supply* of the obturator internus and the superior gemellus comes from the nerve to the obturator internus (L. 5, S. 1 and 2), while the inferior gemellus and the quadratus femoris are supplied by the nerve to the latter muscle (L. 4, 5, S. 1).

Actions. All the foregoing muscles are closely related to the capsular ligament of the hip joint, and, although they may act as lateral rotators of the femur, it is probable that their main function is to control the upper end of the bone and to counteract the medial rotation that would otherwise accompany flexion of the hip joint.

The **Posterior Cutaneous Nerve of the Thigh** (S. 1, 2 and 3) emerges from the greater sciatic foramen below the piriformis and runs downwards, deep to the gluteus maximus and lying on the sciatic nerve. On reaching the origin of the hamstrings, it crosses superficial to the long head of the biceps and is continued down the back of the thigh immediately under the deep fascia, which it pierces in the popliteal fossa.

Branches. (1) Cutaneous, to the skin over the lower and posterior part of the buttock. (2) The *Perineal Branch* arises from the posterior cutaneous nerve in the gluteal region, and winds round the origin of the hamstrings to reach the perineum, where it supplies the skin of the scrotum, or labium majus. (3) Cutaneous, to back of thigh, knee and upper part of leg.

The **Inferior Gluteal Nerve** (L. 5, S. 1 and 2) emerges close to the posterior cutaneous nerve and sinks into the deep surface of the gluteus maximus to supply the muscle.

The **Sciatic Nerve** (L. 4, 5, S. 1, 2 and 3) leaves the pelvis below the piriformis and runs downwards to the thigh. It lies at first on the ischium, and then crosses successively, the gemelli and obturator internus, the quadratus femoris, and the adductor magnus. At first related on its superficial aspect to the posterior cutaneous nerve and the gluteus maximus, it next passes deep to the long head of the biceps (p. 66).

Branches. The nerves of supply to the adductor magnus and the hamstrings may arise while the nerve is still in the gluteal region, but as a rule they arise in the back of the thigh (p. 66).

The **Nerve to Quadratus Femoris** (L. 4, 5 and S. 1) lies between the sciatic nerve and the ischium, and runs downwards deep to the gemelli and obturator internus to reach the quadratus femoris. It also supplies the inferior gemellus.

The **Pudendal Nerve** (S. 2, 3 and 4) and the **Nerve to the Obturator Internus** leave the pelvis below the piriformis, in company with the *internal pudendal artery*, which lies between them. They cross the sacro-spinous ligament or the ischial spine, and enter the ischio-rectal fossa (p. 131) through the lesser sciatic foramen. Their course in the gluteal region, therefore, is very short.

The **Inferior Gluteal Artery** leaves the pelvis at the lower border of the piriformis and at once breaks up into a large number of terminal branches, of which the largest are distributed to the neighbouring muscles. A small branch accompanies the sciatic nerve, and anastomosing branches join the trochanteric and the crucial anastomoses.

The **Gluteus Medius** is overlapped by the gluteus maximus below and behind, but its upper and anterior part is superficial and can be felt when contracting. It arises from the gluteal surface of the ilium over an area limited above by the iliac crest, behind by the posterior gluteal line, and below by the middle gluteal line. The fibres converge to be inserted by a tendon into the lateral aspect of the greater trochanter along a line running downwards and forwards across it.

The **Gluteus Minimus** is covered over by the preceding muscle. It arises from the gluteal surface of the ilium between the middle and the inferior gluteal lines, and the fibres converge to be inserted by a tendon into the anterior surface of the greater trochanter.

The **Tensor Fasciæ Latæ** arises from the anterior part of the outer lip of the iliac crest, and the fibres run downwards and slightly backwards to be inserted into a splitting of the upper part of the iliotibial tract (p. 51). It is partly blended with the anterior fibres of the gluteus medius.

All three muscles are supplied by the *superior gluteal nerve*.

Actions. The gluteus medius and minimus are powerful abductors of the thigh, but their anterior fibres are also medial rotators. *Their most important function, however, is to maintain the balance and poise of the body when the foot of the opposite side is off the ground, as in walking and running. This they do by exerting traction on the hip bone powerful enough to prevent the pelvis from tilting downwards on the unsupported side.*

The tensor fasciæ latæ is an extensor of the knee, acting through the iliotibial tract, and a medial rotator of the thigh.

The **Superior Gluteal Nerve** (L. 4, 5 and S. 1) leaves the pelvis above the piriformis and passes forwards in the interval between the gluteus medius and the gluteus minimus. It supplies both these muscles and ends in the tensor fasciæ latæ.

The **Superior Gluteal Artery,** a branch from the posterior division of the internal iliac artery, emerges from the pelvis at the upper border of the piriformis muscle and at once gives off a *superficial branch*, which is distributed to the gluteal maximus. The remaining *deep branch* breaks up into upper and lower branches, which follow the middle and inferior gluteal lines respectively, in the interval between the gluteus medius and the gluteus minimus.

The *Upper Branch* reaches the anterior superior iliac spine, where it anastomoses with the ascending branch of the lateral circumflex femoral and with branches of the deep circumflex iliac arteries.

The *Lower Branch* terminates in the trochanteric anastomosis. Both branches give off numerous twigs to the neighbouring muscles.

The **Trochanteric Anastomosis** forms one of the anastomoses round the hip joint. Branches from the inferior gluteal and the deep branch of the superior gluteal, both of which are derivatives of the internal iliac artery, gain the trochanteric fossa, where they anastomose with the ascending branch of the medial circumflex femoral artery, which reaches the fossa by running along the tendon of the obturator externus. The trochanteric anastomosis, therefore, is a connexion between the internal iliac on the one hand, and the femoral artery on the other.

The **Crucial Anastomosis** is situated at the upper part of the back of the thigh. The horizontal arms of the cross are formed by the transverse branches of the circumflex femoral arteries, the upper limb is formed by descending branches from the inferior gluteal artery, and the lower limb by an ascending branch from the first perforating artery. Like the trochanteric, the crucial anastomosis establishes a connexion between the internal iliac and the femoral arteries.

THE BACK OF THE THIGH AND THE POPLITEAL FOSSA

The skin on the back of the thigh is supplied by the posterior cutaneous nerve, which has already been described (p. 63).

The *Deep Fascia* is strengthened in the lower part of the thigh, where it forms the roof of the popliteal fossa. In this situation it contains many transverse fibres, and is pierced by the short saphenous vein (p. 69) and the terminal part of the posterior cutaneous nerve.

The *Muscles* in the posterior or flexor compartment of the thigh are frequently termed the "hamstring muscles"; they include the semimembranosus, the semitendinosus and the biceps.

The **Semimembranosus** muscle arises from the back of the ischial tuberosity by a strong tendon, noted for its unusual length. It passes downwards and medially, at first deep to the conjoined origin of biceps and semitendinosus, and subsequently overlapped by the latter muscle. Its tendon of insertion forms the upper and medial boundary of the popliteal fossa, and is inserted into a groove on the postero-medial aspect of the medial condyle of the tibia. From the tendon a strong expansion passes upwards and laterally to strengthen the posterior aspect of the knee joint, forming its oblique posterior ligament (p. 87).

The **Semitendinosus** arises from the ischial tuberosity with the long head of the biceps, and runs downwards on the surface of the semimembranosus to be inserted by a long tendon into the upper part of the medial surface of the tibia just below the gracilis (p. 59).

The **Biceps** arises (1) by a long head, in common with the semitendinosus, and (2) by a short head, from the lateral lip of the linea aspera, the lateral supracondylar line and the lateral intermuscular septum. The two heads unite just above the knee joint in a common tendon, which forms the upper and lateral boundary of the popliteal fossa and can easily be recognised in this situation in the living subject, especially when the knee is actively flexed against resistance. It is inserted into the head of the fibula.

The *Nerve Supply* of all three muscles is derived from the sciatic nerve (tibial nerve portion).

Actions. The hamstrings flex the knee joint and extend the hip. In addition the biceps is a lateral rotator, and the semimembranosus and semitendinosus are medial rotators of the tibia on the femur.

The **Sciatic Nerve** (p. 63) runs downwards in the middle line of the thigh on the posterior aspect of the adductor magnus muscle. Near the upper part of the thigh it is crossed obliquely by the long head of biceps, and in the rest of its course it is overlapped by the contiguous margins of biceps and semimembranosus. It ends near the upper extremity of the popliteal fossa by dividing into the tibial and common peroneal nerves (medial and lateral popliteal nerves).

Branches. In addition to the two terminal branches, the sciatic nerve gives off branches to supply the hamstrings and the ischial fibres of the adductor magnus (p. 58).

The **Popliteal Fossa** is in reality a *region*, which may be opened up by dissection. Above, the biceps laterally and the semimembranosus and semitendinosus medially are not quite in contact; but below the two heads of the gastrocnemius must be artificially separated from each other to form a "fossa" (Plate IV, p. 17).

The *Roof* of the fossa is formed by the deep fascia. The *Floor* consists of (1) the popliteal surface of the femur, (2) the posterior ligament of the knee joint, and (3) the popliteus muscle with its strong covering fascia.

The **Tibial (Medial Popliteal) Nerve** arises from the sciatic nerve as it enters the space at its upper angle. It runs downwards through the fat which fills the fossa, and, although comparatively superficial above, it is placed deeply below, in the interval between the two heads of the gastrocnemius. At first the nerve lies to the lateral side of the popliteal artery, but at the middle of the space it crosses superficial to the vessel, and then continues downwards to its medial side. The popliteal vein intervenes between the nerve and the artery throughout.

At the lower border of the popliteus muscle the nerve passes deep to the tendinous arch of the soleus (p. 75).

Branches. 1. *Cutaneous.* The *sural nerve* branches from the medial popliteal and descends on the surface of the gastrocnemius muscle. It supplies small branches to the skin of the back of the leg, and, in its lower third, is joined by the sural communicating branch from the lateral popliteal nerve. In company with the short saphenous vein, it passes behind the lateral malleolus and gains the foot (p. 69).

2. *Muscular.* The medial popliteal nerve gives branches (*a*) to both heads of gastrocnemius, (*b*) to plantaris, (*c*) to soleus, and (*d*) to the popliteus muscle.

3. *Articular Branches*, usually three in number, supply the knee joint.

The **Common Peroneal (Lateral Popliteal) Nerve** enters the fossa lateral to the tibial nerve, and runs downwards on the medial side of the biceps tendon. It leaves the space by passing between the tendon and the lateral head of the gastrocnemius, and runs downwards behind the head of the fibula. It then turns forwards on the lateral aspect of the neck of the bone, pierces the peroneus longus and divides into (1) the superficial peroneal (musculocutaneous), and (2) the deep peroneal (anterior tibial) nerves. *In this situation the nerve is relatively superficial and can be rolled against the neck of the fibula in the living subject.*

Branches. 1. *Cutaneous.* (*a*) The *peroneal (sural) communicating branch* runs downwards on the lateral head of the gastrocnemius to join the sural nerve (p. 69); (*b*) as it leaves the popliteal fossa, the lateral popliteal nerve gives off a small branch to the skin over the upper part of the antero-lateral aspect of the leg.

2. *Articular Branches*, usually three in number, supply the knee joint.

The **Popliteal Artery** starts at the gap between the adductor magnus and the femur, and runs downwards through the fossa. (On account of the inclination of the long axis of the femur, the artery appears to run downwards and laterally in the detached limb.) At the lower border of the popliteus it ends by dividing into the anterior and posterior tibial arteries.

The *Anterior Relations* comprise the popliteal surface of the femur, the oblique posterior ligament of the knee joint and the popliteus muscle with its covering fascia, *i.e.*, the floor of the fossa.

A fairly thick pad of fat separates the artery from the femur, *but it lies in direct contact with the oblique posterior ligament of the knee joint.*

Posteriorly the artery is separated from the fascial covering of the fossa by its accompanying vein and the tibial nerve (p. 67).

Branches. In addition to its terminal branches, the popliteal artery gives off (1) numerous muscular branches, and (2) articular branches. Of the latter group, the *middle genicular artery* arises from the anterior aspect of the parent trunk and pierces the posterior ligament to supply the intracapsular structures. The others, four in number, wind round to the anterior aspect of the lower end of the femur and upper end of the tibia and take part in an anastomosis round the knee.

The **Popliteal Vein** lies on the lateral side of the artery in the upper part of the fossa, gradually crosses behind it, and in the lower part of the space comes to lie on the medial side. Throughout it is between the artery and the tibial nerve.

The *Anastomosis round the Knee Joint* is anterior to the joint, and the vessels which take part in it run in close contact with the lower end of the femur, the patella and the upper end of the tibia. The descending branch of the lateral circumflex femoral artery (p. 56), the articular branch of the descending genicular artery (p. 58), the articular branches of the popliteal artery and recurrent branches of the anterior tibial artery all unite and re-unite to form an arterial network. The anastomosis thus connects the femoral artery, at the origin of its profunda branch and at its lower end, with the popliteal and anterior tibial arteries, but its primary function is to supply bone.

THE FRONT OF THE LEG AND DORSUM OF FOOT

It is not until this region is reached that revision can be carried out satisfactorily on a detached dissected limb. The student should also provide himself with an articulated skeleton of the limb.

Cutaneous Nerves. The skin over the upper part of the front of the leg is supplied by a branch from the common peroneal nerve. In its lower part it receives branches from the *superficial peroneal nerve*, which, after rising from the common peroneal and supplying the peroneus longus and brevis, pierces the deep fascia in front of the fibula at the junction of the middle and lower thirds of the leg. It then splits into medial and intermediate dorsal branches which continue downwards on to the dorsum of the foot. The *medial branch* gives twigs to the skin of the dorsum and divides into branches, (1) for the medial side of the great toe, and (2) for the second cleft, to supply the adjacent sides of the second and third toes. The *intermediate* *dorsal digital branch* also supplies twigs to the skin of the dorsum and divides into branches for (1) the third cleft, and (2) the fourth cleft. It communicates with the sural nerve.

The *Sural Nerve* (p. 67) runs along the lateral border of the foot and ends by supplying the lateral side of the little toe. It very often takes over a part of the area of supply of the lateral branch of the superficial peroneal nerve.

The *Digital Branch of the Deep Peroneal* pierces the deep fascia over the first interosseous space and supplies the adjacent sides of the great and second toes (p. 72).

Superficial Veins. A well-developed *Dorsal Venous Arch* crosses the foot near the heads of the metatarsal bones. From its medial end the *long saphenous vein* arises and runs upwards *in front of the medial malleolus.* The *short saphenous vein* arises from the lateral side of the arch and, running backwards along the lateral border of the foot with the sural nerve, ascends *behind the lateral malleolus.* It subsequently runs upwards in the superficial fascia of the back of the leg and pierces the fascial roof of the popliteal fossa to end by joining the popliteal vein.

The **Deep Fascia** on the front of the leg is attached to the anterior border of the tibia on the medial side, and laterally is continuous with the fascia covering the peroneal muscles. The *anterior intermuscular septum* passes from its deep aspect to the anterior border of the fibula, between the extensor muscles of the leg from the peronei. The deep fascia is particularly strong in the upper part of the leg, where it gives partial attachment to the tibialis anterior muscle. It is thickened just above the ankle and again on the dorsum of the foot to form the superior and inferior extensor retinacula, which hold down the tendons of tibialis anterior and the extensor tendons.

The *Superior Extensor Retinaculum* is a band of deep fascia, about $1\frac{1}{2}$ inches wide, which is attached laterally to the anterior border of the fibula. At its medial end the ligament splits to enclose the tibialis anterior tendon, which therefore occupies a separate compartment and synovial sheath. To its lateral side the tendons of the extensor hallucis longus, the extensor digitorum longus and the peroneus tertius muscle pass *behind the retinaculum.* They occupy a common compartment, which has no synovial sheath. The anterior tibial vessels and nerve lie posterior to the extensor hallucis longus as they pass behind the retinaculum.

The *Inferior Extensor Retinaculum* is usually a Y-shaped thickening of the deep fascia in the posterior part of the dorsum of the foot. The stem of the Y is attached to the anterior part of the upper surface of the calcaneum, and of the two limbs the upper is attached to the medial malleolus and the lower becomes continuous with the plantar fascia. Individual compartments, each lined by a separate synovial sheath, are provided (1) for the tibialis anterior tendon, (2) for the extensor hallucis longus tendon, and (3) for the tendons of the extensor digitorum longus and the peroneus tertius. These tendons *split the retinaculum into superficial and deep layers.*

The **Tibialis Anterior** arises from the upper half of the lateral surface of the tibia, from the interosseous membrane and from the covering deep fascia. Its tendon begins about the middle of the leg and follows the anterior border of the tibia, crossing the bone immediately in front of the medial malleolus. It passes through the medial compartment of both extensor retinacula, crosses the ankle joint, the talus and the navicular, and is inserted into the antero-inferior part of the medial surface of the medial cuneiform bone and the adjoining part of the base of the first metatarsal.

Its *Nerve Supply* is derived from the deep peroneal nerve.

Actions. The tibialis anterior is a powerful extensor or dorsiflexor of the foot. When the foot is off the ground, it inverts its medial border. When the foot is bearing weight and in the resting position (p. 95), the tibialis anterior assists in maintaining the medial arch, and it may also bend the leg forward on the fixed foot.

The **Extensor Digitorum Longus** arises from the upper three-quarters of the narrow extensor surface of the fibula, from the surrounding deep fascia, and from the upper part of the interosseous membrane. It passes downwards behind the upper and through the lower extensor retinaculum and in front of the ankle joint. On the dorsum of the foot its four tendons separate and pass to the lateral four digits. On the dorsum of the proximal phalanx an expansion is formed to which are attached the lumbrical and interosseous muscles (*cf.* p. 36). The central part of the expansion is inserted into the base of the middle phalanx, while its marginal bands are prolonged down to attachment into the base of the distal phalanx.

Its *Nerve Supply* is derived from the deep peroneal nerve, and its *Action* is indicated by its name. In addition, the extensor digitorum longus dorsiflexes the foot.

The **Peroneus Tertius** arises as part of the previous muscle from the lower part of the extensor surface of the fibula and from the interosseous membrane. It accompanies the extensor digitorum longus, sharing its synovial sheath, and is inserted into the medial side of the base of the fifth metatarsal bone.

The *Nerve Supply* is derived from the deep peroneal nerve.

The *Action* of the peroneus tertius is to dorsiflex the foot and to help the peroneal muscles in eversion.

The **Extensor Hallucis Longus** arises from the middle two-fourths of the extensor surface of the fibula and from the interosseous membrane. At first it lies deep to the extensor digitorum longus, but as it runs downwards it comes to the surface between the tibialis anterior and the extensor digitorum longus. It accompanies the latter behind the upper extensor retinaculum, but it has an independent compartment in the lower retinaculum, lined with an independent synovial sheath. As it passes over the ankle joint it crosses the anterior tibial vessels and nerve, so that its tendon lies medial to the dorsalis pedis artery on the dorsum of the foot. Finally it is inserted into the base of the distal phalanx of the great toe.

Its *Nerve Supply* comes from the deep peroneal nerve. The *Action* of the muscle is indicated by its name and, in addition, it assists in dorsiflexion of the foot.

The **Anterior Tibial Artery** begins on the posterior aspect of the leg, where it arises from the popliteal artery at the lower border of the popliteus muscle. It enters the anterior compartment of the leg by piercing the upper part of the interosseous membrane. In the upper half of its course the artery is very deeply situated, lying on the interosseous membrane between the tibialis anterior and the extensor digitorum longus. In the lower part of its course the artery lies on the tibia and is overlapped by the extensor hallucis longus, but after passing behind the superior extensor retinaculum it becomes superficial in the interval between the tendons of the extensor hallucis longus and the extensor digitorum longus, where its pulsations can be felt in the living subject. In front of the ankle joint the artery becomes the dorsalis pedis artery.

In the upper part of its course the deep peroneal nerve lies to the lateral side of the artery, but for some distance in the middle of the leg it is in front of the vessel, returning to its lateral side near the ankle.

Branches of the anterior tibial artery take part in the anastomoses round the knee and ankle joints.

Venæ Comitantes, usually two in number, accompany the artery and are connected to each other at many points.

The **Deep Peroneal Nerve** arises from the common peroneal nerve *on the lateral side of the neck of the fibula.* It gains the anterior compartment by piercing the anterior intermuscular septum, passing between the extensor digitorum longus and the fibula. It is closely related to the anterior tibial artery, and so bears the same relations as the vessel to the surrounding structures.

On the dorsum of the foot the nerve passes under cover of the extensor digitorum brevis and ends there by supplying twigs to the muscle and to the neighbouring joints. Before doing so, it gives off a *dorsal digital branch*, which accompanies the dorsalis pedis artery on its lateral side, and, piercing the deep fascia, runs to the cleft between the hallux and the second toe, to supply the adjacent margins of those digits. In addition to the terminal distribution, the deep peroneal nerve supplies all the muscles in the anterior compartment of the leg, viz., the tibialis anterior, the extensor digitorum longus, the extensor hallucis longus and the peroneus tertius.

The *Perforating Branch of the Peroneal Artery* (p. 78) pierces the interosseous membrane at its lower end and enters the anterior compartment. It runs downwards behind the superior extensor retinaculum, along the anterior border of the lateral malleolus, to anastomose with branches of the anterior tibial and of the dorsalis pedis artery. This is one of the two anastomoses round the ankle joint, and it establishes a connexion between the peroneal (and therefore the upper part of the posterior tibial artery) and the lower end of the anterior tibial artery and its continuation, the dorsal artery of the foot.

The **Extensor Digitorum Brevis** lies in the lateral part of the dorsum of the foot, where it produces a small elevation when it contracts. It arises from the anterior part of the upper surface of the calcaneum and from the inferior extensor retinaculum. It breaks up into four tendons, which pass to the *medial* four toes. The first tendon is inserted into the dorsal aspect of the base of the proximal phalanx of the great toe, but the other three tendons join the corresponding tendons of the extensor digitorum longus.

Its *Nerve Supply* is derived from the terminal part of the deep peroneal nerve, and its *Action* is indicated by its name.

The **Dorsalis Pedis Artery** begins in front of the ankle joint, runs forwards on the dorsum of the foot and terminates by passing downwards at the posterior end of the first intermetatarsal space to join the plantar arch. It is superficial throughout its course, and is crossed only by the inferior extensor retinaculum and, as a rule, by the first tendon of the extensor digitorum brevis. On its *lateral side* it is accompanied by the digital branch of the deep peroneal nerve and on its *medial side* the tendon of the extensor hallucis longus runs forwards to its insertion. *Inferiorly*, the artery crosses the neck of the talus, the navicular and the intermediate cuneiform bones.

Branches. 1. The *Lateral Tarsal Artery* arises just below the ankle and runs laterally under cover of the extensor digitorum brevis. It gives branches to the skin and the tarsal joints and ends in the anastomosis round the lateral malleolus.

2. The *Arcuate Artery* arises further forwards and passes obliquely across the metatarsals under cover of the tendons of the extensor digitorum brevis. It gives off dorsal metatarsal arteries to the lateral three clefts to supply the dorsal aspects of the digits. It also communicates with the plantar arch.

3. The *First Dorsal Metatarsal Artery* is the apparent continuation of the dorsalis pedis. It supplies branches to both sides of the dorsal aspect of the great toe and the adjacent side of the second toe.

THE PERONEAL REGION

The peroneal muscles occupy the lateral compartment of the leg, being separated from the extensor and flexor compartments by the anterior and the posterior intermuscular septa, respectively.

The **Peroneus Longus** arises from the upper two-thirds of the lateral surface of the fibula and from the adjoining fascia and septa.

The **Peroneus Brevis** arises from the lower two-thirds of the same area, and the upper part of its origin overlaps the lower part of the origin of the peroneus longus.

Both muscles run downwards, the brevis covered by the longus, to the posterior aspect of the lateral malleolus, where the tendon of the brevis is in direct contact with the bone. In this situation the tendons are held down by a thickened band of deep fascia, termed the *superior peroneal retinaculum*, and are provided with a common synovial sheath. Passing below the malleolus, the tendons lie on the lateral surface of the calcaneum and become separated from each other by the peroneal tubercle. Here they are retained in place by the *inferior peroneal retinaculum* and each possesses its own synovial sheath, which is continuous above with the common sheath. The tendon of the peroneus brevis runs forwards above the tubercle to be inserted into the tubercle on the base of the fifth metatarsal bone.

The tendon of the peroneus longus runs below the peroneal tubercle, winds round the lateral aspect of the cuboid and passes medially and forwards across the sole of the foot to be inserted into the lateral surface of the medial cuneiform and the adjoining part of the base of the first metatarsal bone.

Both of these muscles are supplied by the superficial peroneal nerve.

Actions. When the foot is not under load, *e.g.*, when it is off the ground, the peroneal muscles produce eversion, but also to be noted is the part played by the peroneus longus in maintaining the transverse arch of the foot and in helping to accentuate it when the resting posture is changed for one of activity. By their tendency to draw the foot to the lateral side, the peroneal muscles balance the medial pull exerted by the tibialis posterior and the long flexors of the toes, so that in the movements of walking, running, etc., the foot is held in the midway position.

The **Superficial Peroneal Nerve** arises from the common peroneal nerve on the lateral side of the neck of the fibula. It runs downwards and forwards, at first in the substance of the peroneus longus and then between the peroneus brevis and the anterior intermuscular septum. At the junction of the middle and lower thirds of the leg it pierces the deep fascia to become subcutaneous.

Branches. The superficial peroneal nerve supplies the peroneus longus and brevis. Its cutaneous and communicating branches are described on p. 69.

THE BACK OF THE LEG

The skin of this region draws its nerve supply from a variety of sources. (1) The *saphenous nerve* and the *medial cutaneous nerve of the thigh* supply branches to the medial part of the area. (2) The terminal branches of the *posterior cutaneous nerve of the thigh* and the *sural nerve* supply the central part. (3) The *peroneal communicating branch of the common peroneal* and the *sural nerve* supply branches to the lateral part of the region.

The *Deep Fascia* invests the superficial muscles and becomes thickened below, where it forms the *flexor retinaculum*, which stretches between the calcaneus and the medial malleolus. A second layer of deep fascia separates the superficial from the deep muscles, and is attached to the posterior border of the fibula and the medial border of the tibia. Below, it reinforces the flexor retinaculum. A third layer of deep fascia covers the surface of the tibialis posterior, and separates it from the flexor hallucis longus, the flexor digitorum longus and the posterior tibial vessels and nerve. As the muscle gives place to its tendon the fascia blends with it, and consequently is absent in the lower part of the leg.

The **Gastrocnemius** arises (1) by a lateral head, from the lateral aspect of the lateral femoral condyle, and (2) by a medial head, from the popliteal surface of the femur just above the articular surface of the medial condyle. The two fleshy bellies do not unite, but each is separately continued into a broad common tendon, the *tendo calcaneus*, which narrows below and is inserted into the posterior surface of the calcaneus. A bursa is interposed between the tendon and the upper part of the posterior surface of the bone.

The **Plantaris** has a small fleshy belly, which arises from the lateral supracondylar line of the femur and runs downwards, inclining medially under cover of the lateral head of the gastrocnemius. Its short belly gives rise to a very long, narrow tendon, which runs deep to the medial head of the gastrocnemius to be inserted into the posterior surface of the calcaneus.

The **Soleus** arises (1) from the upper fourth of the posterior surface of the shaft of the fibula, extending upwards on to the head of the bone; (2) from a tendinous arch over the posterior tibial vessels and tibial nerve; and (3) from the soleal line on the posterior surface of the tibia, extending downwards for 2 or 3 inches along the medial border of the bone.

In its upper half this muscle is covered by the gastrocnemius but, where the common tendon of the latter begins, the belly of the soleus projects beyond its margins and can be identified in the living subject when it is thrown into contraction (Plate IV, p. 17).

The tendon develops on the superficial aspect of the muscle, and joins the deep surface of the tendo calcaneus.

All three muscle bellies are supplied by the tibial nerve at the level of the knee, but the soleus receives an additional branch from it lower, in the leg.

Actions. All three act as plantar flexors of the foot. The gastrocnemius supplies the propulsive force in walking, running, etc., but the soleus probably functions rather as a postural muscle, steadying the leg on the foot in the upright attitude.

The **Deep Muscles of the Back of the Leg** include the popliteus above, and the flexor digitorum longus, the tibialis posterior and the flexor hallucis longus, in that order from the medial to the lateral side, but in the upper part of the leg the tibialis posterior is overlapped by the other two muscles. In the lower part of the leg the tendon of the tibialis posterior is crossed by the flexor digitorum longus, and occupies the groove on the posterior aspect of the medial malleolus.

The **Popliteus** arises by a cord-like tendon from the lateral surface of the lateral condyle of the femur, *within the capsular ligament of the knee joint*, and is inserted into the posterior surface of the tibia above the soleal line. The most medial fibres of the muscle arise from the posterior aspect of the capsular ligament of the knee joint where it blends with the peripheral border of the lateral semilunar cartilage. Its tendon passes downwards and backwards, separating the lateral semilunar cartilage from the lateral ligament of the joint, and emerges through the infero-lateral part of the posterior portion of the capsular ligament.

The **Flexor Digitorum Longus** arises from the medial part of the posterior surface of the tibia, below the soleal line. It crosses superficial to the tendon of the tibialis posterior, and lies to its lateral side as they pass forwards into the sole of the foot. This muscle corresponds to the flexor digitorum profundus in the hand and has a similar mode of insertion. Bases distal phalanges. *

The **Tibialis Posterior** arises from the lateral part of the posterior surface of the tibia, the interosseous membrane, and the adjoining part of the fibula. At first the muscle lies very deeply, but its tendon becomes more superficial, and, as it is being crossed by the tendon of the flexor digitorum longus, it grooves the posterior surface of the lower end of the tibia just behind the medial malleolus. It then passes forwards under cover of the flexor retinaculum into the sole of the foot, where its principal attachment is to the tuberosity of the navicular (p. 421).

The **Flexor Hallucis Longus** arises from the posterior surface of the fibula in its lower two-thirds, *i.e.*, below the fibular origin of the soleus. It is the bulkiest of the deep muscles and overlaps the tibialis posterior and hides the peroneal artery. Its tendon lies lateral to the tendon of the flexor digitorum longus as it passes under cover of the flexor retinaculum, but is crossed by it in the sole of the foot (p. 80) and then runs forwards to be inserted into the plantar surface of the base of the distal phalanx of the great toe.

With the exception of the popliteus, the deep muscles are all supplied by the *tibial nerve*. The *nerve to the popliteus* arises in the popliteal fossa, runs downwards across the popliteal vessels to reach the lower border of the muscle, and then ascends to enter its deep surface. It supplies the superior and inferior tibia-fibular joints.

Actions. The popliteus acts as a flexor of the knee and as a medial rotator of the tibia on the femur. It is brought into play at the commencement of flexion of the fully-extended knee, and its rotatory effect "unlocks" the joint (p. 89).

Although, when the foot is raised off the ground, the flexor digitorum longus and the flexor hallucis longus carry out the action indicated by their names, their effective use occurs when the heel is raised and the body weight is transferred to the heads of the metatarsal bones and the digital pads of the toes. The pressure which the latter are capable of exerting on the ground is due to the action of the flexors, and it can only be exerted to the full when the great toe is extended a little at the metatarsophalangeal joint and flexed at the interphalangeal joint, and when the other toes are extended at the metatarsophalangeal and distal interphalangeal joints, but are flexed at the proximal interphalangeal joints (*see also* p. 80).

The tibialis posterior is a powerful invertor of the foot and can assist in plantar flexion.

The effect of the tonus of the deep muscles in supporting the longitudinal arch of the foot is just as important as the movements which they produce by active contraction. As the tendons run forwards in the sole of the foot, they lie below and in close relationship with the *plantar calcaneonavicular* ("*spring*") *ligament*, which supports the head of the talus. Neither the ligament, nor the other structures which support the longitudinal arch of the foot are equal to the task when the tonus of the deep muscles on the back of the leg is subnormal, nor is the ligament springy.

The **Tibial Nerve** continues downwards beyond the lower border of popliteus (p. 67) to pass deep to the tendinous arch of the soleus. Covered by that muscle and the gastrocnemius, it runs downwards between the flexor digitorum longus and the flexor hallucis longus and on the surface of the tibialis posterior muscle. In the lower part of the leg it lies on the posterior surface of the tibia between the tendons of the flexor digitorum longus and flexor hallucis longus. With the same relations the nerve passes under the flexor retinaculum and divides into the lateral and medial plantar nerves.

Throughout its course in the leg the nerve is closely related to the posterior tibial vessels. Lying at first to their medial side, it crosses superficially to reach their lateral side, along which it continues into the foot.

Branches. 1. *Muscular*, to soleus, flexor hallucis longus, tibialis posterior and flexor digitorum longus.

2. *Cutaneous.* The *Medial Calcaneal Branches* arise near the termination of the posterior tibial nerve and pierce the flexor retinaculum to supply the skin in the neighbourhood, including the plantar surface of the heel.

The **Posterior Tibial Artery** is one of the terminal branches of the popliteal artery. It begins at the lower border of the popliteus under the contiguous borders of the two heads of the gastrocnemius and the tendinous arch of the soleus. It is, therefore, deeply situated at its origin. The artery runs downwards on the surface of the tibialis posterior in close relationship with the tibial nerve and, in the lower part of the leg, comes to lie on the posterior surface of the tibia. In the latter part of its course the posterior tibial artery is superficial, being covered only by the skin and fasciæ. Accompanying the nerve under cover of the flexor retinaculum, the vessel terminates by dividing into the lateral and medial plantar arteries.

Branches. 1. The *Peroneal Artery* is the largest and most important branch. It arises a short distance below the termination of the popliteal artery and runs downwards closely associated with the flexor hallucis longus muscle. As a rule, the artery lies deep to the muscle and close to the medial crest of the fibula, which separates the origin of the flexor hallucis longus from that of the tibialis posterior. In the lower part of the leg it gives off a *perforating branch*, which pierces the interosseous membrane and joins the anastomosis round the lateral malleolus (p. 72). The terminal part of the peroneal artery takes part in the same anastomosis.

2. A small *Communicating Artery* connects the lower ends of the peroneal and the posterior tibial arteries.

3. Numerous unnamed branches supply muscles and skin, as do the above.

Two *Venæ Comitantes*, draining the plantar veins, accompany the posterior tibial artery. At the lower border of the popliteus they join the venæ comitantes of the anterior tibial artery and form the popliteal vein.

The **Flexor Retinaculum** is attached to the medial malleolus and to the medial border of the posterior surface of the calcaneum. Above, it is continuous both with the investing deep fascia and with the fascial layer which covers the deep muscles. Below, it gives origin to the abductor hallucis and is continuous with the thin layer of fascia which covers that muscle. Under cover of the retinaculum, the tendons of the deep muscles, the posterior tibial vessels and nerve, and their terminal branches, pass forwards behind the medial malleolus into the sole of the foot.

The tendon of the tibialis posterior lies close to the malleolus, with the tendon of the flexor digitorum longus on its lateral side. The posterior tibial vessels, with the corresponding nerve to their lateral side, occupy the interval between the flexor digitorum longus and the flexor hallucis longus tendon, which passes under cover of the lateral portion of the retinaculum. Not infrequently there is practically no interval between these tendons, and the vessels and nerve then lie superficial to them.

THE SOLE OF THE FOOT

The skin of the sole of the foot is supplied by (1) the *medial calcaneal branches* (p. 77), which are distributed to the posterior and medial portion; (2) branches from the *medial plantar nerve*, and (3) branches from the *lateral plantar nerve*. (4) The *plantar digital nerves* (p. 83) are similar in distribution to the digital nerves of the hand. Those which supply the medial three toes and the medial side of the fourth toe are derived from the medial plantar nerve; the others are branches of the lateral plantar nerve.

The **Deep Fascia** of the sole of the foot presents the same plan as the deep fascia of the palm of the hand. It consists of weak lateral and medial portions, covering respectively the abductor digiti minimi and the abductor hallucis, and a greatly strengthened central portion, termed the plantar aponeurosis.

The *Plantar Aponeurosis* forms a dense fibrous sheet, attached posteriorly to the medial and lateral tubercles of the calcaneus. It widens out anteriorly and divides into *five* slips, one for each toe, which behave like the corresponding slips in the hand (p. 30). The great toe, therefore, bears a different relation to the deep fascia of the sole from that borne by the thumb to the deep fascia of the palm, and the diminished mobility of the great toe as compared with the thumb is partly accounted for in this way.

The function of the plantar aponeurosis is primarily to fix the skin of the sole, which is strongly attached to it. It also provides additional attachment for the long muscles of the sole, and it has some protective value. Its role in maintaining the arches is uncertain.

Fibrous Flexor Sheaths, as in the hand (p. 31), retain the flexor tendons in place on the toes.

The **Muscles of the Sole of the Foot.** The muscles and tendons of the sole are arranged in four layers, but only the most superficial layer covers the whole extent of the sole, so that in certain situations the muscles of the first and third layers are in contact with one another.

The *First Layer* includes the abductor hallucis, the flexor digitorum brevis and the abductor digiti minimi. These three muscles all extend from the posterior part of the calcaneus to the toes.

The **Flexor Digitorum Brevis** divides into four tendons which pass to the lateral four toes, where they behave in the same way as the tendons of the flexor digitorum superficialis in the hand (p. 32).

The **Abductor Hallucis** is inserted into the medial side of the base of the proximal phalanx of the great toe, and the **Abductor Digiti Minimi** into the lateral side of the base of the proximal phalanx of the little toe.

Actions. When the foot is not under load, these muscles act as their names imply, but when it is under load they are not able to do so. Instead, *like all the muscles of the sole, they act synergically to help to brace the arches of the foot and give them additional and important support.*

The abductor digiti minimi is supplied by the *lateral plantar nerve*, and the two other muscles of this layer by the *medial plantar nerve*.

The *Second Layer* includes the flexor digitorum accessorius, the lumbricals and the tendons of the flexor digitorum longus and the flexor hallucis longus.

The **Flexor Digitorum Accessorius** arises by two heads, one from each side of the calcaneus. The medial head, which is fleshy and much the larger of the two, occupies the deep hollow on the medial surface of the calcaneus, and is joined by the tendinous lateral head, which runs forwards and medially across the long plantar ligament. About the middle of the sole the muscle is inserted into the tendon of the flexor digitorum longus. It is covered by the flexor digitorum brevis.

The **Lumbricals** are four in number. They arise from the tendons of the flexor digitorum longus and proceed to the four lateral toes, where each is inserted chiefly into the tibial side of the dorsal expansion of the corresponding extensor tendon.

The **Tendon of the Flexor Digitorum Longus** runs forwards and laterally from the flexor retinaculum. It lies first on the medial surface of the sustentaculum tali and *then crosses superficial to the flexor hallucis longus tendon, which separates it from the plantar calcaneonavicular ligament* (p. 93). As it receives the insertion of the flexor accessorius, it divides into four tendons for the lateral four toes. These tendons behave similarly to the tendons of the flexor digitorum profundus in the hand.

The **Tendon of the Flexor Hallucis Longus** grooves the posterior aspect of the talus and then occupies a continuation of the groove on the inferior surface of the sustentaculum. Immediately in front of this it crosses deep to the tendon of the flexor digitorum longus and lies below the lateral part of the plantar calcaneonavicular ligament (p. 93). In this situation, it gives a strong slip to the tendon of the flexor digitorum longus, by which it is carried to the second and third toes. It then runs forwards to be inserted into the base of the distal phalanx of the great toe.

The *Nerve Supply* of the flexor digitorum accessorius and the lateral three lumbricals is derived from the lateral plantar nerve, but the first lumbrical is supplied by the medial plantar nerve. The flexor digitorum longus and the flexor hallucis longus receive their supply on the back of the leg from the tibial nerve.

Actions. When the foot is under load, the flexor digitorum accessorius maintains the tendons of the flexor digitorum longus taut, enabling the tibial belly of that muscle to relax (p. 77) as the leg bends forwards in walking. The lumbricals counteract the tendency of the toes to "buckle" under the pull of the digital flexors in running, etc. (p. 77). This they do by preventing too great a degree of extension at the metatarsophalangeal joints and of flexion at the proximal interphalangeal joints.

It will be observed that the muscles of the second layer are all connected to the flexor digitorum longus tendon and that they form an X-shaped figure, so that on each border of the foot the first and third layers come into contact with each other.

The *Third Layer of Muscles* comprises the flexor hallucis brevis, the oblique and transverse heads of the adductor hallucis, and the flexor digiti minimi brevis, *i.e.*, it includes two short flexors and two adductors. It is limited to the anterior part of the foot.

The **Flexor Hallucis Brevis** covers the plantar aspect of the first metatarsal, and its fleshy belly divides into two heads. Of these the medial is inserted, in common with the abductor hallucis, into the base of the proximal phalanx of the hallux, and the lateral is inserted into the lateral side of the same bone, in common with the adductor. A sesamoid bone is developed in each tendon of insertion.

The **Adductor Hallucis,** like the adductor pollicis, consists of an oblique and a transverse head. The *oblique head* lies along the lateral border of the preceding muscle. It arises from the plantar aspects of the bases of the second, third and fourth metatarsal bones, and is inserted in common with the lateral head of the flexor hallucis brevis.

The *transverse head* is a small muscle, which is placed under the *heads* of the metatarsal bones. It arises from the plantar ligaments of the third, fourth and fifth metatarsophalangeal joints, and is inserted in common with the preceding muscle.

The **Flexor Digiti Minimi Brevis** covers the plantar surface of the fifth metatarsal bone and is inserted into the base and lateral border of the proximal phalanx of the little toe.

The *nerve supply* of the flexor hallucis brevis is derived from the medial plantar nerve; the remaining two muscles are supplied by the lateral plantar nerve.

Actions. When the foot is not under load, these muscles act as their names imply, but, in addition, the oblique head of the adductor hallucis flexes the great toe at the metatarsophalangeal joint. When the foot is under load these muscles brace the plantar aspects of the joints with which they are related and resist flattening of the arches of the foot.

The *fourth layer of muscles* includes the interossei, both plantar and dorsal, and the tendons of peroneus longus and tibialis posterior.

N.B. As in the hand, the dorsal interossei are abductors and the plantar interossei are adductors, but the line of reference passes through the *second* digit and not the third as is the case in the hand.

The **Plantar Interossei,** three in number, arise from the plantar aspects of the third, fourth and fifth metatarsal bones, and are inserted into the tibial sides of the bases of the proximal phalanges of the corresponding toes, and also into the tibial side of the dorsal extensor expansion.

The **Dorsal Interossei,** four in number, arise from the adjoining sides of the metatarsal bones. Each takes origin by two heads, which unite to form a small tendon of insertion. It is attached to the base of the proximal phalanx and the adjoining part of the dorsal extensor expansion. The first dorsal interosseous is inserted on the tibial side of the second toe, and the three others are inserted on the fibular sides of the second, third and fourth toes respectively.

All the interossei are supplied by the *lateral plantar nerve.*

All the small muscles of the foot are called into action in a synergic capacity, whenever the foot is in active use under load; by their increased tone they maintain the stability of the foot as an arched lever and so serve to increase the efficiency of the prime movers, viz.: the gastrocnemius and the long digital flexors and extensors.

The **Peroneus Longus** tendon runs obliquely across the sole, and is held in place by a strong fibrous sheath, which is derived from the long plantar ligament. Placed at first in the groove on the plantar surface of the cuboid, the tendon crosses the lateral and intermediate cuneiform bones to be inserted into the lateral aspect of the base of the first metatarsal and the adjoining part of the medial cuneiform bone.

Actions. The peroneus longus accentuates the transverse arch of the foot and so enables the inverted foot to remain plantigrade in the active, erect posture, when it is under load. When its insertion is fixed, the tone of the muscle helps to steady the leg on the foot. In addition, in the erect posture, it helps to maintain the lateral longitudinal and the transverse arches of the foot, for it is below the cuboid and the transverse arch near the bases of the metatarsal bones. When the foot is raised from the ground the peroneus longus is an evertor.

The **Tibialis Posterior Tendon** has already been referred to (p. 76). In addition to being inserted into the tuberosity of the navicular, the tendon gives off slips which pass to the calcaneus, the cuboid, the three cuneiform bones, and the bases of the second, third and fourth metatarsals. These additional slips assist in the maintenance of the arches of the foot.

Having revised the arrangement of the muscles in the sole of the foot, the student can now pass on to the nerves and vessels.

The **Medial Plantar Nerve** arises from the tibial nerve under cover of the flexor retinaculum, and it runs forwards into the sole under the abductor hallucis muscle, with the medial plantar vessels to its medial side. Reaching the abductor hallucis, the nerve runs forwards in the interval between this muscle and the flexor digitorum brevis.

Branches. (*a*) *Muscular*, to the abductor hallucis and the flexor digitorum brevis, and to the flexor hallucis brevis and the first lumbrical.

(*b*) *Cutaneous*, to both sides of the hallux, the second and the third toes, and the tibial side of the fourth toe.

When the distribution of this nerve is compared with that of the median nerve in the palm of the hand, the similarity is very striking.

The **Lateral Plantar Nerve** also arises from the posterior tibial nerve under the flexor retinaculum, and runs forwards and laterally into the sole of the foot in the direction of the base of the fifth metatarsal bone. Here it divides into superficial and deep branches. The latter bends sharply medially and ends by supplying the adductor hallucis (oblique head), and the first dorsal interosseous muscle.

At first the nerve is covered by the abductor hallucis and the flexor digitorum brevis and rests on the flexor digitorum accessorius and the long plantar ligament. It then continues in the interval between the flexor digitorum brevis and the abductor digiti minimi.

Branches. (*a*) *From Main Trunk.* (1) *Muscular*, to flexor accessorius and abductor digiti minimi; (2) *Cutaneous*, to skin of sole.

(*b*) *From the Superficial Branch.* (1) *Muscular*, to flexor digiti minimi brevis and the muscles in the fourth interosseous space; (2) *Cutaneous*, digital branches to the adjacent sides of the fourth and fifth toes and to the fibular side of the fifth toe.

(*c*) *From the Deep Branch.* (1) *Muscular*, to the remaining interossei, the lateral three lumbricals, and both heads of the adductor hallucis.

Compare the distribution of this nerve with the ulnar nerve in the hand, as regards its motor and sensory branches.

The **Lateral Plantar Artery** is the principal artery of the sole of the foot. It arises from the posterior tibial artery under cover of the flexor retinaculum and runs in company with the lateral plantar nerve, which lies to its medial side. Like the nerve, its course towards the base of the fifth metatarsal bone runs between the muscles of the first and second layers. The terminal part of the artery bends medially across the foot in company with the deep branch of the nerve, and this portion of the vessel is termed the *plantar arch.* At the proximal end of the first intermetatarsal space the artery passes upwards to join the dorsalis pedis artery.

Branches. (*a*) In the first part of its course the artery gives off:

(1) calcaneal branches, to the skin of the heel; (2) muscular; and (3) cutaneous branches to the skin of the sole of the foot.

(*b*) *The Plantar Arch* gives off (1) perforating branches which pass upwards through the lateral three intermetatarsal spaces; (2) plantar digital arteries, to the lateral three clefts and the lateral side of the little toe.

The **First Plantar Metatarsal Artery** (*Arteria Magna Hallucis*), supplying the first cleft between the great toe and the second toe and gives a branch to the medial side of the former, is derived from the dorsalis pedis artery at its point of union with the plantar arch.

The **Medial Plantar Artery** is a small vessel which arises from the posterior tibial under cover of the flexor retinaculum and runs forwards medial to the medial plantar nerve. It gives off small muscular and cutaneous branches, and communicates with the digital branches to the medial three clefts. It ends by joining the branch from the first plantar metatarsal artery which supplies the medial side of the great toe.

THE JOINTS OF THE LOWER LIMB

The **Hip Joint** is a synovial joint of the ball-and-socket variety, so constituted as to give the maximum strength, together with a sufficient range of movement. The *Acetabulum* is a deep cup-shaped hollow on the lateral aspect of the hip bone. It presents a horseshoe-shaped articular surface, lined with hyaline cartilage. The antero-inferior part of the rim is deficient, and the gap is termed the *acetabular notch.* The floor of the acetabulum, termed the *acetabular fossa,* is occupied by a small pad of fat which is covered by synovial membrane. The cartilaginous strip is widest at its upper part, where the weight of the body is transmitted from the hip bone to the head of the femur.

The cavity of the acetabulum is deepened and its opening is narrowed by the presence of a fibrocartilaginous rim, termed the *acetabular labrum.* Inferiorly the labrum bridges across the acetabular notch, and is here termed the *transverse ligament.*

The *Head of the Femur* forms rather more than half a sphere, and is gripped by the labrum beyond its maximum diameter, an arrangement which strengthens the joint. A little below and behind its centre there is a small depression, free from cartilage, to which the *ligament of the head of the femur* is attached.

The **Capsular Ligament** of the joint is attached to the acetabular labrum and to the bone above and behind the acetabulum. It extends far beyond the articular margins of the head of the femur and is attached to the intertrochanteric line in front, and half-way along the posterior aspect of the neck of the bone behind. As a result, the whole of the anterior surface of the neck of the femur is intracapsular, as well as the medial half of its posterior surface.

The *Iliofemoral Ligament*, which is particularly strong and dense, is a thickened part of the anterior aspect of the capsular ligament. Above, it is attached to the anterior inferior iliac spine immediately below the origin of the straight head of the rectus femoris. As it passes downwards it divides into two bands, separated by a narrow interval. Of these, the upper runs to the upper part of the intertrochanteric line and the lower to the lower part of the same line.

The *Pubofemoral Ligament* supports the infero-medial aspect of the joint. It consists of a number of fibres which pass from the iliopubic eminence and obturator membrane to blend with the lower and anterior part of the capsular ligament.

The *Ischiofemoral Ligament* is a thickening of the posterior aspect of the capsular ligament, passing from the ischium just below the acetabulum.

A number of circular fibres are present in the capsular ligament, and they are collected together on the posterior aspect, where they form the *zona orbicularis*.

The *Ligament of the Head of the Femur* is a vestigial structure, which passes from the pit on the head of the femur to the transverse ligament and the margins of the acetabular notch. It lies within the joint, and is therefore invested with synovial membrane.

The *Synovial Membrane* lines the capsular ligament, and is reflected at its femoral attachment to cover the intracapsular portions of the neck of the femur. As it lines the transverse ligament the synovial membrane is carried into the joint (1) to cover the fat which occupies the acetabular fossa, and (2) to enclose the ligament of the head.

Active Movements. Flexion is limited, when the knee is flexed, by the contact of the femoral head with the acetabular labrum. When the knee is extended the tension of the hamstrings limits flexion at the hip joint. *Extension* consists in the restoration of the flexed thigh to its position in the erect attitude. Hyperextension is limited by the tension of the strong iliofemoral ligament. In the erect attitude the weight of the body falls a little behind the transverse axis of the hip joint and tends to cause hyperextension. This tendency is normally overcome by the balanced tone of the flexor and extensor muscles. It may be noted that the apparent hyperextension of the thigh which occurs in running and walking is really attributable to movements of the vertebral column.

Abduction is limited by the tension of the pubofemoral ligament and the adductors, and *adduction* by contact with the opposite limb.

Medial rotation tightens the ischiofemoral ligament, and *lateral rotation* has a similar effect on the iliofemoral ligament, as well as the rotator muscles.

Owing to the character of the joint, no appreciable accessory movements are possible.

The *Nerves* of the joint are derived from (1) the femoral (branch to rectus femoris), (2) the obturator, and (3) the nerve to the quadratus femoris.

Relations. The lateral edge of the pectineus, the ilio-psoas and the straight head of the rectus femoris are in direct contact with the *anterior aspect* of the capsular ligament and separate it from the femoral vessels and nerve. The obturator externus tendon lies at first *below* the capsule, and then in contact with its *posterior aspect.* In addition, the upper and medial part of the quadratus femoris, together with its nerve and vessels, the obturator internus tendon and the gemelli are in immediate relationship with the posterior aspect. In this way the sciatic nerve and its neighbouring structures are separated from the joint. The piriformis and the gluteus minimus, near its insertion, lie above the joint.

The **Knee Joint** is a synovial joint of the ginglymus, or hinge variety, but in addition a small amount of rotation and gliding takes place between the tibia and the femur. The arrangement of the synovial membrane and the intra-articular ligaments is by no means simple, and the complexity is due to the fact that the knee joint represents three joints, originally separate, which have become thrown into one, viz., the femoropatellar and two femorotibial joints.

The articular surface of the femur is shaped like a very short, and relatively broad, inverted Y. The stem of the Y lies on the anterior aspect of the bone and is grooved longitudinally in conformity with the shape of the articular surface of the patella. When the knee is extended, the lower facets on the patella articulate with this surface. As the limb is flexed, the middle, and finally the upper, patellar facets come into contact with it.

The two limbs of the Y cover the inferior and posterior surfaces of the two femoral condyles and are separated from each other by the intercondylar notch. They articulate with the articular areas on the superior surfaces of the tibial condyles. When the knee is extended, the tibia is in contact with the inferior surfaces of the condyles, but on full flexion it articulates with their posterior aspects.

The *Articular Capsule* of the knee joint is a very thin fibrous layer, closely associated with the synovial membrane. Anteriorly it is, of necessity, absent over the area occupied by the patella, but on each side of that bone it is considerably strengthened by expansions from the tendons of vasti lateralis and medialis, and it is still further strengthened on the lateral side by the iliotibial tract. Posteriorly, it forms a thin layer behind the condyles of the femur, but opposite the intercondylar notch it is strengthened by the oblique posterior ligament.

The **Ligamentum (Tendo) Patellæ** is attached above to the lower border of the patella and below to the tubercle of the tibia. It constitutes the insertion of the quadriceps extensor into the tibia.

The **Fibular Collateral (Lateral) Ligament** is a cord-like extra-capsular band, attached above to the lateral aspect of the lateral condyle of the femur just above the groove for the popliteus. Below, it is attached to the head of the fibula, just in front of the styloid process.

As this ligament crosses the lateral aspect of the joint, the tendon of the popliteus intervenes between it and the lateral semilunar cartilage.

Near its lower attachment the tendon of the biceps passes superficial to the ligament, and its insertion into the head of the fibula is split into anterior and posterior portions by the ligament.

The **Tibial Collateral (Medial) Ligament** is a thin band which extends downwards on the shaft of the tibia for 2 inches. Above, it is attached to the medial surface of the medial condyle of the femur below the adductor tubercle. Below, it crosses the medial condyle of the tibia and is attached to the upper part of the subcutaneous surface of the bone, near its posterior border.

As the medial ligament crosses the knee joint, it is firmly attached to the circumference of the medial semilunar cartilage and is here capsular in nature.

This ligament is crossed by the tendons of sartorius, gracilis and semitendonosus as they pass to their insertions.

The **Oblique Posterior Ligament** of the knee joint forms a prominent oblique band of fibres, which is derived from the tendon of the semi-membranosus and runs upwards and laterally to reach the lateral condyle. Its deep surface blends with the posterior aspect of the articular capsule.

This ligament possesses great strength. Relaxed when the knee is flexed, it becomes taut in extension and helps to prevent hyper-extension. *It is very closely related to the popliteal artery.*

Intracapsular Structures. The **Medial Meniscus (Semilunar Cartilage)** is C-shaped which probably helps lubrication of the joint and adapts the upper surface of the medial condyle of the tibia to the curvature of the medial condyle of the femur. It is much broader behind than in front, and, while its peripheral border is thick, its central border thins off into a fine edge.

Attachments. The anterior end is attached to the anterior part of the intercondylar area of the tibia, and is connected to the lateral semilunar cartilage by a few fibres, which constitute the *transverse ligament.* The posterior end is attached to the posterior part of the intercondylar area of the tibia, immediately in front of the posterior cruciate ligament. *The peripheral border is adherent to the fibrous capsule and, particularly, to the medial ligament of the joint.*

The **Lateral Meniscus (Semilunar Cartilage)** is more circular in outline. It also may help in lubrication of the joint and it certainly adapts the upper surface of the lateral condyle of the tibia to the curvature of the lateral condyle of the femur.

Attachments. Its anterior end is attached to the top of the tibia behind the anterior cruciate ligament and in front of the lateral intercondylar tubercle, which separates it from the attachment of its posterior end. In addition, a fibrous band leaves the posterior end and runs up along the posterior cruciate ligament to the medial condyle of the femur. The tendon of the popliteus intervenes between the peripheral border of the cartilage and the lateral ligament and fibrous capsule of the joint. As a direct result, the lateral semilunar cartilage is *less fixed in position and is more easily able to adapt itself to sudden twisting movements of the joint.* In addition, the traction exerted by the medial fibres of the popliteus muscle during lateral rotation of the femur draws the posterior part of the cartilage backwards out of harm's way. On the other hand, the *fixation of the medial semilunar cartilage renders it much more liable to injury.*

In flexion and extension the cartilages move with the tibia, but in rotatory movements they move with the femur.

The **Anterior Cruciate Ligament** is a strong fibrous band attached to the anterior part of the intercondylar area of the tibia behind the anterior end of the medial semilunar cartilage. It passes upwards, backwards and laterally to the posterior part of the medial surface of the lateral femoral condyle. When the knee is flexed these two points of attachment are approximated and the ligament is therefore relaxed. In extension, however, the reverse occurs, and the tension of the anterior cruciate ligament helps to limit hyper-extension.

The **Posterior Cruciate Ligament** passes upwards, forwards and medially from the posterior part of the intercondylar area of the tibia to be attached to the anterior part of the lateral surface of the medial condyle of the femur. Its anterior fibres become relaxed in extension of the knee, but become taut in flexion.

The **Synovial Membrane** of the knee joint forms a large and complicated sac. On the anterior aspect of the joint it is continued upwards for at least two inches above the patella, forming the so-called *suprapatellar bursa.* On each side it extends for $\frac{3}{4}$-inch beyond the articular margin of the femoral condyle.

From the upper part of the deep surface of the ligamentum patellæ a triangular fold of synovial membrane, containing a little fat between its two layers, passes backwards to the anterior margin of the intercondylar notch of the femur, where its apex is attached. This fold is termed the *infrapatellar synovial fold*, and it is well seen in median sagittal sections of the knee joint. Its base is related to the fat covering the deep surface of the ligamentum patellæ and its borders are free, constituting the *alar folds.*

The relationship of the synovial membrane to the cruciate ligaments is somewhat complicated. It is as if the two ligaments had been introduced into the joint from behind, carrying the synovial membrane with them. The posterior cruciate ligament therefore has no covering on its posterior aspect, although the anterior cruciate ligament is covered anteriorly. A small pocket of synovial membrane is intruded between the two ligaments from the medial side and acts as a bursa during the movements of the joint.

The *active movements* at the knee joint include flexion, extension and rotation. Flexion of the knee is usually accompanied by some degree of flexion of the hip joint, and the movements of the tibia and femur on one another are a combination of gliding, rolling and rotation. In the resting upright posture the knee joints are *not quite fully extended* (a statement which the student can easily verify for himself) and the attitude is maintained *by the balanced tone of the flexor and extensor muscles and not by the tension of the ligaments.* The movement of extension can be completed by a movement of medial rotation of femur on tibia, which hyper-extends the joint and renders all the ligaments tense except the anterior fibres of the posterior cruciate ligament. *This so-called locking enables the fully extended knee to withstand severe strain.* No further rotation is possible when the knee is fully extended, and any action tending to produce pure rotation is liable to injure one or other of the ligaments. The movement of flexion is accompanied in its initial stages by lateral rotation of the femur on the tibia, when the foot is on the ground.

When the knee is flexed to a right angle a considerable range of rotation is possible, and when it is slightly flexed, a small amount of abduction and adduction can be effected, *provided the foot is on the ground.*

Passive Accessory Movements. When the knee is flexed to a right angle, the tibia can be moved backwards and forwards on the femur. In slight flexion, a small amount of abduction and adduction can be obtained.

Numerous *Bursæ* occur around the knee joint, though only a few of these are clinically important. Four are associated with the anterior aspect of the joint, and of these only the first communicates with the joint cavity. (1) *The suprapatellar bursa* (p. 89 is in effect an extension of the joint). (2) The *subcutaneous prepatellar bursa* lies between skin and patella. Variable in extent, it extends down in front of the ligamentum patellæ. (3) A small *subcutaneous infrapatellar bursa* lies between the skin and the lower end of the ligamentum patellæ. (4) The *deep infrapatellar bursa* separates the deep aspect of the lower end of the ligamentum patellæ from the tibia.

Three bursæ are associated with the postero-lateral aspect of the joint. Of these the first always, and the second sometimes, communicates with the joint cavity. (1) As the tendon of the popliteus lies within the capsular ligament it is covered on its medial aspect by the synovial membrane of the joint, which is continued downwards on the deep surface of the tendon, after it has pierced the capsule. (2) A bursa is interposed between the lateral head of origin of the gastrocnemius and the lateral femoral condyle. (3) A small bursa separates the tendon of the biceps from the lateral ligament of the joint.

Three bursæ are associated with the postero-medial aspect of the knee joint, and of these the first frequently communicates with the cavity of the joint. (1) A bursa lies deep to the medial head of the gastrocnemius and separates it from the medial condyle above and the semimembranosus tendon below. (2) The *tibial intertendinous* bursa is associated with the tendons of the sartorius, gracilis and semitendinosus at their insertions. (3) A third bursa is associated with the semimembranosus tendon at its insertion.

Nerve Supply. The knee joint is well supplied with nerves. It receives three branches from the femoral, three from the common peroneal and three from the tibial, and an additional twig from the obturator nerve.

Its *blood supply* is relatively rich, and is derived from the anastomosis round the joint, which primarily supply the epiphyses.

The **Superior Tibiofibular Joint** is a small synovial joint of the plane variety, possessing a capsular ligament lined with synovial membrane, and strengthened by anterior and posterior ligaments.

The **Interosseous Membrane** stretches from the interosseous border of the fibula to that of the tibia. It is widest above and narrows rapidly below, where it blends with the interosseous ligament of the inferior tibiofibular joint. A large opening is present at its uppermost part for the passage of the anterior tibial vessels, and a much smaller opening near its lower end transmits the perforating branch of the peroneal artery (p. 72).

The **Inferior Tibiofibular Joint** is unique amongst the articulations of the limbs in that it is a syndesmosis and therefore belongs to the fibrous group. The opposed bony surfaces are roughened and give attachment to a strong *interosseous ligament*, which prevents separation of the two bones from each other. Anterior and posterior ligaments hide the interosseous ligament from view. The *transverse tibiofibular ligament* runs from the upper part of the depression on the medial surface of the lateral malleolus to the posterior border of the lower end of the tibia. It is partly blended with and obscured by the posterior ligament of the ankle joint.

The **Ankle Joint** is a synovial joint of the hinge variety. The lower surface of the tibia and the lateral surface of the medial malleolus articulate with the upper surface of the body and the medial surface of the talus, respectively. In addition, the medial surface of the lateral malleolus articulates with the lateral surface of the talus. As a result of this arrangement, the talus is a close fit between the malleoli.

The *Articular Capsule* surrounds the joint and is attached to the various bones close to their articular margins, except below and in front, where it passes well forwards on to the dorsal aspect of the neck of the talus.

The *Anterior* and *Posterior Ligaments* are scarcely worth naming, being merely slight thickenings of the capsule.

The *Deltoid Ligament*, placed on the medial side of the joint, is a strong triangular sheet, attached by its blunted apex to the margins and tip of the medial malleolus. Below, its attachment is more extensive and stretches from the medial surface of the posterior part of the talus, along the sustentaculum tali of the calcaneus, to the neck of the talus and the dorsal aspect of the navicular. It is closely related to the tendons of the tibialis posterior and the flexor digitorum longus, as they pass forwards into the sole of the foot.

The *Lateral Ligament* consists of three separate bands: (1) The *anterior talofibular ligament* is a flattened band which runs from the anterior border of the lateral malleolus to the lateral surface of the talus. It is put on the stretch during plantar flexion of the foot. (2) The *calcaneofibular ligament* is rounded and cord-like. It is attached just in front of the tip of the lateral malleolus above, and runs downwards and backwards to a slight elevation on the lateral surface of the calcaneus. Its superficial aspect is crossed by the tendons of the peroneus longus and brevis. It is taut in dorsiflexion and inversion of the foot. (3) The *posterior talofibular ligament* is directed *medially* from the pit on the medial side of the lateral malleolus to the posterior tubercle of the talus. It is taut in dorsiflexion of the foot. Any one of these bands may be damaged in sprains of the ankle joint.

The *Synovial Membrane* lines the capsular ligament and clothes the intracapsular portion of the neck of the talus. In addition it may pass upwards for a short distance between the lower ends of the tibia and the fibula.

The *active movements* of the ankle joint are limited to dorsiflexion and plantar flexion. As will be seen below, the movements of eversion and inversion occur at the tarsal joints.

Accessory Movements. When the foot is placed in plantar flexion, slight side to side gliding movement, rotation, abduction and adduction can be obtained in the passive patient.

Relations. Anteriorly, the joint is related to the tendons of the tibialis anterior and extensor hallucis longus, to the anterior tibial vessels and nerve, and to the tendons of the extensor digitorum longus and peroneus tertius, in that order from the medial to the lateral side.

Medially, it is related to the tibialis posterior and flexor digitorum longus tendons. *Posteriorly*, it is related to the same tendons and also, more laterally, to the posterior tibial vessels and nerve and the flexor hallucis longus.

Laterally, the peroneal tendons cross the calcaneofibular ligament.

The Tarsal Joints. 1. The *Talocalcaneal* joint is formed by the inferior surface of the body of the talus and the convex facet on the middle of the upper surface of the calcaneus. It is a joint of the synovial variety, and possesses a capsular ligament, which is attached to the margins of the articular areas of the two bones. Anteriorly the capsule blends with the *interosseous ligament*, which connects the talus to the calcaneus. This ligament is attached to the deeply notched inferior surface of the neck of the talus above, and below to the upper surface of the calcaneus immediately in front of the talocalcaneal joint.

2. The *Talocalcaneonavicular Joint* is formed by the head of the talus, the upper surface of the sustentaculum tali and the posterior surface of the navicular bone. It is a joint of the synovial variety and possesses an independent joint cavity, surrounded by a capsular ligament and lined with synovial membrane in the usual way. Since the sustentaculum tali does not articulate with the navicular bone, the joint is closed inferiorly by the capsule, *which is specially strengthened in this situation by the plantar calcaneonavicular ligament.* This ligament is of great strength and is always in

PLATE XIII. ANTERO-POSTERIOR RADIOGRAPH OF THE ANKLE REGION IN A YOUNG ADULT.

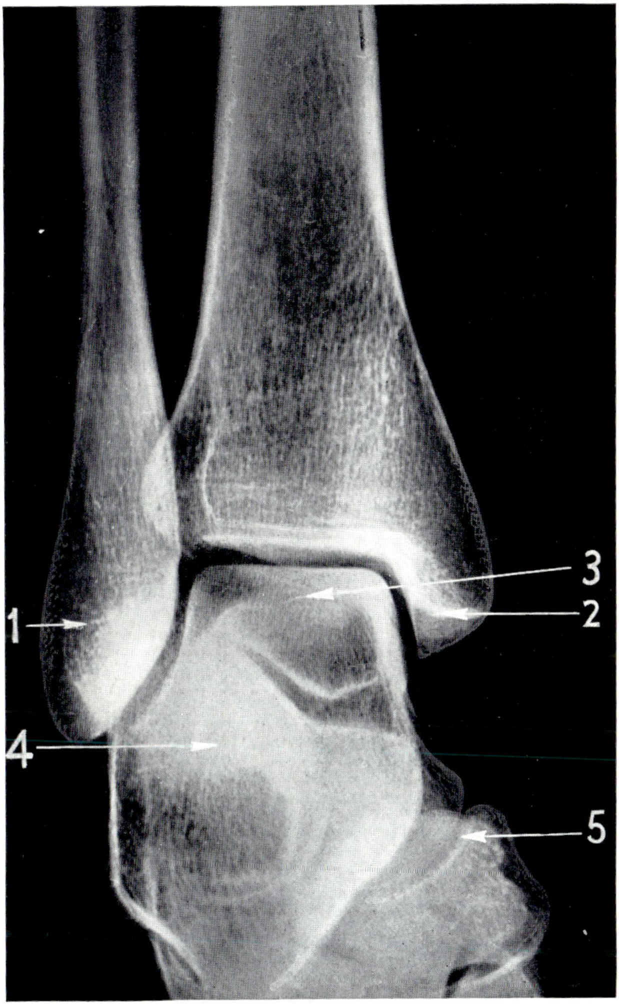

1. Lateral malleolus.
2. Medial malleolus.
3. Body of talus.
4. Posterior surface of calcaneum.
5. Talonavicular joint.

Observe how the talus is mortised in between the two malleoli to ensure the stability of the ankle joint, and note that the lateral malleolus descends to a much lower level than the medial malleolus.

To face p. 92

Plate XIV. Lateral Radiograph of Ankle and Foot in a Young Adult.

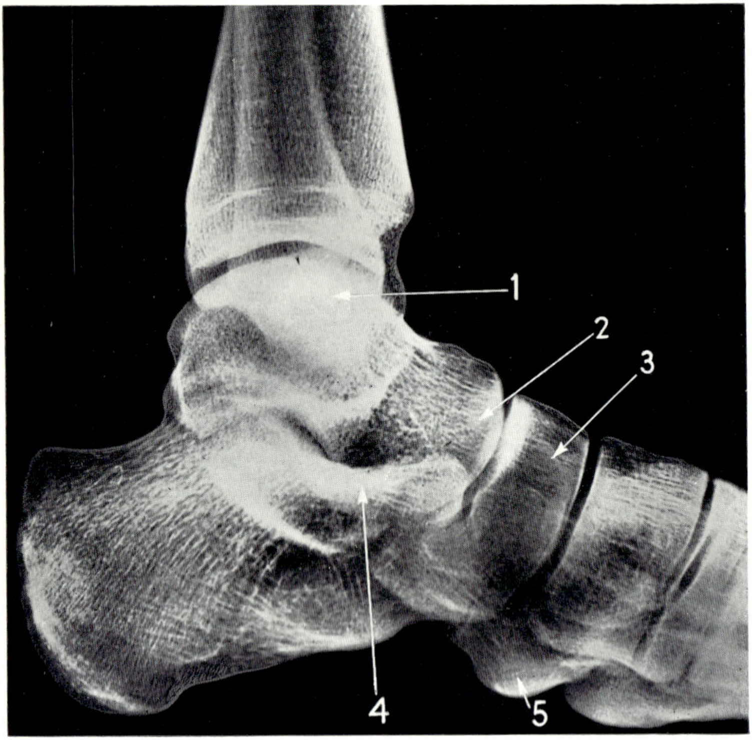

1. Body of talus, partially obscured by the shadows of the two malleoli.
2. Head of talus, articulating distally with the navicular bone.
3. Navicular bone.
4. Sustentaculum tali of calcaneum.
5. Ridge on plantar surface of cuboid.

The foot is in the position of slight plantar flexion so that the obliquity of the long axis of the calcaneum is diminished. Note the trabeculæ in the calcaneum.

part fibrocartilaginous. It is attached posteriorly to the front of the sustentaculum tali, and anteriorly to the tuberosity and inferior surface of the navicular bone. Superiorly, it supports the head of the talus, and is therefore possibly *a factor in resisting extreme flattening of the medial longitudinal arch of the foot.* Inferiorly, it is related to the tendons of the tibialis posterior, the flexor digitorum longus and the flexor hallucis longus, which provide the active support on which the integrity of the arch depends (p. 95).

3. The *Calcaneocuboid Joint* is also an independent joint lined by its own synovial membrane. The capsular ligament is strengthened inferiorly by the *long and the short plantar ligaments.* The latter is attached to the anterior tubercle of the calcaneus and to the posterior part of the inferior surface of the cuboid.

The *Long Plantar Ligament* lies superficial to the short plantar ligament. It is attached posteriorly to the plantar surface of the calcaneus as far forwards as its anterior tubercle. In front it is, for the most part, attached to the ridge on the cuboid, but some fibres are continued onwards to the bases of the third, fourth and fifth metatarsal bones, and bridge over the groove in which the tendon of the peroneus longus lies.

Both of these ligaments may assist in maintaining the longitudinal arch of the foot.

The talocalcaneonavicular and the calcaneocuboid joints constitute the *transverse tarsal joint.* This articulation, together with the talocalcaneal joint, is involved in the movements of inversion and eversion of the foot. When the foot is off the ground during these movements, the talus is fixed and the calcaneus and navicular swing round it, carrying the other bones of the foot with them. The range of movement is increased by the simultaneous movement of the cuboid on the calcaneus, but the amount of movement at this joint is very slight, and the movements of inversion and eversion are in no way dependent on it. The chief factors which limit inversion of the foot are the tension of the peronei and a strong band of fibres which passes from the infero-lateral aspect of the neck of the talus to the adjoining part of the upper surface of the calcaneus. This band is continuous with the interosseous talocalcaneal ligament.

When the foot is on the ground and under load, movements of inversion and eversion are more limited and it is the talus that moves on the calcaneus and the navicular, the movements being imposed on the foot by the body weight acting through the tibia. This occurs when one is walking across a sloping surface and both feet are thus able to remain plantigrade, although the higher one is everted and the lower one inverted.

4. The *Cuneonavicular Joint* is formed by the navicular bone behind and the three cuneiform bones in front. Its capsular ligament is strengthened by dorsal and plantar ligaments. The joint cavity is continuous with that of the intercuneiform joints, and, passing forwards between the medial and intermediate cuneiform bones, becomes continuous with the joint cavity of the metatarsocuneiform and the corresponding intermetatarsal joints. In addition, when the navicular and cuboid bones come into contact, the cubocuneiform joint cavity is also continuous with the joint cavity of the cuneonavicular joint.

5. The *Cubometatarsal Joint* is placed between the cuboid bone behind and the bases of the fourth and fifth metatarsal bones in front. The joint cavity is projected forwards between the contiguous surfaces of the bases of the fourth and fifth metatarsals.

6. The *Tarsometatarsal Joint* of the great toe is, like the corresponding joint in the hand, an independent joint with a separate synovial lining.

In addition to the dorsal and plantar ligaments, strong interosseous ligaments connect the opposed non-articular surfaces of the cuboid and the three cuneiform bones to one another, and the base of the second metatarsal to the medial and lateral cuneiform bones.

The *Tarsometatarsal Joints* follow an oblique line, which runs backwards and laterally across the foot, from the first to the fifth joint. Owing to the shortness of the intermediate cuneiform bone the base of the second metatarsal projects backwards between the medial and lateral cuneiform bones and for this reason is the least mobile.

The **Arches of the Foot.** In addition to supporting the body weight in the erect attitude, the foot is required to act as a lever for the forward propulsion of the body in walking, running, etc. For this purpose the foot must be converted into a resilient lever and, owing to the number of its constituent joints, this can only be effected by its arrangement in an arched form. *In the child* at rest in the upright posture, the foot is flat and this condition is normal, but, when the posture is changed for one of activity, the flattening disappears at once and the foot becomes arched. *In the adult*, although the arching is more pronounced in activity, it is a permanent feature.

Both a longitudinal and a transverse arch have to be considered.

The *Longitudinal Arch* involves the whole of the tarsus and metatarsus, but it is higher on the medial side of the foot where it forms the instep. This *medial arch* consists of a short posterior pillar, formed by the calcaneus and the body of the talus; a 'keystone', formed by the head of the talus; and a long anterior pillar, formed by the navicular, cuneiforms and the corresponding metatarsals. The critical point in the arch is the 'keystone', and this is supported by (1) the tendons of the deep muscles on the back of the leg (p. 93); (2) the small muscles in the sole of the foot; (3) the plantar aponeurosis and the plantar ligaments of all the joints concerned, including the plantar calcaneonavicular ligament (p. 93). It must be emphasised that the muscles are the principal support and that the ligaments are only called on when extreme flattening occurs. The *lateral arch* is lower. It consists of a short posterior pillar—the calcaneus—and an anterior pillar formed by the cuboid and the fourth and fifth metatarsals. It is supported by the peroneus longus and the short muscles of the little toe and, in extreme flattening, by the long and short plantar ligaments (p. 93).

The *Transverse Arch* is situated in the region of the cuboid and cuneiform bones and the bases of the metatarsals. It is produced by the shape of the bones and is maintained by the peroneus longus and the tibialis posterior and, under conditions of strain, by the strong interosseous ligaments.

In the resting upright posture the body weight acting on the talus flattens both the longitudinal and transverse arches. When the posture is changed to one of activity, the simultaneous contraction (or increased tone) of the tibiales, the long flexors of the toes, the peronei and the small muscles of the foot restore and accentuate the arches, converting the foot into an almost rigid but slightly resilient lever. It is important to note that if the muscles are weakened none of the connective tissue supports are adequate; they are at the most merely auxiliary to the muscles.

THE LYMPH VESSELS OF THE LOWER LIMB

The superficial lymph vessels of the dorsum of the foot, the front of the leg, and the thigh end in those *superficial inguinal lymph nodes* which lie along the terminal part of the long saphenous vein (p. 51). A few of the deep lymph vessels of the dorsum of the foot and the front of the leg end in the *anterior tibial lymph node*, which lies on the upper part of the interosseous membrane. Efferents from this node pass through the membrane with the anterior tibial vessels and join the *popliteal lymph nodes*, which lie in the fat of the popliteal fossa.

The superficial and deep lymph vessels from the sole of the foot, the back of the leg and the knee joint terminate in the popliteal nodes, which send their efferents to the deep inguinal lymph nodes.

The *Deep Lymph Vessels of the Thigh* and the efferents from the

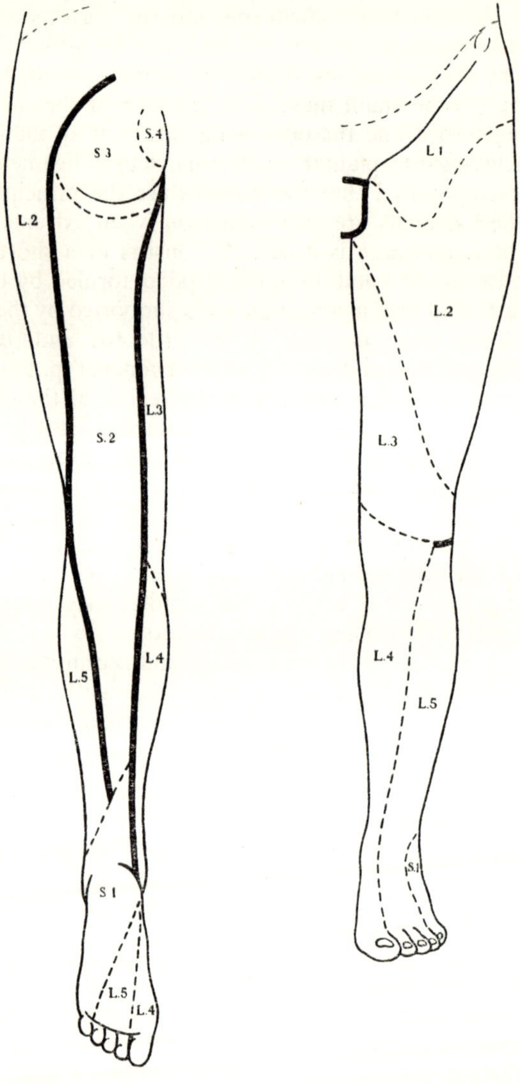

FIG. 2. The segmental distribution of the cutaneous nerves of the lumbar and sacral plexuses to the skin of the lower limb.

Note.—The individual nerve areas overlap one another across the interrupted lines but across the heavy black (axial) lines the overlap is minimal. The ventral axial line starts at the medial end of the inguinal fold and soon curves round the medial side of the limb to descend on the medial side of its posterior aspect. The dorsal axial line sends a short extension forwards at about the level of the knee joint.

superficial inguinal lymph nodes join the *deep inguinal lymph nodes* (p. 51), which lie on the medial side of the upper end of the femoral vein, one of them occupying the femoral canal. The efferents from these nodes pass to the external iliac lymph nodes (p. 202).

The lymph vessels of the buttock join the lateral nodes of the *superficial inguinal group*, which lie in the superficial fascia along the inguinal ligament. These same nodes also receive afferents from the adjoining part of the anterior abdominal wall. The medial nodes of the group receive afferents from the perineum. The efferents from the whole group join the deep inguinal lymph nodes (Plate XII, p. 65).

THE SEGMENTAL INNERVATION OF THE LOWER LIMB

Like the upper limb (p. 49) the lower limb develops as an outgrowth from the lateral aspect of the trunk. In its early stages it resembles the upper limb bud, but as the three parts of the limb (thigh, leg and foot) become defined and the bud lengthens, the growth changes are accompanied by a process of *medial* rotation around its long axis. As a result, the extensor surface of the thigh becomes its ventral or anterior surface, the tibia becomes the medial bone of the leg, and the great toe the most medial digit.

The innervation of the skin of the lower limb is derived from the segments L.1–S.3, but the pre- and post-axial borders of the limb (p. 49) are not so easy to trace as in the upper limb. Broadly speaking, the pre-axial border commences above at the middle of the inguinal ligament, descends to the knee and is then continued obliquely downwards and medially to the medial side of the great toe, so that L.2 is distributed to the front of the thigh, L.3 to the front and medial side of the thigh, L.4 to the medial side of the leg and *great toe* and L.5 to the lateral side of the leg and dorsum of the foot. S.1 supplies the little toe and the lateral side of the foot, S.2 the back of the leg and, with S.3, the back of the thigh (Fig. 2, p. 96).

Section III

THE THORAX

THE THORACIC WALL

The superficial structures of the chest wall have been considered in connexion with the upper limb. While revising the thorax, the student must have frequent access to dissections.

Each **External Intercostal** muscle extends as far forwards as the junction of ribs with costal cartilages. In the anterior part of the intercostal space the muscle becomes an *anterior intercostal membrane*, which is a fine aponeurotic layer continued to the border of the sternum. The fibres of the muscle and the membrane are directed downwards, forwards and medially, from the lower border of the rib above to the upper border of the rib below.

Each **Internal Intercostal** muscle, placed on a deeper plane, extends forwards to the sternum, but posteriorly the muscular fibres are replaced by a *posterior intercostal membrane*. The fibres proceed downwards, backwards and laterally from the floor of the subcostal groove of the rib above to the upper border of the rib below.

Both muscles are supplied by the corresponding intercostal nerve, and said to be elevators of the rib below, though some consider the internal intercostals to be depressors. All that is certain is that these muscles have a respiratory function, their precise contribution being still undetermined.

The **Transversus Thoracis** forms the third and deepest layer of the thoracic wall and probably corresponds to the transversus abdominis. It consists of three portions, more or less distinct from one another, viz.: (1) the subcostales; (2) the intercostales intimi; and (3) the transversus proper (sternocostalis).

The *Subcostal Muscles* are present only in the lower part of the thorax, where they cover the inner surfaces of the ribs between their tubercles and their angles.

The *Intercostales Intimi* are absent or poorly developed in the first and second spaces, but increase progressively in their antero-posterior extent from above downwards. In each space the intercostalis intimus is partly blended with the corresponding internal intercostal inferiorly, but superiorly it is attached to the inner surface of the rib, above the subcostal groove, and the two muscles are separated by the intercostal vessels and nerve.

The Transverus thoracis itself is a thin musculo-tendinous sheet passing from the back of the lower end of the sternum to be inserted by a number of processes into the costal cartilages of the sixth to the second ribs. Its lower border is horizontal and marches with the upper border of the transversus abdominis. It probably acts as a depressor of the costal cartilages into which it is inserted.

The *Nerve Supply* of all the parts of the transversus thoracis group is derived from the corresponding intercostal nerves.

The **Intercostal Nerves** are the anterior primary rami of the first to eleventh thoracic nerves. After emerging from the intervertebral foramina they pass between the intercostalis internus and intimus, and, as they travel round the chest wall, they lie below the intercostal vessels, which occupy the subcostal groove. Having supplied the intercostal muscles, each nerve reaches the anterior edge of the intercostalis intimus and then runs medially on the pleura, from which it is separated near its termination by the sternocostalis muscle. Finally, it crosses in front of the internal mammary artery, and turning forwards, pierces the internal intercostal muscle, the anterior intercostal membrane, the pectoralis major and its covering fascia to supply the skin.

Each intercostal nerve gives off a *lateral cutaneous branch*, which reaches the surface near the mid-axillary line in the intervals between the digitations of the serratus anterior muscle. It divides into anterior and posterior branches, which overlap, respectively, the perforating branch in front and the posterior primary ramus behind.

The first intercostal nerve is very small, because most of the anterior ramus of T. 1 joins the brachial plexus. It gives off only trivial cutaneous branches, and the skin over the first intercostal space is supplied by the descending branches of the cervical plexus (p. 2).

The lateral cutaneous branch of the second intercostal nerve is distributed to the skin over the axillary floor and to the skin of the upper arm. It is termed the intercostobrachial nerve (p. 6).

The lower five intercostal nerves cross the costal margin and enter the abdominal wall to supply its muscles and skin (p. 142).

The **Internal Thoracic (Mammary) Artery** arises in the neck from the first part of the subclavian artery and descends on the pleura behind the termination of the subclavian vein, crossing, or being crossed by, the phrenic nerve. It then passes downwards behind the first costal cartilage, half-an-inch from the sternum, and ends behind the anterior extremity of the sixth costal cartilage by dividing into the musculophrenic and the superior epigastric arteries. As it runs down the chest wall, it lies *behind* the costal cartilages, intercostal muscles and nerves, and *in front* of the pleura and the slips of the sternocostalis muscle. Its course is almost vertical, and is placed half-an-inch from the edge of the sternum.

Opposite each of the upper six spaces the internal thoracic artery gives off *perforating branches*, which accompany the terminal branches of the corresponding intercostal nerves. In female subjects the second and third perforating branches are usually much enlarged, and take part in the blood supply of the mammary gland.

In addition, the internal mammary gives off numerous small branches to supply the lymph nodes of the mediastinum, the remains of the thymus, the pericardium, etc.

Of the two terminal branches, (1) the *superior epigastric* runs downwards behind the rectus abdominis muscle to anastomose with the inferior epigastric (p. 143), and (2) the *musculophrenic* passes downwards and laterally, behind the costal margin, supplying the diaphragm and lower intercostal muscles.

THE THORACIC CAVITY

The **Mediastinum** lies between the two pleuræ and consists of the pericardium, heart, great vessels, œsophagus, trachea, thoracic duct, and a number of smaller structures. Below the mediastinum reaches to the diaphragm. It is customary to divide this visceral mass into four parts.

The *Superior Mediastinum* is bounded below by an imaginary plane drawn from the lower border of the manubrium sterni to the lower border of the fourth thoracic vertebra. It contains the arch of the aorta and its branches, the innominate veins and the commencement of the superior vena cava, trachea, œsophagus, etc.

The *Anterior Mediastinum* lies immediately below the superior mediastinum and is placed between the sternum in front and the pericardium behind. It contains a few lymph nodes and a little areolar tissue.

The *Middle Mediastinum* lies below the superior and behind the anterior mediastinum. It contains the pericardium, the heart and the roots of the great vessels, and the roots of the lungs. It is level with the middle four thoracic vertebrae.

The *Posterior Mediastinum* lies behind the pericardium and extends upwards to the lower limit of the superior mediastinum. It descends behind the diaphragm in front of the lower four thoracic vertebrae. It contains the œsophagus, the descending thoracic aorta, the vagus nerves, etc.

The **Pleuræ** are two distinct serous membranes. Each forms a closed double-walled sac, which invests the lung and lines the walls of the space in which it lies. The pleura thus has visceral and parietal layers, and the latter may be subdivided further into costal diaphragmatic, mediastinal and cervical regions, which are in fact continuous.

The *Costal Pleura* lines the inner surfaces of the ribs, the sides of the vertebral bodies and the back of the sternum. It is directly continuous, above, with the cervical pleura, which covers the apex of the lung, below, with the diaphragmatic pleura, which covers the upper surface of the diaphragm, and medially, both in front and behind, with the mediastinal pleura.

It is essential for the student to be familiar with the outline of the pleural sac as projected on to the surface skin. As the costal pleura is traced medially behind the sternum, it will be found to pass backwards, to form the mediastinal pleura, along a line which can be related to the surface and which is not identical on the two sides of the body. This line begins at the sternoclavicular joint and runs downwards and medially to the middle of the manubrium. From this point, on the right side, it runs downwards behind the sternum practically in the median plane until it reaches its junction with the xiphoid process. On the left side a similar arrangement is found above the level of the fourth costal cartilage, but at that point the line of reflection deviates laterally until the left margin of the sternum is reached, where it turns sharply downwards to the sternal end of the sixth cartilage.

The lower limit of the pleural sac can be traced laterally from behind the xiphoid process, gradually descending, so that in the mid-clavicular line it crosses the *eighth* rib. In the mid-axillary line it reaches its lowest level, and it here crosses the *tenth* rib. The posterior portion of the line ascends slightly as it passes medially, crosses the eleventh and twelfth ribs and reaches the vertebral column at the lower border of the *twelfth thoracic vertebra*. It should be noted that the intersection of the twelfth rib and the costodiaphragmatic line of reflection occurs opposite the lateral border of the sacrospinalis muscle (Plate III, p. 16).

On the left side the line of reflection begins behind the sixth costal cartilage, but otherwise, for all practical purposes, the levels to which it extends are the same as on the right side.

The *Mediastinal Pleura* forms the lateral boundary of the mediastinum. It is interrupted by the root of the lung, on the anterior, superior and posterior aspects of which it is carried laterally to become continuous with the visceral layer. Below the root of the lung the two enclosing layers are continued downwards for a short distance to constitute the *pulmonary ligament*, which stretches from the mediastinal pleura behind the pericardium to the mediastinal surface of the lung. The arrangement is precisely as if the root of the lung, surrounded by a tube of pleura, had originally been deeper and had subsequently shrunk without the shrinkage affecting the pleura. Such a shrinkage would allow the layers of pleura to come into contact with each other below the root of the lung.

The *Cervical Pleura* rises above the sternal end of the clavicle and so appears to bulge upwards into the neck. This appearance is due to the obliquity of the first rib, and it will be found that the pleura never rises above the oblique plane of the thoracic inlet, *i.e.*, it never rises above the head of the first rib. It can be mapped out on the surface of the body by drawing a curved line, convex upwards, from the sternoclavicular joint to the junction of the *medial and intermediate thirds* of the clavicle, reaching from 1 to 1½ inches above the clavicle.

The upper aspect of the cervical pleura is covered by an aponeurotic derivative of the scalene muscles, termed the *suprapleural membrane*. This fibrous sheet is attached to the transverse process of the seventh cervical vertebra, the cupola of the pleura, and is attached to the inner border of the first rib. It separates the pleura from the first part of the subclavian artery, the phrenic nerve, etc., and it *contains* the apex within the thorax.

Posteriorly, the cervical pleura covers the first thoracic nerve and the sympathetic trunk (p. 127).

The *Visceral Pleura* covers the lung, dipping into its fissures and covering the opposed surfaces of its lobes, and is everywhere closely adherent to it.

The two pleuræ approach each other very closely in the anterior mediastinum, and again in the posterior mediastinum, between the lower end of the œsophagus and the descending thoracic aorta.

The **Lungs** lie within the pleural sacs, but during ordinary respiration they do not fill all of the available space. Each lung possesses a blunt apex, which projects above the sternal end of the first rib, and a hollowed-out base, which is in contact with the upper surface of the diaphragm. The margins of the basal surface are thin and, except in forced inspiration, they do not reach the costodiaphragmatic line of reflection. In quiet respiration, the costal and the diaphragmatic pleuræ are in apposition with each other below the lower border of the lung, over an area which is 1 to 3 inches deep. This is known as the *costodiaphragmatic recess*. It is into this recess that the thin margins of the base of the lung descend as they expand during deep inspiration.

In addition to a base and an apex, the lung possesses a very extensive costovertebral surface and a much smaller mediastinal surface.

The **Apex** of the lung, owing to the obliquity of the thoracic inlet, can be examined in the lower part of the neck, as it projects for about 1 inch above the sternal end of the clavicle. It is always in close contact with the cervical pleura, and therefore presents the same relations (p. 102).

The **Base** of the lung rests on the diaphragm, which separates it from the right lobe of the liver on the right side, and from the left lobe of the liver, the stomach and the spleen on the left side. In adaptation to the convexity of the dome of the diaphragm, the base presents a corresponding concavity, the margins of which are thin and sharp except on the medial side.

The **Medial Surface** of each lung is divisible into a *mediastinal part*, on which the hilum is situated, and a *vertebral part.* Both parts present very different relationships on the two sides of the body. *On the Right Side* the hilum is occupied by the eparterial and hyparterial bronchi, the right pulmonary artery, and upper and lower right pulmonary veins, together with lymph nodes and antonomic nerves. Below and in front of the hilum, the mediastinal aspect of the right lung is hollowed out in adaptation to the *right atrium* of the heart and the overlying pericardium and phrenic nerve. The superior vena cava lies in contact with the right lung in front of the hilum and, in the preserved lung, produces a deep groove which flows into the cardiac depression below and is continuous above with the the groove made by the right innominate vein. In preserved lungs another groove curves forwards above the hilum to flow into the groove for the superior vena cava. This is produced by the vena azygos.

The cardiac hollow is limited posteriorly by the hilum and the attachment of the pulmonary ligament, and behind those structures the right side of the œsophagus comes into contact with the mediastinal surface.

The *vertebral part* of the medial surface of the right lung is related to the heads of the ribs and the sympathetic trunk, the sides of the vertebral bodies, the splanchnic nerves and the right posterior (aortic) intercostal arteries and veins.

On the Left Side the hilum is occupied by the single left bronchus, the left pulmonary artery, the upper and lower left pulmonary veins, lymph nodes, nerves, etc. Below and in front of the hilum, the heart (*ventricular part*) produces a very deep hollow. Immediately above the cardiac hollow the mediastinal aspect is in contact with the pulmonary trunk and the ascending aorta. The arch of the aorta passes backwards above the root of the lung producing a deep groove in preserved lungs, which is continuous, behind the hilum, with the groove produced by the descending thoracic aorta. Above the groove for the arch of the aorta the subclavian artery runs upwards in contact with the lung, and then turns laterally in the neck in front of the apex.

The *vertebral part* of the medial surface of the left lung is grooved deeply by the descending thoracic aorta, which separates the viscus from the bodies of the fourth to the eighth or ninth thoracic vertebræ. Otherwise the relations are similar to those already described for the right lung.

The **Costal Surface** of each lung is related to the inner surfaces of the ribs and costal cartilages, the intercostal spaces, and to a slight extent, to the back of the sternum.

Below the apex the lung possesses a thin *anterior border*, which lies in contact with the costomediastinal line of pleural reflection. On the right side, the same line may be taken as corresponding both to the pleural reflection and to the anterior border of the lung. On the left side, however, the two by no means correspond below, although they do so above the fourth costal cartilage. Below that point the *cardiac notch* on the anterior border of the lung is very much deeper than the cardiac notch on the pleural line of reflection, and on this account there is a comparatively large area of the pericardium which is intimately related to the chest wall (p. 107).

Movements. In quiet respiration expansion affects the thin inferior and anterior borders and the superficial portion of the lung substance. In deep respiration these parts are further affected together with the deeper part of the lung substance. On account of the limitations imposed on the apex by the suprapleural membrane, expansion upwards is negligible, but it occurs very freely in a downward direction (p. 102), and very appreciably from side to side and in an antero-posterior direction.

The **Lymph Vessels** of the lungs consist of (1) a superficial set, which forms a plexus under the visceral pleura, and (2) a deep set, which accompanies the branches of the pulmonary vessels. Both groups end in the bronchial lymph nodes in the hilum of the lung, efferents from which join the thoracic duct on the left side and the right lymphatic duct on the right side.

The **Root of the Lung** is a short, broad pedicle consisting of the pulmonary artery and veins, the bronchus (or bronchi on the right side), lymph vessels, bronchial vessels and nerves. It is covered in front, above, and behind by pleura.

Anteriorly, it is crossed by the superior vena cava and the phrenic nerve on the right side, and by the phrenic nerve on the left side. The *anterior pulmonary plexus*, a vagosympathetic plexus, lies in front of the root of the lung and sends numerous branches into the hilum.

Superiorly, the vena azygos arches forwards on the right side; the aortic arch curves backwards on the left side.

Posteriorly, the vena azygos on the right side, and the descending thoracic aorta on the left side, are related to the root of the lung. The *posterior pulmonary plexus* is another vagosympathetic plexus. It lies behind the root of the lung and sends many branches along the vessels into the interior of the lung.

Lobes and Fissures. The left lung is divided into an *upper* and a *lower lobe* by an *oblique fissure*, which cuts deeply into the lung, leaving the two lobes connected to each other only by the branches of the pulmonary vessels and the bronchi. The oblique fissure cuts the posterior border of the lung about 2½ inches below the apex, and from there it can be traced downwards and forwards across the medial and costal surfaces until it cuts the inferior border a little behind (lateral to) the cardiac notch. The opposed walls of the fissure are lined with visceral pleura.

The *upper lobe* of the left lung lies above and in front of the oblique fissure, and comprises the apex, substantial portions of the costal and medial surfaces and the whole of the anterior border, including the cardiac notch. The lower part of the notch may show a small projection, termed the *lingula*, which has some importance clinically. The *lower lobe* lies below and behind the oblique fissure and comprises the remainder of the lung. Clinically the upper lobe is accessible from the front and in the upper part of the axilla, and the lower lobe from behind and from the side.

The right lung is divided into three lobes and consequently has two fissures. Of these fissures one exactly corresponds to the oblique fissure of the left lung: the other, termed the *horizontal fissure*, cuts off a wedge-shaped portion from the lower part of the upper subdivision of the lung. This fissure meets the oblique fissure in the mid-axillary line and cuts horizontally across the costal surface of the lung on a level with the fourth costal cartilage. In this way the right lung is divided into upper, middle and lower lobes. The lower lobe is the exact counterpart of the lower lobe of the left lung, and the upper and middle lobes together are the equivalent of the upper lobe of the left lung. Clinically, the middle lobe is accessible only from in front, below the level of the fourth costal cartilage.

The **Phrenic Nerves** (C. 3, 4 and 5) differ from each other in their thoracic relationships. The *right nerve* enters the thorax behind the first costal cartilage on the right side of the right brachiocephalic vein, and throughout its course is closely related to the mediastinal pleura. It accompanies the superior vena cava, which lies on its medial side in front of the root of the lung, and then descends on the *pericardium*, by which it is separated from the right atrium of the heart. As it reaches the diaphragm it comes into contact with the right side of the short intrathoracic part of the inferior vena cava, and its terminal branches pass through the opening in the diaphragm for that vessel.

The *Left Phrenic Nerve* runs downwards behind the left brachiocephalic vein and crosses the left side of the aortic arch to gain the anterior surface of the root of the left lung. From there it passes downwards over the left side of the pericardium and reaches the diaphragm. Except where it runs behind the left brachiocephalic vein, the left phrenic nerve is in contact with the left mediastinal pleura throughout its course.

THE PERICARDIUM AND HEART

The **Pericardium** is a fibroserous sac which encloses the heart and the roots of the great vessels. It is situated in the middle mediastinum.

The *serous pericardium* forms a closed sac similar to the pleura, and possesses visceral and parietal layers. The *fibrous pericardium* supports the outer surface of the parietal layer, to which it is everywhere firmly adherent. It is a fibrous sheet of very considerable strength and blends inferiorly with the central tendon of the diaphragm. Superiorly, it blends with the outer coats of the great vessels as they leave or enter the pericardium. It is through the outer fibrous coat of the arch of the aorta that the fibrous pericardium becomes connected with the pretracheal fascia.

The *visceral layer* of the serous pericardium is integral with the heart and is usually termed the *epicardium*. It covers the anterior and inferior surfaces of the heart and ascends on the back of the left atrium before it is reflected downwards as the *parietal layer*. This reflection forms the upper limit of a *cul-de-sac*, which is termed the *oblique sinus of the pericardium*. The roots of the aorta and of the pulmonary trunk are completely enclosed in a single tube of epicardium for a distance of about 1 inch, and the posterior part of the tube becomes reflected on to the left atrium to line the posterior wall of a short passage, termed the *transverse sinus*. Thus, the transverse sinus is bounded in front by the aorta and pulmonary trunk and behind by the superior vena cava and the left atrium. When one finger is placed in the transverse sinus and another in the oblique sinus, the two are separated from each other by a narrow strip of the left atrium and a double reflection of the serous pericardium.

The great veins which enter the heart are covered by the serous pericardium anteriorly and on each side, but not posteriorly.

At an early stage in the development of the human embryo the heart is tubular and is connected to the dorsal wall of the pericardium by a dorsal mesocardium. This fold breaks down and the gap so formed persists as the transverse sinus of the pericardium.

The **Relations of the Pericardium,** which is tantamount to saying the relations of the heart, are of great importance to the physician.

Inferiorly, the pericardium rests on the diaphragm, by which it is separated from the liver and the stomach (Plate XVI, p. 124).

On the right side the right phrenic nerve is in close apposition with the pericardium, which occupies the hollowed-out area on the mediastinal aspect of the right lung and pleura.

On the left side similar relationships are presented to the left phrenic nerve, lung and pleura.

Posteriorly, the œsophagus and the descending thoracic aorta are in intimate relationship.

Superiorly, the pericardium is related to the great vessels.

Anteriorly, the relations to be noted are more numerous. The heart and pericardium are so situated that about one-third lies to the right and two-thirds to the left of the median plane. They are placed behind the body of the sternum and the medial ends of the third, fourth, fifth and sixth costal cartilages and the corresponding intercostal spaces. To the right of the median plane the mediastinal pleura and the thin anterior border of the right lung are interposed between the pericardium and the chest wall. Owing to the cardiac notch on the left costomediastinal line of pleural reflection, the pericardium is in direct contact with the posterior surface of the left half of the sternum below the fourth costal cartilage. Lateral to this area, owing to the greater size of the cardiac notch of the lung, the pericardium is separated from the fourth and fifth spaces, the fifth and sixth cartilages, and the internal mammary vessels only by the costal and mediastinal layers of the pleura, which are in apposition with each other in this region. The remainder of the anterior surface of the pericardium is separated from the chest wall by the pleura and the anterior border of the left lung.

The **Heart** lies within the pericardium in the middle mediastinum. Its precise position, relative to the vertebral column, varies with posture and with respiration. With the body in the recumbent position the base of the heart lies opposite to the fifth, sixth, seventh and eighth thoracic vertebræ, but when the body is upright it sinks downwards at least the depth of one vertebral body.

The *sternocostal surface* of the heart can be examined when the pericardium is opened from in front. It includes portions of all of its chambers, but its auricle is the only part of the left atrium visible from this aspect. The right and left auricles lie one on each side of the root of the pulmonary trunk, which itself obscures the root of the aorta.

The right atrium forms the right boundary of this surface of the heart, and the right part of the coronary (atrio-ventricular groove), which separates it from the right ventricle, runs obliquely downwards and to the right behind the lower part of the sternum.

The left ventricle, which constitutes the convex left surface of the heart (Plate XVI, p. 124), forms a strip along the left side of the anterior aspect. On its right side it is separated from the right ventricle by the anterior interventricular groove.

The *inferior* surface of the heart rests on the diaphragm. It consists almost entirely of the ventricular portion, and the two ventricles are separated from each other by an inferior interventricular groove. That portion of the right atrium into which the inferior vena cava opens also constitutes a part of the diaphragmatic surface.

The *base* of the heart is directed backwards and is formed by the two atria, the left participating to a much greater extent than the right.

The *apex* of the heart lies at the lower part of its left border, separated from the chest wall by the pericardium, the pleura and the thin margin of the cardiac notch of the left lung. It is situated on the left ventricle. The *apex-beat*, which can be felt in the fifth intercostal space, in the mid-clavicular line, lies a little above the true anatomical apex.

With the heart *in situ*, and the lungs retracted so as to expose the sterno-costal surface completely, it is possible to recognise that, when the heart is outlined on the anterior chest-wall, (1) the right profile is formed by the right atrium and extends from the upper border of the right third costal cartilage about half an inch from the sternal margin down to the sixth costal cartilage, being gently convex to the right; (2) the lower profile is formed by the right ventricle and a small portion of the left ventricle and extends from the apex to the lower end of the right border; (3) the left profile is formed by the left ventricle and extends upwards and medially, with a gentle convexity to the left, to the lower border of the left second costal cartilage, half an inch from the sternal margin.

The **Coronary Arteries** open from the root of the aorta and supply the muscular wall of the heart.

The *Right Coronary Artery* arises from the anterior aortic sinus and passes forwards between the right side of the pulmonary trunk and the right auricle. It descends in the right coronary groove, giving off branches to the right atrium and ventricle, and then winds round on to the posterior aspect, where it anastomoses with its fellow of the opposite side, continuing as the posterior interventricular artery.

The *Left Coronary Artery* arises from the left (posterior) aortic sinus and passes forwards between the pulmonary trunk and the left auricle. It gives off a large anterior interventicular branch which runs downwards in the anterior interventricular groove. It then winds round the left border of the heart in the coronary groove closely associated with the coronary sinus, and ends by anastomosing with the right coronary artery.

The interventricular arteries anastomose at the apex.

The *Veins* of the heart accompany the arteries. The largest is found in the left part of the atrioventricular groove, posteriorly, and is termed the *coronary sinus*. It begins at the left margin of the heart (where it is continuous with the *great cardiac vein*, which ascends in the anterior interventricular groove), and it runs to the right in company with the left coronary artery. It receives tributaries from the walls of the heart and ends in the right atrium. The coronary sinus represents part of the modified body and left horn of the sinus venosus and it is therefore not surprising to find that its muscular coat consists of cardiac muscle. The *oblique vein*, which joins the coronary sinus from the back of the left atrium, represents the left duct of the sinus venosus (duct of Cuvier).

The *Nerves* of the heart are derivatives of the vagosympathetic cardiac plexuses (p. 127). The branches, which have several small ganglia associated with them in the atrial region, are, for the most part, distributed in company with the branches of the coronary vessels.

The **Right Atrium.** When the interior of the right atrium is examined, the *musculi pectinati*, which form a series of transverse ridges, are striking features of the anterior and lateral walls. Posteriorly, they end on a longitudinal elevation, which runs from the right side of the orifice of the superior vena cava to the right side of the orifice of the inferior vena cava. This ridge constitutes the *crista terminalis*, and it indicates the boundary line between the primitive atrium and what was originally the right horn of the sinus venosus. Its position is marked on the outer surface by a shallow groove, termed the *sulcus terminalis*, which, however, is only visible in a well-fixed heart.

The posterior wall of the right atrium is formed by the *interatrial septum*, and when the thumb is introduced into the right atrium and a finger into the left atrium—a procedure which it is always advisable to adopt in dealing with the atrial portion of the detached heart—it can be identified at once. Its central portion is thinner than the rest of the septum and constitutes the *fossa ovalis*, which occupies the site of the fœtal *foramen ovale* (*secundum*). The margins of the fossa form a recognisable rim, termed the *limbus of the fossa ovalis*, which is continuous below and in front with the valve of the inferior vena cava. The thin floor of the fossa ovalis represents a persistent part of the septum primum of the heart of the embryo, while the limbus is formed from the septum secundum, with which the rest of the septum primum and the left venous valve of the orifice of the sinus venosus are incorporated.

The interior of the auricle is roughened by many muscular ridges. It should be observed that the whole of the interior of the right atrium and of the other chambers of the heart is lined by an endothelial layer, which is termed the *endocardium*.

The *Superior Vena Cava* opens into the uppermost part of the right atrium (sinus venosus portion), and its orifice is devoid of any valve. The *Inferior Vena Cava* opens into the same part of the chamber at its lower limit, and a thin, crescentic fold of endocardium is connected to the anterior margin of the orifice, forming the *valve of the vena cava*.

The *Coronary Sinus* opens into the right atrium between the orifice for the inferior vena cava and the right atrioventricular opening. A small fold of endocardium obscures the orifice and is termed the *valve of the coronary sinus*.

The right venous valve of the orifice of the sinus venosus disappears in its cranial portion, but the crista terminalis marks the line of its attachment. The caudal half of the valve forms most of the valve of the inferior vena cava and the valve of the coronary sinus.

The **Right Atrioventricular (Tricuspid) Orifice** occupies the lower part of the anterior wall of the right atrium and lies behind the right half of the body of the sternum opposite the fourth intercostal space. It is so placed that the blood, driven into the right ventricle by the contraction of the atrium, passes forwards and to the left and slightly downwards. The opening is large enough to admit the tips only of three fingers. It is guarded by the tricuspid valve.

The **Right Ventricle.** The interior of the right ventricle of the heart is characterised by numerous elevations, the precise arrangement of which is open to considerable variation. These are the *trabeculæ carneæ*, and they differ from the musculi pectinati of the right atrium by their varying size and inconstant arrangement.

The flaps of the tricuspid valve are anchored to the ventricular walls by fine tendinous bands, termed the *chordæ tendineæ*. A few of these spring directly from the ventricular septum, which forms the left wall of the right ventricle, but most are attached to the *papillary muscles*, which are small conical muscular elevations. Two of these are fairly constant. The *anterior papillary muscle* springs from the anterior wall of the ventricle, and its base is connected to the ventricular septum by a rounded bundle, termed the *septomarginal trabecula* (*moderator band*). The *inferior papillary muscle* springs from the inferior wall of the chamber.

A curved muscular ridge, termed the *supraventricular crest*, arches across the upper and anterior part of the cavity of the ventricle, extending between the anterior wall and the upper part of the right side of the ventricular septum. This ridge forms the lower and posterior boundary of the *infundibulum*, which constitutes the outflowing part of the ventricle as it leads upwards to the pulmonary orifice. The importance of the infundibulum depends on the fact that its muscular walls maintain their tonus during ventricular diastole and provide support for the relatively fragile cusps of the pulmonary valve in order to enable it to sustain the backward pressure of the blood in the pulmonary trunk. It represents the persistent ventral part of the bulbus cordis of the embryo. Occasionally it is congenitally stenosed.

The *Tricuspid Valve* guards the atrioventricular opening. It consists of three incompletely separated cusps or flaps, which are attached by their bases to a fibrous *atrioventricular ring*. The margins and outer surfaces of the flaps receive the chordæ tendineæ, by which they are brought under the control of the papillary muscles. Each cusp consists of a double layer of endocardium containing a little fibrous tissue. The cusps are anterior, inferior and medial in position, the last-named being related to the ventricular septum.

The **Left Atrium.** The interior of this chamber is smooth-walled except in the auricle, where the condition is similar to that found in the right auricle. The anterior, or right, wall is formed by the atrial septum, while the left atrioventricular opening is placed in front and to the left. The pulmonary veins, usually two from each lung, open through the posterior wall. Their orifices are not provided with valves. Originally two pulmonary veins issue from each developing lung rudiment and unite to form a single vein on each side. These two, in turn, join to form a single vessel, which opens into the left atrium. In the course of development, this single trunk and the right and left trunks all become absorbed into the cavity of the left atrium, so that the four veins open independently in the adult. This process may be arrested on one or both sides, reducing the number of veins opening into the atrium to three or two, as the case may be.

The Left Ventricle. The walls of this chamber are provided with trabeculæ carneæ as in the right ventricle, and these are especially numerous near the apex of the heart. There are two strong papillary muscles, of which one is attached to the inferior wall and one to the antero-lateral wall, and both are connected by chordæ tendineæ to the cusps of the mitral valve.

The **Left Atrioventricular (Mitral) Orifice** lies in the lower and back part of the ventricle and is placed behind the left half of the body of the sternum opposite the fourth costal cartilage. When examined from the interior of the left atrium, it will be found large enough to admit the tips of two fingers. The *mitral valve*, which guards the opening, comprises two cusps, each consisting of a double layer of endocardium with a little fibrous tissue between. The *anterior cusp* is much the larger and intervenes between the mitral and the aortic orifices. Owing to its position both surfaces come into contact with the blood stream and both are smooth, the chordæ tendineæ being confined mainly to the margins of the cusp. In its mode of attachment and in its action the mitral valve is similar to the tricuspid valve.

The *Aortic Orifice* lies in the upper and back part of the ventricle, on a slightly higher level and nearer to the chest wall than the mitral orifice. The portion of the ventricle which lies below and in front of it has comparatively thin walls, consisting for the most part of fibrous and elastic tissue, and is known as the *aortic vestibule*.

The *Ventricular Septum* is a muscular partition which completely separates the two ventricles from each other. As already stated, the moderator band (p. 110) and some chordæ tendineæ are attached to its right, or anterior, surface. The upper and posterior part is devoid of muscle fibres over a small area which lies immediately below the aortic orifice, and is obscured, from the right side, by the medial cusp of the tricuspid valve. It is known as the *membranous part of the septum*.

Before passing on to the consideration of the greater vessels, examine, if possible, a cross-section of the ventricular portion of the heart. It will then be seen that, though the walls of the right ventricle are thick and muscular, the walls of the left ventricle are nearly three times as thick. Further, the ventricular septum tends to bulge into the cavity of the right ventricle, and is set very obliquely, so that the pulmonary orifice of the right ventricle lies to the left side of the aortic orifice of the left ventricle.

Structure. Between the epicardium on its outer surface and the endocardium on its inner surface the heart wall consists almost entirely of cardiac muscle, but a restricted amount of fibrous tissue is present at the base of the ventricles and forms a fibrous skeleton for the attachment of the muscular fibres.

With the exception of the atrioventricular bundle (p. 114) there is no continuity between the atrial and the ventricular muscle, and the walls of the atria are connected to the base of the ventricles by two fibrous rings, one of which surrounds each atrioventricular orifice. Similar rings surround the orifices of the aorta and pulmonary trunk and the aortic ring is connected to the adjoining margins of both atrioventricular rings by a small mass of fibrous tissue, termed the *trigonum fibrosum dextrum.* On its opposite side the aortic ring is connected to the pulmonary ring by a flattened, fibrous band, termed the *tendon of the infundibulum.* All this cardiac fibrous tissue is derived from the endocardial cushion tissue of the embryonic heart and serves to give attachment to muscle fibres both of the atria and of the ventricles.

In the atria the superficial, transverse fibres are common to both chambers, but the deeper, looped fibres are confined to each. Attached to their respective atrioventricular rings both in front and behind, the looped fibres arch over the roof between their two attachments. Annular fibres surround the orifices of the great veins and the two auricles.

In the ventricular wall the superficial fibres form a series of spirally twisted V-shaped loops which spring from the fibrous skeleton at the ventricular base and sweep with a spiral twist to the region of the apex of the heart where they form a whorl with the corresponding contralateral fibres. The ascending limbs of the V's are placed more deeply and run upwards and backwards to end, some in the papillary muscles and others in the fibrous skeleton. The deeper fibres form modified figures of 8. Arising in a papillary muscle they run in the ipsilateral ventricular wall to the septum, traverse the septum, and run in the contralateral ventricular wall to end in a papillary muscle of that side.

The superficial fibres constitute a modified longitudinal coat and the deeper fibres a modified circular coat.

It is to be noted that the attachment of many of the ventricular fibres to the papillary muscles ensures synchronicity between the closure of the atrioventricular valves and ventricular systole, the valves being retained in the closed position until diastole begins.

The **Conducting System** of the heart consists of specialised cardiac muscle and comprises the sinu-atrial node, the atrioventricular node, the atrioventricular bundle and its two limbs and their terminal subendocardial plexuses of Purkinje fibres.

The *sinu-atrial node* lies at the upper end of the sulcus terminalis and in this situation forms the whole thickness of the wall of the right atrium between the epicardium and the endocardium. It consists of a network of specialised cardiac muscle fibres, rather narrower than the atrial muscle fibres and completely cross-striated. The fibres branch and are directly continuous with neighbouring atrial fibres. The node has been termed the "pace-maker" of the heart, for it is the site of origin of cardiac contraction.

The *atrioventricular node* lies in the lower part of the atrial septum, just above the orifice of the coronary sinus. It is identical in structure with the sinu-atrial node, but its fibres are continued onwards as the *atrioventricular bundle*, which crosses the right atrio-ventricular ring under cover of the medial cusp of the tricuspid valve to gain the ventricular septum. The bundle follows the lower border of the membranous part of the septum and then divides into right and left limbs, which straddle the upper border of the muscular septum, and then descend, each on its own side of the septum, close to the endocardium. The *right limb* can be traced to the septal end of the moderator band, which carries it to the base of the anterior papillary muscle, where it forms a plexus of Purkinje fibres and these are distributed to the papillary muscle and the ventricular myocardium. The *left limb* soon divides into two or more branches and these subdivide into smaller branches which traverse the trabeculæ carneæ and reach the papillary muscles where they too form plexuses of Purkinje fibres.

A specialised conducting system is necessary because the heart beats more rapidly than it could if the impulse were propagated by direct spread through the cardiac muscle, which is in any case not continuous from atria to ventricles. Although conduction through the atrioventricular node imposes some delay on the passage of the impulse, the higher rate of conductivity of the Purkinje fibres in the atrioventricular bundle and its limbs ensures the requisite speed of propagation throughout the walls of the ventricles. The impulse, initiated at the sinu-atrial node, is conducted by the atrial musculature to the atrioventricular node and the delay which occurs there and in conduction through its ramifications enables the atria to fill the ventricles before the latter contract.

Cardiac muscle has a lower rate of rhythmicity than nodal tissue and this explains the fact that, when the ventricles are isolated by a complete lesion of the stem of the a.-v. bundle (the condition known as "heart block"), they beat at a slower rate than the atria, which are still under the control of the sinu-atrial node.

The **Pulmonary Orifice** lies behind the upper border of the left third costal cartilage near its junction with the sternum. It is guarded by a valve, consisting of three semilunar cusps. These cusps are attached to the arterial wall by their lower curved borders, and bound little pockets, the mouths of which are directed upwards. Each cusp consists of a double layer of endocardium with a little fibrous tissue in between. The action of such valves is purely automatic and is devoid of any nervous or muscular control. During ventricular systole the flaps are pressed against the arterial wall by the outrushing blood and the pockets are obliterated. On the conclusion of ventricular systole blood endeavours to pass back into the ventricle, but the reflux opens up and fills the pockets so that the cusps overlap into the centre of the lumen and close the orifice completely.

The **Aortic Orifice** is placed behind the left half of the sternum on a level with the lower border of the third left costal cartilage. It is guarded by a valve, similar in every way to the pulmonary valve except as regards the position of the three cusps. Opposite each cusp the aortic wall is bulged outwards, and these localised dilatations are termed the *aortic sinuses*. It is from the anterior and left (posterior) sinuses that the right and left coronary arteries arise, respectively.

The cusps of the pulmonary and aortic valves are derived from the distal bulbar swellings, four in number, which develop at the single orifice of the truncus arteriosus in the embryonic heart. The fusion of the right and left swellings separate the single orifice into an anterior, or pulmonary, and a posterior, or aortic opening.

THE GREAT VESSELS

The **Superior Vena Cava** commences opposite the lower border of the sternal end of the *right first costal cartilage*, where it is formed by the union of the two brachiocephalic veins. It runs downwards to the uppermost part of the right atrium, which it reaches on a level with the sternal end of the right third costal cartilage. Its course can be mapped out as a strip, half-an-inch broad, projecting beyond the right margin of the sternum.

Anteriorly, the superior vena cava is separated from the chest wall and the internal mammary vessels by the anterior margin of the right lung and pleural sac. In its lower half the vessel is covered anteriorly by the visceral layer of the serous pericardium. *Laterally*, the phrenic nerve is closely applied to the vessel, and both are related to the pleura and the mediastinal surface of the lung in front of the hilum. *Posteriorly*, the vessel is related to the structures constituting the root of the right lung. *Antero-medially*, it is closely related to the ascending aorta.

Tributaries. The *Vena Azygos* arches forwards from the posterior mediastinum, above the root of the right lung, and joins the posterior aspect of the superior vena cava just before it enters the pericardium.

Not only is there no valve at the mouth of the superior vena cava, but there are none throughout its whole extent. Nor are there any in the brachiocephalic veins. *The nearest venous valve to the heart in the superior caval area is in the internal jugular vein, half-an-inch above its termination* and this is not usually functional. When it is, the venous pulse transmitted from the heart is limited to the lower part of the vein.

Above the point where it is joined by the vena azygos, the superior vena cava represents the right anterior cardinal vein. Below that point it represents the persistent right duct of the sinus venosus.

The **Inferior Vena Cava** has a very short intrathoracic course. It pierces the central tendon of the diaphragm level with the ninth thoracic vertebra in the erect attitude and enters the lowest part of the right atrium. As it does so it comes into relation, on its lateral side, with the mediastinal aspect of the right lung, and a notch can frequently be seen in the fixed lung in that position.

The **Right Brachiocephalic (Innominate) Vein** is formed behind the sternal end of the right clavicle by the union of the right subclavian and internal jugular veins. It runs downwards in the superior mediastinum and, on a level with the lower border of the right first costal cartilage, joins with the left brachiocephalic vein to form the superior vena cava.

The vein, with the right phrenic nerve on its right side, grooves the mediastinal surface of the right lung. It has the brachiocephalic artery and the trachea to its left side.

The **Left Brachiocephalic (Innominate) Vein** has a corresponding origin, but its course passes obliquely across to the right behind the manubrium sterni to reach the right brachiocephalic vein.

Superficially, it is related to the remains of the thymus and to the upper part of the manubrium sterni. Behind it the large branches of the aortic arch ascend to the neck, separating the vein from the trachea, and the left phrenic and vagus nerves run downwards to cross the aortic arch. The summit of the aortic arch lies below the vein.

Tributaries. (*a*) The *Inferior Thyroid Veins* run downwards in front of the trachea (p. 120), and end in the brachiocephalic veins. Frequently both join the left brachiocephalic vein. (*b*) The *Vertebral* and (*c*) the *Internal Thoracic* (*Mammary*) *Veins* join the brachiocephalic vein of the same side.

The **Aorta** arises from the base of the left ventricle and runs at first upwards, forwards and to the right as far as the right border of the manubrium opposite the second costal cartilage. This part of the vessel is the *ascending aorta.* The *arch* turns backwards and to the left until it reaches the left side of the body of the fourth thoracic vertebra, where it turns downwards as the *descending thoracic aorta.* (The arch is thus the part of the aorta in the superior mediastinum.)

The **Ascending Aorta** is much nearer to the surface of the body at its termination than it is at its commencement. It is separated from the sternum at its origin by the pulmonary trunk and the left lung and pleura. *To its right side,* but on a more posterior plane, lies the superior vena cava. *Posteriorly,* it is related to the right pulmonary artery, the right atrium and the right bronchus, and *on its left side* lie the termination of the pulmonary trunk and the left lung and pleura.

In its proximal part the ascending aorta, together with the pulmonary trunk, is enclosed in a tube of serous pericardium and lies in front of the transverse sinus of the pericardium; above this level it obtains a thick investment from the fibrous pericardium.

Owing to the curvature of the aorta, the blood entering from the left ventricle impinges on the right wall of the ascending part of the vessel. As a result this wall becomes bulged outwards, so that the vessel is not circular on transverse section in this part of its course.

Branches. The right coronary artery, springing from the anterior aortic sinus, and the left coronary artery, springing from the left (posterior) sinus, have already been described (p. 108).

The **Arch of the Aorta** is directed backwards and to the left, but the principal inclination is backwards. On this account it lies chiefly behind the lower half of the manubrium sterni, projecting a little beyond its left margin. This projection, which is convex to the left, can be recognised in X-ray photographs and is known as the aortic "knuckle" (Plate XVI, p. 124). At its commencement the arch is separated from the right half of the manubrium only by the thin anterior margin of the right lung and pleura, but at its termination it is deeply placed.

To its left side, the arch is related to the pleura and mediastinal surface of the left lung, which it grooves above the hilum (p. 105). The left phrenic and vagus nerves and the nerves to the superficial part of the cardiac plexus cross this surface of the vessel and intervene between it and the pleura.

To its right side, the arch is related to the trachea, the *left recurrent laryngeal nerve,* the œsophagus, the thoracic duct and the fourth thoracic vertebra.

Inferiorly, the arch overhangs the bifurcation of the pulmonary trunk and the root of the left lung, and it is related to the superficial part of the cardiac plexus, the *left recurrent laryngeal nerve* and the ligamentum arteriosum.

Superiorly, the arch is related to the left brachiocephalic vein and it gives off from its convexity three large branches (v. infra).

The arch of the aorta is formed from the right and left aortic sacs, the left fourth aortic arch and the adjoining portion of the primitive left dorsal aorta.

Branches. 1. The **Brachiocephalic (Innominate) Artery** arises from the aorta as it lies in front of the trachea and passes upwards, backwards and to the right to the posterior aspect of the sterno-clavicular joint, where it divides into the right subclavian and common carotid arteries.

Anteriorly, the artery is separated from the manubrium sterni by the remains of the thymus and the left brachiocephalic vein, by which it is crossed near its origin. *To its right side*, lie the right brachiocephalic vein and the superior vena cava, which intervene between the artery and the right pleura and lung. *Posteriorly*, the artery lies on the trachea below, and the longus cervicis above, and the right vagus constitutes a postero-lateral relation. *To its left side*, it is related to the left common carotid at its origin, and to the right side of the trachea at a higher level.

2. The **Left Common Carotid Artery** branches from the aortic arch immediately to the left side of the brachiocephalic artery, and runs upwards and to the left to enter the neck behind the left sterno-clavicular joint. At their origins the left common carotid and the brachiocephalic artery lie side by side in front of the trachea, but they diverge as they ascend, so that they come to lie one on each side of that structure.

Anteriorly, the artery is crossed by the left brachiocephalic vein, and the remains of the thymus intervene between it and the manubrium. *On its left side*, it is related to the left phrenic and vagus nerves and the left lung and pleura. *Posteriorly* it is successively in contact with the trachea, the left recurrent laryngeal nerve and the œsophagus.

3. The **Left Subclavian Artery** arises from the aortic arch behind the left common carotid and arches upwards and laterally to enter the neck. Except at its origin, where it is crossed by the left brachiocephalic vein, the artery lies in a groove on the surface of the left lung, with the left common carotid in front and to the right, and the trachea and œsophagus to its right side.

The **Pulmonary Trunk** arises from the infundibulum of the right ventricle and runs upwards, backwards and to the left. Placed at first in front of the ascending aorta, it inclines to its left side and terminates in the concavity of the aortic arch by dividing into right and left branches. The trunk of the artery is therefore quite short, being not more than 2 inches long. It is related anteriorly to the sternal end of the left second intercostal space, from which, however, it is separated by the thin anterior margin of the left lung and the pleura. *Posteriorly*, the artery is related to the commencement of the aorta and the left coronary artery below, and to the left atrium above.

The first inch of the pulmonary trunk is enclosed, together with the aorta, in a common tube of serous pericardium (p. 106), and for the rest of its course the artery is invested with the fibrous pericardium.

The *Ligamentum Arteriosum* is a fibrous band which runs from the bifurcation of the pulmonary trunk upwards and to the left, to become attached to the lower aspect of the aortic arch. It is the vestige of the ductus arteriosus of the fœtus (p. 120), a vessel which short-circuits the blood from the pulmonary circulation into the aorta and represents the dorsal end of the left sixth aortic arch. The left recurrent laryngeal nerve hooks round the left side of the ligamentum arteriosum at its attachment to the aortic arch.

The **Right Pulmonary Artery** runs horizontally to the right behind the ascending aorta and the superior vena cava, and in front of the œsophagus and the hyparterial bronchus. It then enters the root of the right lung.

The **Left Pulmonary Artery** runs to the left, behind the upper left pulmonary vein and in front of the descending aorta and the left bronchus, to enter the hilum of the left lung.

Circulation through the Fœtal Heart. In the fœtus oxygenated blood enters the heart from the inferior vena cava, the valve of which directs the flow through the foramen ovale into the left atrium, while the deoxygenated blood from the superior vena cava passes into the right ventricle. Probably a small amount of intermingling of the two streams occurs, but the effect is negligible. As the inflow to the left atrium from the pulmonary veins is very limited in amount in the fœtus, the chamber is filled from the inferior vena cava.

From the left atrium the oxygenated blood passes into the left ventricle and so to the aorta. From the right ventricle the pulmonary trunk carries the deoxygenated blood to the ductus arteriosus, which is relatively a wide vessel and in direct continuity with the pulmonary trunk. The right and left pulmonary arteries are small vessels in the fœtus, so that most of the blood carried by the pulmonary trunk passes through the ductus into the aortic arch distal to the origin of the left subclavian artery. Hence, deoxygenated blood enters the aorta beyond the origins of the great vessels to the fore part of the body, which is growing more rapidly than the rest.

When respiration begins, the right and left pulmonary arteries enlarge to convey the extra blood required by the pulmonary circulation. This change is aided by functional closure of the ductus arteriosus due to contraction of the smooth muscle in its wall. In the ensuing months proliferation of the intima leads to permanent obliteration of the ductus and its walls become converted into fibrous tissue.

Ligature of the umbilical cord arrests the flow of blood through the umbilical vein and the ductus venosus (p. 167) into the inferior vena cava and, as a result, the pressure in the right atrium drops, while at the same time the increased inflow from the pulmonary veins raises the pressure in the left atrium, so that equilibrium is reached between the two atria. As a result the foramen ovale (secundum) is kept closed by the apposition of the upper free margin of the floor of the fossa ovalis (septum primum) to the left side of the annulus ovalis. Later, fusion of the apposed surfaces is usually complete, but the presence of a small valvular communication between the two atria is by no means infrequent, although it has little functional significance.

The **Trachea** begins in the neck opposite the lower border of the sixth cervical vertebra, and runs downwards into the thorax in front of the œsophagus. In the superior mediastinum it maintains the same relationship, and it terminates opposite the upper border of the fifth thoracic vertebra, slightly to the right of the median plane, by dividing into the right and left principal bronchi. In the male adult subject it is 4 to $4\frac{1}{2}$ inches in length; in the female it is $\frac{1}{2}$ inch shorter. The tube is kept patent by the presence in its wall of a series of horseshoe-shaped cartilages, which support its lateral and anterior aspects but are deficient posteriorly, where the wall is consequently flattened.

Anteriorly, in the neck, the isthmus of the thyroid gland covers the second, third and fourth tracheal rings. From its lower border the inferior thyroid veins descend in front of the trachea.

A little above its bifurcation the trachea is crossed by the arch of the aorta, and the roots of the brachiocephalic and left common carotid arteries lie in front of it and separate it from the left brachiocephalic vein. As these two arteries ascend they diverge to the right and left respectively, and in the interval between them the trachea is related anteriorly to the remains of the thymus and to the inferior thyroid veins. Throughout its course in the thorax the trachea lies behind the manubrium sterni and, since it contains air, it is recognisable in antero-posterior X-ray photographs of the chest (Plate XVI).

Posteriorly, the trachea is related to the œsophagus, by which it is separated from the longus cervicis muscle and vertebral bodies.

To the left side, the trachea, from its commencement to the sixth ring, is related to the left lobe of the thyroid gland. Below that level it is successively related to the left common carotid, the left subclavian artery, and the aortic arch. The left recurrent laryngeal nerve lies in the groove between the trachea and the œsophagus, both in the thorax and in the neck.

To the right side, the trachea is related to the right vagus nerve and the vena azygos, which arches forwards above the root of the right lung to join the superior vena cava. Above the vena azygos the right side of the trachea is closely related to the right vagus nerve and the mediastinal pleura and, near the thoracic inlet, to the brachiocephalic artery. In the neck, the right lobe of the thyroid gland and the right recurrent laryngeal nerve occupy positions similar to those on the left side.

Numerous tracheobronchial lymph nodes and the deep part of the cardiac plexus are associated with the trachea at its bifurcation, and the paratracheal lymph nodes lie on each side of it in the superior mediastinum.

The trachea is developed from the caudal part of the laryngo-tracheal groove, which forms in the ventral wall of the foregut. The groove becomes separated off from the gut, the process beginning at the level of the tracheal bifurcation and extending headwards. The communication of the larynx with the laryngeal part of the pharynx indicates the derivation of the larynx and trachea from the foregut.

The **Principal Bronchi** diverge from each other to reach the roots of the lungs. They differ in size, length and inclination. The *right principal bronchus* is the *shorter and also the wider of the two, and is more nearly vertical in direction.* On this account foreign bodies sucked into the trachea usually pass into the right bronchus. After a short course, about 1 inch in length, it gives off an eparterial bronchus to the upper lobe and continues as the hyparterial bronchus. This gives off a branch to the middle lobe and the trunk then enters the lower lobe, to which it is distributed. Behind the right bronchus the right vagus nerve gives off numerous pulmonary branches (posterior pulmonary plexus) and the vena azygos ascends to arch forwards over its upper border. Anteriorly the right pulmonary artery crosses the hyparterial bronchus.

The *Left Principal Bronchus* reaches the hilum of the lung before it divides into branches for the upper and lower lobes. *The arch of the aorta runs backwards above it and the descending thoracic aorta runs downwards behind it*, a relationship of considerable practical importance. Anteriorly the left pulmonary artery crosses in front of the left bronchus above the point of origin of its first branch.

It may be noted that the first branch given off by the left bronchus divides almost at once into two branches, one of which corresponds closely in pattern to the eparterial bronchus and the other to the bronchus of the middle lobe of the right lung.

The divisions of the bronchi and the pulmonary lobules which they supply constitute self-contained and functionally independent units, known to the clinician as *broncho-pulmonary segments.*

The segments of the right upper lobe and the upper part of the left upper lobe are: (1) apical, (2) posterior, and (3) anterior. The right middle lobe has lateral and medial segments, and those of the corresponding (lower) part of the left upper lobe are termed superior and inferior lingular segments. Both lower lobes have a similar pattern of five divisions: (1) apical, (2) subapical, (3) anterior basal, (4) lateral basal, and (5) posterior basal. In addition, the right lower lobe has a medial basal (cardiac) segment.

The intrapulmonary bronchi divide and subdivide and their smallest branches are known as *terminal bronchioles.* The walls of the larger branches contain a layer of circular muscle (broncho-constrictor) fibres and are prevented from collapsing by the presence of irregular plates of hyaline cartilage. The walls of the terminal bronchioles are devoid of cartilage and at the point where a terminal bronchiole opens into a group of air-sacs (*alveoli*) there is a marked thickening of its circular muscle coat. Vagal fibres from the pulmonary plexuses supply the broncho-constrictor muscle.

The **Œsophagus** begins opposite the lower border of the sixth cervical vertebra, where it is continuous with the laryngeal part of the pharynx.

In the neck, it lies in front of the vertebral column and the longus cervicis muscles. On each side of it is the corresponding lobe of the thyroid gland, and its left border is in contact with the thoracic duct (p. 125). Anteriorly, the œsophagus is in direct contact with the trachea and the recurrent laryngeal nerves.

In the thorax, the œsophagus does not remain strictly in the median plane. As it passes through the thoracic inlet it lies a little to the left, but opposite the fifth, sixth, seventh and eighth thoracic vertebræ it is usually median in position. In the lower part of the thorax it again inclines to the left, and at the same time passes forwards from the vertebral column to pierce the muscular part of the left dome of the diaphragm at the level of the tenth thoracic vertebra.

Posteriorly, in the upper two-thirds of its intrathoracic course, the œsophagus is closely related to the bodies of the vertebræ, but the thoracic duct, the azygos and hemiazygos veins, the right posterior (aortic) intercostal arteries and part of the œsophageal plexus intervene. In the posterior mediastinum the œsophagus is separated from the vertebral column by a recess of the right pleural sac (p. 101) and, at its lower end, by the descending thoracic aorta.

Anteriorly, in the upper part of the thorax, the œsophagus is related to the trachea and the left recurrent laryngeal nerve. Opposite the fifth thoracic vertebra it is crossed by the left bronchus (the bifurcation of the trachea being situated a little to the right of the median plane). Below that level the pericardium separates the œsophagus from the left atrium.

The *right edge* of the œsophagus is intimately related to the mediastinal surface of the right lung (p. 103), except at its upper and lower ends.

The *left edge* is related to the thoracic duct and the left subclavian artery in the superior mediastinum. Opposite the fourth thoracic vertebra it is crossed by the arch of the aorta. Below that level it is related to the descending thoracic aorta and, at its lower end, to the mediastinal surface of the left lung.

Below the level of the roots of the lungs the two vagus nerves emerge from the posterior pulmonary plexus, and come into close relationship with the œsophagus. Together with sympathetic nerves they constitute the *œsophageal plexus*, which surrounds the œsophagus. From the plexus the right vagus nerve descends on the posterior surface of the œsophagus and the left vagus on its anterior surface. An interchange of fibres occurs in the plexus, and fibres from the left vagus accompany the right vagus into the abdomen, and vice versa.

The *Blood Supply* of the œsophagus is derived from branches of the inferior thyroid artery in the neck, and from the descending thoracic aorta in the thorax. Branches of the left gastric (p. 160) ascend from the abdomen through the œsophageal opening in the diaphragm. The *œsophageal veins* join the vena azygos, but those at the lower end of the œsophagus communicate freely with tributaries of the left gastric vein, which joins the portal vein. *This venous* anastomosis is an important connection between the portal and the systemic venous systems and may become widely opened up when the portal channels through the liver are obstructed.

The **Right Vagus Nerve** enters the thorax on the postero-lateral aspect of the innominate artery, and runs downwards and medially to reach the right side of the trachea, where it is crossed by the vena azygos as it runs forwards to reach the superior vena cava. It continues downwards with a backward inclination and passes on to the posterior aspect of the right bronchus, and so reaches the posterior surface of the root of the right lung. There it takes part in the formation of the posterior pulmonary plexus (p. 105). On emerging from the plexus the right vagus passes on to the œsophagus, where, together with its fellow of the opposite side, it forms the œsophageal plexus. Finally, it descends on the posterior aspect of the œsophagus, passes through the œsophageal opening of the diaphragm, and reaches the posterior aspect of the stomach.

The **Left Vagus Nerve** enters the thorax on the lateral side of the left common carotid artery and passes behind the left brachiocephalic vein. It then crosses the left side of the aortic arch, below which it turns backwards to reach the posterior surface of the root of the left lung. There it helps in the formation of the posterior pulmonary plexus and then proceeds downwards to the œsophageal plexus, from which it descends on the anterior surface of the œsophagus.

In their course through the thorax both vagus nerves give off branches to the lungs and to the œsophagus. In addition the right vagus supplies some cardiac branches, and the left recurrent laryngeal nerve branches from the left vagus.

The **Left Recurrent Laryngeal Nerve** arises from the left vagus as that nerve crosses the arch of the aorta and passes backwards below the *ligamentum arteriosum.* It then ascends in close contact with the right side (often described as the posterior aspect) of the aortic arch, and gains the groove between the left side of the trachea and the œsophagus. In the thorax it gives off a few cardiac branches, but its great importance is due to the fact that it supplies all the muscles which act on the left vocal fold, with the exception of its tensor (cricothyroid, external laryngeal nerve, p. 299).

The **Descending Thoracic Aorta** commences on the left side of the body of the fourth thoracic vertebra and runs downwards, inclining to the right and forwards relative to the vertebral column, so that, opposite the twelfth thoracic vertebra, it comes to lie in the median plane. At this level the vessel passes behind the diaphragm and enters the abdomen. Throughout its course it is closely related to the left mediastinal pleura and the left lung. As it descends, it passes behind the root of the left lung and then behind the heart. In this situation it is crossed obliquely in front by the œsophagus, which gradually passes from its right to its left side. In the lower part of its extent part of the diaphragm intervenes between the vessel and the liver.

On its right side the descending aorta is first related to the bodies

PLATE XV

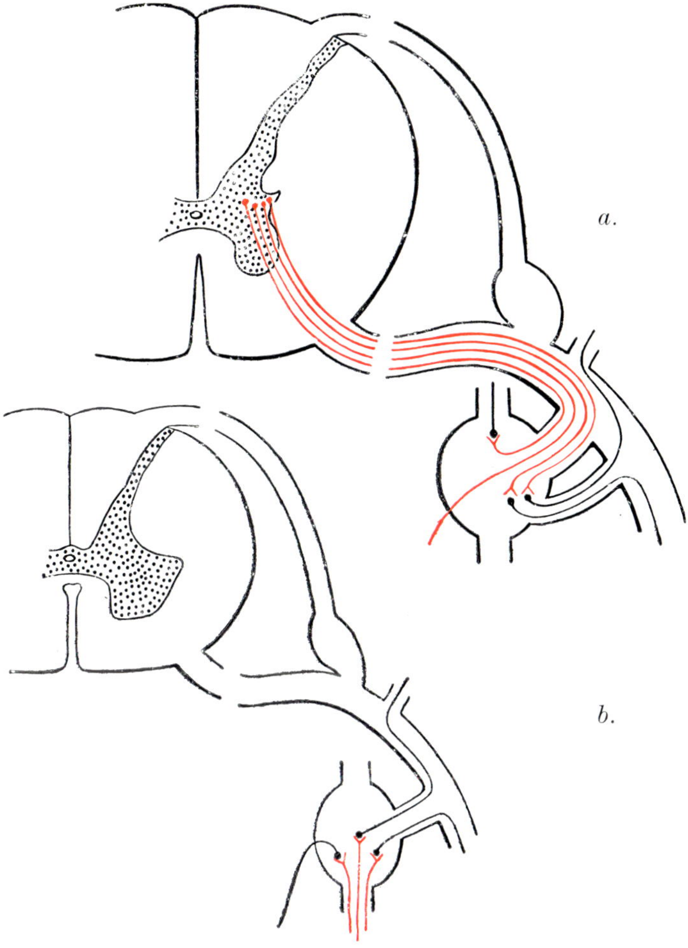

a.

b.

The Connexions of the Ganglionated Trunk of the Sympathetic with the Spinal Nerves.

a. Mid-thoracic region. The preganglionic fibres, shown in red, arise in the lateral column, and travel by the anterior nerve root, the spinal nerve and its ventral ramus before traversing the white ramus communicans to reach the corresponding sympathetic ganglion. The postganglionic fibres, shown in black, traverse the grey ramus communicans for the most part and reach the ventral ramus. Some are distributed by the ventral ramus and some by the dorsal.

b. The cervical region. No preganglionic fibres are present in the anterior nerve root and there is no white ramus communicans. Some preganglionic fibres are ascending in the ganglionated trunk. Most of the postganglionic fibres pass *viâ* the grey ramus communicans to the ventral ramus, where they diverge.

To face p. 124

PLATE XVI. ANTERO-POSTERIOR RADIOGRAPH OF CHEST IN A FEMALE SUBJECT AGED 20.

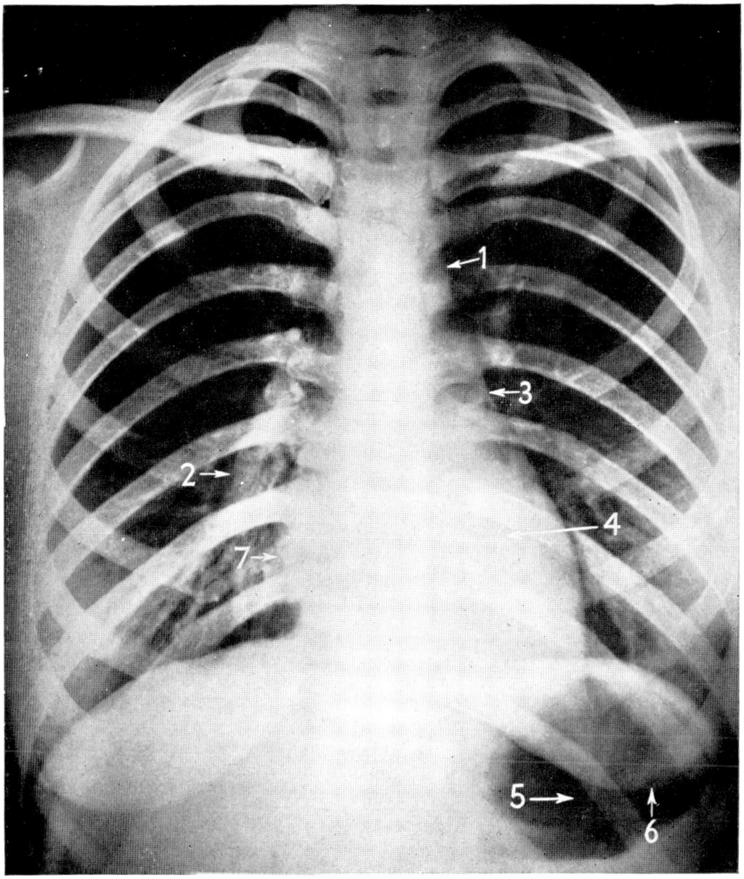

1. Aortic "knuckle," less conspicuous than it is in elderly subjects.
2. Right pulmonary vessels.
3. Pulmonary trunk.
4. Left ventricle.
5. Bubble of gas in fundus of stomach.
6. Lower margin of shadow of left breast.
7. Margin of right atrium.

The air-containing trachea forms a less opaque band in the median plane above the suprasternal notch, the position of which can be identified from the medial ends of the clavicles.

Owing to distortion caused by the divergence of the rays in the peripheral parts of the large field shown, the lower border of the heart *appears* to lie at or near the upper border of T.11, and other structures in the periphery are affected in a similar manner.

PLATE XVII. LATERAL RADIOGRAPH OF CHEST OF A YOUNG ADULT.

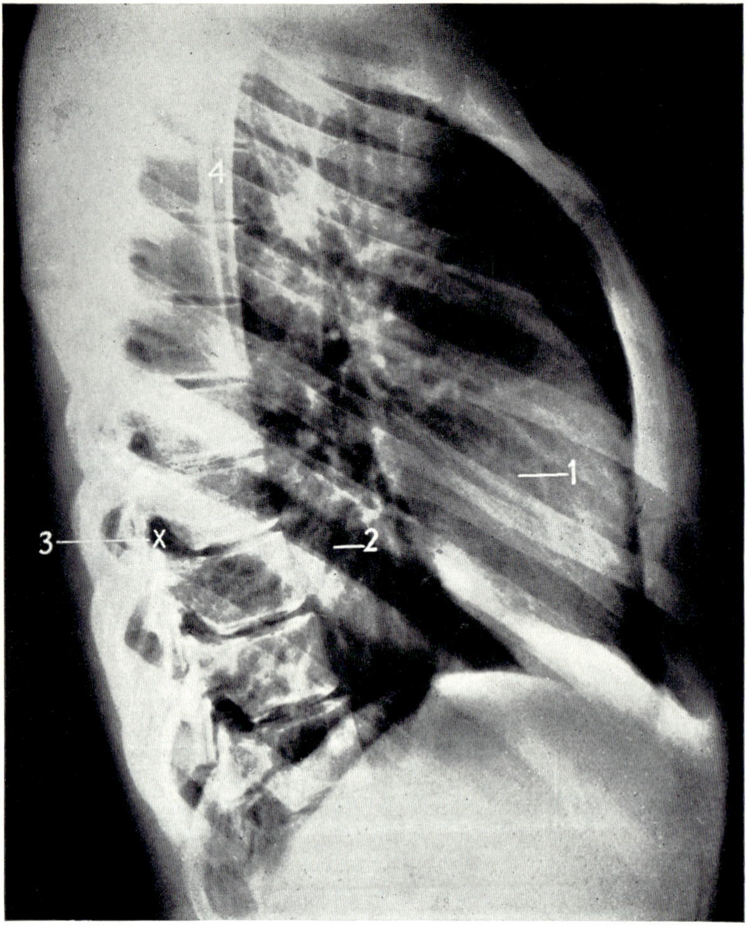

1. Shadow of heart.
2. Retrocardial space, which contains the œsophagus and the descending thoracic aorta, etc.
3. The eighth thoracic intervertebral foramen.
4. Body of T.4. Note that its lower border is on the same horizontal plane as the manubriosternal joint.

Note.—The linear shadows which cross the bodies of T.3–T.6 anteriorly are caused by the lateral borders of the two scapulæ.

Observe how narrow the intervertebral discs are in the thoracic region and compare with Plate XX.

of the thoracic vertebræ, and subsequently to the œsophagus, the vena azygos and the thoracic duct. In the lower part of the thorax it comes into contact with the right mediastinal pleura.

Posteriorly, the vessel is related to the left mediastinal pleura and the lung above, and to the bodies of the vertebræ below, its own intercostal branches and the hemiazygos veins intervening.

Branches. (*a*) Nine pairs of *posterior intercostal arteries* are given off to the lower nine intercostal spaces. The upper arteries run upwards and laterally to reach the spaces for which they are destined. Those of the right side cross the vertebral bodies and pass behind the œsophagus. On both sides, the arteries are crossed by the sympathetic trunk. Each artery, on gaining the intercostal space, takes up a position in the costal groove between the vein above and the corresponding nerve below. Opposite the angle of the rib the artery gives off a collateral branch, which follows the lower border of the space. The vessels anastomose with the *anterior* intercostal arteries from the internal thoracic and musculophrenic arteries. The lower two, however, are exceptional in that they pass forwards into the anterior abdominal wall in company with the corresponding nerves.

Each posterior intercostal artery gives off a posterior branch, which passes backwards below the transverse process of the corresponding vertebra. It sends a spinal branch through the intervertebral foramen to supply the spinal cord and its membranes, and then accompanies the posterior primary ramus of the corresponding nerve to supply the muscles and superficial tissues of the back.

The origin, course and distribution of the posterior intercostal arteries indicate that, like the lumbar arteries in the abdomen, they are persistent intersegmental arteries.

(*b*) Two *subcostal arteries* arise in series with the intercostals. Each runs along the lower border of the twelfth rib and ends in the abdominal wall.

(*c*) Œsophageal, pericardial and bronchial arteries are small branches which are distributed to the œsophagus, pericardium and bronchi.

The **Thoracic Duct** begins in the abdomen at the upper end of the *cisterna chyli*, which is an elongated sac placed behind the right crus of the diaphragm and in contact with the right side of the bodies of the first and second lumbar vertebræ. The duct enters the thorax on the right side of the descending aorta and on the left side of the vena azygos, and ascends through the posterior mediastinum in company with those vessels. At first it lies behind the right pleural sac, but it soon comes to lie behind the œsophagus. As it ascends, it gradually crosses the median plane and gains the left border of the œsophagus. In the superior mediastinum it emerges from the angle between the aortic arch and the œsophagus, and runs upwards along the left edge of the œsophagus in contact with the left mediastinal pleura, the left subclavian and common carotid arteries in turn intervening. Its course in the neck is described on p. 247.

The thoracic duct returns lymph from both lower limbs, the abdomen (except for the upper surface of the right lobe of the liver), the left side of the thorax, the left side of the head and neck, and the left upper limb emptying at or near the junction of left jugular and subclavian veins.

On the right side a *right lymphatic duct* is usually found terminating in the angle between the internal jugular and the subclavian vein. It is formed by the union of the jugular, subclavian and right bronchomediastinal lymph trunks. The last-named returns lymph from the upper surface of the right lobe of the liver, the right lung and pleura, and the right side of the heart.

The **Vena Azygos** begins in the abdomen, where it is connected to the posterior aspect of the inferior vena cava opposite the point of entry of the renal veins. At its commencement it is very minute, but it attains a much greater size on being joined by a large vein formed by the union of the ascending lumbar and the subcostal vein of the right side. (These two veins are often considered the formative tributaries of the azygos.) Entering the thorax on the right side of the thoracic duct and the descending aorta, it runs upwards in front of the vertebral bodies and is overlapped by the right edge of the œsophagus. At the upper border of the root of the lung the vein emerges from under cover of the œsophagus and arches forwards above the right bronchus, crossing the right vagus and the right side of the trachea to reach the superior vena cava, in which it terminates. Its horizontal terminal portion is related to the mediastinal surface of the right lung and pleura. The terminal part of the vena azygos represents the cephalic end of the right posterior cardinal vein.

Tributaries. In addition to numerous small veins (œsophageal, pericardial, etc.), the vena azygos receives the two hemiazygos veins, the lower eight posterior intercostal veins of the right side and the right superior intercostal vein. The last-named is a common trunk formed by the veins from the second and third intercostal spaces and runs downwards to join the azygos vein as it arches forwards above the root of the right lung.

The *Inferior Vena Hemiazygos* collects the blood from the lower intercostal spaces of the left side and crosses the median plane under cover of the aorta and thoracic duct to join the vena azygos.

The *Superior Vena Hemiazygos* is formed by some of the upper left intercostal veins. It may join the inferior hemiazygos vein, or it may cross the median plane at a slightly higher level to terminate in the vena azygos.

The *Superior Intercostal Artery* is a branch of the subclavian artery (p. 249). It descends in front of the neck of the first rib, where it lies between the sympathetic trunk on the medial side and the anterior primary ramus of the first thoracic nerve on the lateral side. It has already been observed that the posterior intercostal arteries of the lower nine spaces are derived from the descending thoracic aorta. The corresponding arteries in the upper two spaces are given off by the superior intercostal.

The **Thoracic Part of the Sympathetic Trunk** is continuous above with the cervical and below with the lumbar parts of the trunk. It is situated on the heads of the ribs, against which it is plastered by the parietal pleura. Although, on morphological grounds, it would be reasonable to expect to find twelve thoracic ganglia, there are, in fact, usually eleven, and the number is frequently diminished by the fusion of neighbouring ganglia with one another.

Each ganglion is connected to the corresponding spinal nerve by a *grey* and a *white ramus communicans* (Plate XIII, p. 128), the latter containing the efferent preganglionic fibres from the spinal cord. As a rule, the highest white ramus communicans is an outflow from the first thoracic nerve.

In addition to these lateral branches, the thoracic ganglia give medial branches to the aorta (upper five ganglia), to the posterior pulmonary plexus (second, third and fourth ganglia), to the deep part of the cardiac plexus (second, third, fourth and fifth), and to the abdominal viscera. The latter branches are termed the *splanchnic nerves*, and are usually three in number.

(*a*) The *Greater Splanchnic Nerve* arises from the fifth, sixth, seventh, eighth and ninth ganglia, and runs downwards and forwards on the sides of the vertebral bodies into the posterior mediastinum. It leaves the thorax by piercing the crus of the diaphragm to join the *cœliac ganglion* (p. 190).

(*b*) The *Lesser Splanchnic Nerve* arises from the ninth and tenth (sometimes tenth and eleventh) ganglia and pierces the crus to terminate in a similar manner.

(*c*) The *Lowest Splanchnic Nerve* arises from the lowest thoracic ganglion and pierces the crus to join the sympathetic plexus on the renal artery.

The **Cardiac Plexus** (pp. 109, 117 and 124) is vagosympathetic in constitution and is formed, for the most part, by cervical branches of both nerves (pp. 236, 239). It consists of a *superficial part*, placed below the aortic arch and in front of the right pulmonary artery, and a *deep part*, placed in front of the bifurcation of the trachea. The vagus fibres are *inhibitory*, and the sympathetic are *accelerator* in function, the former being functionally more effective.

THE INTERVERTEBRAL JOINTS

The **Intervertebral Joints** of the thorax include (*a*) the joints of the vertebral bodies, and (*b*) the joints of the vertebral arches.

(*a*) The *Joints of the Vertebral Bodies* are placed between the opposed bodies of adjacent vertebræ and are cartilaginous in character. The opposed surfaces are covered by hyaline cartilage, and these cartilage-covered surfaces are connected to one another by an intervertebral disc of fibrocartilage. The deformability of the disc, which has a pulpy core (*nucleus pulposus*) in its substance, permits a small degree of movement between any two adjoining vertebræ.

Certain ligaments, which do not completely surround the joint, act as additional connecting media. (1) The *anterior longitudinal ligament* is placed on the anterior aspects of the vertebral bodies and extends from the atlas above to the first sacral segment below. (2) The *posterior longitudinal ligament* is similarly disposed on the posterior aspects of the vertebral bodies. Above, it becomes continuous with the membrana tectoria (p. 285), and so reaches the skull.

(*b*) The *Joints of the Vertebral Arches* are placed between the articular processes of adjacent vertebræ, and are synovial in gliding joints character. The joints receive additional support from (1) the ligamenta flava, (2) the supraspinous, (3) the interspinous, and (4) the intertransverse ligaments. These terms explain themselves, with the exception of (1). The ligamenta flava are attached in pairs to the anterior surface of the lamina above and to the upper border of the lamina below. They are composed of yellow elastic tissue, and probably have a part to play in maintaining the curvatures of the vertebral column and in restoring the flexed column to the erect posture.

The **Costovertebral Joints** include (*a*) the joints between the heads of the ribs and the bodies of the vertebræ, and (*b*) the joints between the tubercles of the ribs and the transverse processes of the vertebræ. Both groups are synovial joints. In the upper five or six costotransverse joints the articular surfaces are reciprocally curved and each permits rotatory movements of the corresponding rib around the long axis of its neck. In the lower joints the surfaces are plane and only gliding movement occurs.

Radiate Ligaments connect the heads of the ribs to the vertebral bodies with which they articulate, and *costotransverse ligaments* extend from the neck and the non-articular part of the tubercle to the transverse processes of the numerically corresponding vertebra and of the vertebra above.

The **Sternocostal Joints** are simple synovial joints of the plane variety, with the exception of the first, in which the costal cartilage is directly implanted on to the manubrium sterni.

Section IV

THE ABDOMEN

THE PERINEUM

The perineum can only be revised satisfactorily from a part in process of dissection. It is essential also for the student to have by him a dried pelvis in which the ligaments are intact.

It is convenient to subdivide the region into anterior or urogenital and posterior or anal parts, triangular on the surface, and for this purpose a line is drawn from the anterior part of one ischial tuberosity, in front of the anus, to the anterior part of the other

THE ANAL TRIANGLE

The **Anal Triangle** is bounded behind by the coccyx, and on each side by the ischial tuberosity and the sacrotuberous ligament, overlapped by the lower border of the gluteus maximus muscle. In the median plan the underlying region contains the lower part of the anal canal and the external sphincter muscle, and on each side of the median plane it includes the ischiorectal fossa.

The skin around the tip of the coccyx is supplied by the coccygeal plexus. Around the anus and over the ischiorectal fossa it is supplied by the inferior hæmorrhoidal nerve (S. 2, 3 and 4).

The *External Sphincter* muscle of the anus is attached posteriorly to the coccyx. The fibres run forwards on both sides of the anal canal to blend with the perineal body (p. 194). It is supplied by the perineal branch of S. 4 and also by the inferior hæmorrhoidal nerve.

The **Ischiorectal Fossa** lies below the lateral part of the pelvic diaphragm (p. 192). Its *medial wall* is formed by the levator ani and the anal canal, and the origin of the muscle from the fascia covering the parietal pelvic muscles (p. 192) shuts off the fossa from the pelvic cavity. The *lateral wall* is formed by the part of the obturator internus muscle and its covering fascia below the origin of the levator. In the posterior part of this wall the fascia shuts off communication with the gluteal region through the lesser sciatic foramen. *Posteriorly*, the fossa is limited by the sacrotuberous ligament, and, *anteriorly*, the base of the perineal membrane (p. 134) intervenes between the fossa and the urogenital triangle. The walls thus meet above at a sharp angle, the fossa being wedge-shaped.

The ischiorectal fossa contains a dense pad of fat, through which pass the branches of the internal pudendal vessels and nerve and the perineal branch of S. 4.

The **Internal Pudendal Artery** enters the perineum from the gluteal region by passing through the lesser sciatic foramen. Together with its accompanying vein and the pudendal nerve, it is enclosed at once in connective tissue closely applied to the fascia covering the obturator internus. Embedded in this fascial *pudendal canal*, the artery runs forwards in the lateral wall of the ischiorectal fossa, and then enters the urogenital triangle.

In this part of its course the internal pudendal artery gives off its *inferior rectal branch.* This vessel runs medially and downwards across the fossa and, having pierced the wall of the anal canal, ramifies in the submucous coat, where it anastomoses with the middle and superior rectal arteries.

The **Pudendal Nerve** is closely associated with the corresponding vessels. As it traverses the pudendal canal it divides into the dorsal nerve of the penis (or clitoris), which lies above the vessels, and the perineal nerve, which lies below them. From the latter the *inferior rectal nerve* arises. It crosses the ischiorectal fossa in company with the corresponding vessels, and is distributed (1) to the external sphincter, and (2) to the skin around the anus.

The *Inferior Rectal Vein* begins in the submucous tissue of the anal canal, where its radicles communicate freely with those of the superior and middle rectal veins (pp. 174 and 205). It terminates in the internal pudendal vein.

The *Perineal Branch of the Fourth Sacral Nerve* pierces the coccygeus muscle and enters the fossa at its posterior end. It runs forwards to be distributed to the skin and to the external sphincter muscle.

The *Lymph Vessels* of the lower half of the anal canal and of the skin of the anal triangle join the medial lymph nodes of the superficial inguinal group.

THE UROGENITAL TRIANGLE

This triangle overlies the anterior, or urogenital, part of the perineum. It is bounded in front by the pubic symphysis, on each side by the rami of the pubis and ischium, and posteriorly by a line drawn between the anterior parts of the ischial tuberosities.

The skin of this area includes the skin of the scrotum and penis. The *superficial nerves* which supply it are derived from three sources:

1. The terminal branches of the *ilio-inguinal nerve* (L. 1) supply the skin of the uppermost part of the scrotum (or labium majus).

2. The *Perineal* branch from the posterior cutaneous nerve of the thigh (p. 63) supplies the skin of the posterior part of the scrotum (or labium majus) and perineum.

3. (*a*) The *Scrotal* (*Labial*) *Nerves* arise from the perineal branch of the pudendal, and run forwards in the urogenital triangle to supply the skin of the perineum and scrotum (or labium majus).

(*b*) The *Dorsal Nerve of the Penis* (*or Clitoris*) is one of the terminal branches of the pudendal nerve. It is distributed to the skin of the penis (p. 135) or clitoris (p. 138).

Small superficial branches from the internal pudendal artery supply the skin of the perineum and scrotum (or labium majus).

The *Dartos Muscle* is a thin sheet of involuntary muscle which replaces the fatty superficial fascia over the scrotum. Over the penis the superficial fascia is devoid of fat, but elsewhere in the perineum the usual fatty covering is present.

The deepest layer of the superficial fascia is membranous in character and contains no fat. It is continuous with a similar layer of fascia in the lower part of the anterior abdominal wall (p. 139).

The arrangement and attachments of this layer of fascia are quite definite, and they are of importance, because they determine the directions in which extravasated urine will spread after rupture of the spongy portion of the urethra.

Anteriorly, where it becomes continuous with the fascia of the abdominal wall, the sheet is narrow and is attached at its borders to the bodies of the pubic bones. In the median plane, however, it is free. This portion of the fascia gives off to the penis a tubular investment, which is continuous behind with a sac-like investment given to the scrotum.

On reaching the pubic arch the fascial sheet widens out and is attached on each side to the margins of the pubic and ischial rami. Posteriorly, it blends with the base of the perineal membrane (p. 134).

The **Superficial Perineal Space** contains the spongy portion of the urethra, the structures forming the root of the penis, and the associated muscles. Its superficial limit is the fascial layer described above, while its deep boundary is the perineal membrane. The space is closed behind by the fusion of the roof with the floor, and on each side by the attachments of the walls to the margins of the pubic arch. In front, however, this pouch-like region is open. Urine, extravasated following rupture of the spongy portion of the urethra, fills the posterior part of the pouch and then spreads into the scrotum and penis. If allowed to go further, it will ascend in front of the pubic symphysis and so reach the anterior abdominal wall.

The **Superficial Perineal Muscles.** The *Superficial Transverse Perineal Muscle* arises from the medial aspect of the ischial ramus immediately in front of the tuberosity and is inserted into the perineal body (p. 194).

The *Ischiocavernosus* arises close to the preceding muscle and covers the free surface of the crus, into which it is inserted anteriorly.

The *Bulbospongiosus* arises from the perineal body and from a median raphe which separates the two halves of the muscle on the inferior surface of the bulb. The fibres are inserted in three groups: (1) The posterior fibres cover the bulb and are inserted into the perineal membrane. (2) The intermediate fibres pass round the posterior part of the corpus spongiosum penis and are inserted into a common aponeurosis on its dorsal surface. (3) The anterior fibres diverge from one another, cross the corpora cavernosa and wind round them to be inserted into a common aponeurosis on the dorsum of the penis.

All the superficial perineal muscles are supplied by the *perineal branch of the pudendal nerve.*

Actions. The two transverse muscles act together to steady the perineal body (p. 194) during defæcation and to fix it during contraction of the external sphincter and bulbospongiosus.

The actions of the ischiocavernosus muscles are by no means obvious. They may, and probably do, play some part in connexion with erection of the penis (p. 136), possibly by helping the fibrous envelope of the corpora cavernosa to withstand overdistension.

The bulbospongiosus compresses the bulb against the perineal membrane and constricts the corpus spongiosum penis, thus assisting in the evacuation of the last drops of urine or seminal fluid from the urethra. The muscle also plays some part in penile erection.

The **Roots of the Penis** comprise the bulb and the two crura. The *bulb* is the expanded posterior end of the corpus spongiosum. It is closely applied to the inferior aspect of the perineal membrane, and its deep surface is pierced by the urethra. Superficially it is covered by the bulbospongiosus muscle.

The *Crus* is the tapering posterior end of the corpus cavernosum penis. It is closely attached to the medial aspect of the corresponding side of the pubic arch, and its free surface is covered by the ischiocavernosus muscle. The internal pudendal artery and the dorsal nerve of the penis pierce the perineal membrane under cover of the anterior end of the crus.

Both the bulb and the crura, like the corpora cavernosa, the corpus spongiosum and the glans penis, consist of erectile tissue, which is characterised by a sponge-work of cavernous spaces, filled with venous blood and capable of considerable distension.

The **Perineal Branch of the Pudendal Nerve** runs forwards in the pudendal canal and terminates in the superficial perineal pouch.

Branches. (*a*) *Muscular*, to levator ani and the superficial perineal muscles.

(*b*) *Cutaneous*—the scrotal (labial) nerves (p. 132).

(*c*) A branch to the bulb.

The **Urogenital Diaphragm (Perineal Membrane)** is above the superficial perineal space, and is mostly hidden by the structures of root of the penis and by the superficial perineal muscles. It fills up the gap of the pubic arch, to which it is attached on each side. Posteriorly, its base blends with the fascial roof of the pouch and with the perineal body (p. 194). Anteriorly, however, it does not reach the symphysis pubis, but leaves a gap for the passage of the unpaired *deep dorsal vein of the penis* into the pelvis. The dorsal nerve of the penis passes through the lateral part of the same gap on each side.

Several structures pierce the perineal membrane to enter the superficial perineal pouch.

1. The urethra pierces it in the median plane, 1 inch below the symphysis pubis, and is accompanied, on each side, by the small duct of the bulbo-urethral gland, which opens into the spongy portion.

2. The artery to the bulb of the penis pierces the diaphragm a little to the lateral side of the urethra.

3. The internal pudendal artery pierces the diaphragm close to its lateral attachment, and under cover of the anterior part of the crus.

4. The vagina, in addition, in the female.

The **Deep Perineal Space** is separated from the superficial by the urogenital diaphragm, and from the anterior part of the pelvis by the fibrous tissue which forms the sheath of the prostate and contributes to the formation of the perineal body. It contains (1) the sphincter urethræ and the deep transverse perineal muscles; (2) the membranous part of the urethra; (3) the bulbo-urethral glands; (4) the internal pudendal artery and the artery to the bulb of the penis; and (5) the dorsal nerve of the penis (or clitoris).

1. The *sphincter urethræ* muscle arises from the pubic arch on a level with the urethra, and its fibres diverge as they pass medially to surround it. They are inserted into a median raphe both on its superior and on its inferior aspect. The *nerve supply* is derived from the perineal branch of the pudendal nerve, and the *action* of the muscle is indicated by its name.

2. The *Membranous Part of the Urethra* is $\frac{1}{2}$ inch long and lies

1 inch below the pubic symphysis. *It is the shortest and most fixed part of the tube*, and is surrounded by the sphincter urethræ. Above, it is continuous with the prostatic urethra; below, it is continuous with the spongy urethra. The prostatic and membranous parts are directed downwards and forwards, but the spongy part curves upwards and forwards in the bulb of the penis before it turns downwards in the corpus spongiosum. A circular muscle coat surrounds the membranous part of the urethra and is continuous above with the muscle fibres of the prostate.

3. The *Bulbo-urethral Glands* are two small pea-like bodies which lie postero-lateral to the membranous urethra and under cover of its sphincter muscle. Their ducts pass through the urethral opening in the perineal membrane and open into the floor of the spongy portion of the urethra.

4. The *Internal Pudendal Artery* passes forwards from the pudendal canal above the urogenital diaphragm. It lies under cover of the pubic arch and has the dorsal nerve of the penis on its lateral side. Under cover of the anterior part of the crus it pierces the perineal membrane, and enters the superficial pouch, where it at once divides into (*a*) the dorsal artery of the penis (or clitoris), and (*b*) the deep artery of the penis (or clitoris).

Branches. (i) The *Artery to the Bulb* runs medially on the surface of the deep transverse perineal muscle, and pierces the perineal membrane to end in the bulb.

(ii) The *Dorsal Artery of the Penis* runs forwards in the interval between the corpus cavernosum and the corpus spongiosum penis and so reaches the dorsum of the penis. Here the two arteries lie one on each side of the deep dorsal vein, which is median in position. The dorsal nerve lies lateral to the artery, and both vessels and nerves are enclosed between the two layers of the *suspensory ligament* of the penis. This is a triangular, fibrous band which passes from the front of the symphysis pubis to the proximal part of the dorsum of the penis, where it splits into right and left layers which blend with the fascial sheath of the organ. The vessel supplies the body of the penis and terminates in the glans. The *dorsal artery of the clitoris*, though much smaller, has a like distribution.

(iii) The *Deep Artery of the Penis* pierces the medial aspect of the anterior part of the crus and runs forwards in the corpus cavernosum penis, to which it supplies the *helicine arteries* (p. 136). The *deep artery of the clitoris* is similar.

5. The *Dorsal Nerve of the Penis* (*Clitoris*) arises from the pudendal nerve in the pudendal canal and accompanies the internal pudendal and the dorsal arteries, which lie to its medial side. It supplies

branches to the corpus cavernosum, glans and skin of the penis or clitoris.

The **Penis** consists of two *corpora cavernosa penis*, placed side by side on its dorsal aspect, and the *corpus spongiosum penis* closely applied to their ventral surface. Posteriorly, the corpora cavernosa penis taper off into the crura and the corpus spongiosum expands into the bulb. Distally, the latter is continued as the acorn-like *glans penis*, and both are traversed by the urethra. In the latter situation the urethra has an elongated dilatation, termed the *fossa terminalis* (fossa navicularis).

The two corpora cavernosa are enclosed in strong, fibrous envelopes, the density of which accounts for the fact that, when the contained cavernous spaces of the erectile tissue become distended with blood, the flaccid penis is converted into the firm, erect organ.

The corpus spongiosum is surrounded by a much thinner fibrous covering, and all three corpora are in turn surrounded by the *fascia penis*, which is directly continuous with the membranous layer of the superficial fascia of the perineum (p. 132). The superficial dorsal vein of the penis lies in the loose areolar tissue between the fascia penis and the skin; the *deep dorsal vein* and the dorsal nerves and arteries lie between the fascia penis and the fascial envelope of the corpora cavernosa.

The factors which contribute to produce erection of the penis are (1) dilatation of the small, tortuous *helicine arteries* (branches of the deep arteries of the penis), which pour an increased amount of blood directly into the cavernous spaces; (2) retardation of the outflow from the veins of the penis, due to the pressure of the engorged corpora cavernosa and possibly also to the contraction of the ischio-cavernosi muscles (p. 133), and (3) the strong, fibrous envelope of the corpora cavernosa (*vide supra*).

The *prepuce* is a retractible fold of skin which more or less completely hides the glans and is connected to the notch on its margin just below the urethral orifice by a fold, termed the *frenulum*. The outer covering of the glans is a thin layer of modified skin.

The penis is developed from the genital tubercle, which develops in both sexes at the headward end of the cloacal membrane. After the partition of the cloaca, the urogenital membrane breaks down, and in both sexes the urogenital orifice lies in the perineum caudal to the genital tubercle, which has enlarged to form the phallus. In the male, however, the orifice is continuous with a groove along the ventral aspect of the phallus. The original orifice becomes closed and the borders of the groove fuse from behind forwards, so that a new orifice is formed which moves progressively forwards to the base of the developing glans. In this way the penile portion of the urethra is formed by the fusion of folds which are homologous with the labia minora in the female. The fossa terminalis is the last part of the urethra to be completed and it is formed by bilateral extensions of the glans in a ventral direction.

The prepuce develops as an almost circular ridge in the epithelium covering the phallus and extends distally to cover the dorsal aspect of the glans completely and the sides partially. As already indicated the lateral parts of the preputial fold grow ventrally with the corresponding parts of the glans and, when they fuse, the frenulum persists as a permanent glandulo-preputial connexion. Prior to birth the epithelial cells between the surface of the glans and the covering prepuce begin to desquamate, but the preputial space so formed is not complete until towards the end of the first year, when, in most cases the prepuce can be retracted.

The **Scrotum** is a rugose pouch of very thin skin, which encloses the testes and the lower ends of the spermatic cords. Its rugosity, which varies with temperatures, mood, and health, is attributable to the presence immediately under the skin of a layer of plain muscle, termed the *dartos muscle*, which replaces the superficial fascia. This muscle sends a median vertical partition between the testes. A median raphe forms a slightly raised ridge on the surface of the scrotum and indicates the development of the scrotum from two lateral labioscrotal swellings, which become fused in the male but remain separate as the labia majora in the female.

THE FEMALE PERINEUM

The Anal Triangle needs no special description (p. 130).

The structures underlying the Urogenital Triangles in male and female possess many features in common, but the external genital organs require a separate description.

The *Mons Pubis* is a rounded hairy surface projection lying in front of the pubes. It is caused by an underlying pad of dense fat.

The *Labia Majora* are two elongated skin folds, which form the lateral boundaries of the pudendal cleft. They are united to each other in front below the mons pubis to form the *anterior commissure*. Similarly, a *posterior commissure* connects the posterior ends of the labia majora in front of the anus. The inner surfaces of the labia are covered with modified skin, which possesses numerous sebaceous glands.

The *Labia Minora* are two similar but shorter folds which lie within the pudendal cleft. The posterior ends are connected by a short transverse fold, termed the *frenulum labiorum*. Their anterior extremities split each into two layers, the lateral of which meet above the clitoris and form its *prepuce*. The medial layers are attached to the inferior aspect of the glans of the clitoris and constitute its *frenulum*.

The *Vestibule of the Vagina* lies between the labia minora and in front of the frenulum labiorum. In it the urethral orifice is placed, immediately in front of the opening of the vagina. A small depression, termed the *vestibular fossa*, lies behind the orifice of the vagina.

The *Clitoris* lies at the front or apex of the vestibule. It is homologous with the penis, and has a similar structure. The glans is hidden by the prepuce.

The *Superficial Perineal Space* is formed in the way already described for the male subject (p. 132). It contains the crura of the clitoris, the bulb of the vestibule, the superficial perineal muscles, and the terminal parts of the urethra and the vagina.

The *Crus of the Clitoris* corresponds to the crus penis in position, relations, structure and function. Like the male structure, but much smaller it is covered by an ischiocavernosus muscle.

The *Bulb of the Vestibule* corresponds to the bulb of the penis but, owing to the presence of the vagina, it is a bilateral structure. Each half lies below the urogenital diaphragm in contact with the lateral wall of the vagina. It is covered by the bulbospongiosus muscle. The bulb consists of erectile tissue and its two halves are united to each other in front of the urethra by a venous plexus, termed the *bulbar commissure*. Anteriorly, the commissure joins the glans clitoridis and so corresponds to the corpus spongiosum penis.

The *Ischiocavernosus* and the *Transversus Perinei Muscles* require no special description.

The *Bulbospongiosus* is attached behind to the perineal body, and its fibres diverge to surround the vagina and to cover the bulb of the vestibule. In front they are attached to the body of the clitoris. The muscle acts as a sphincter for the vagina.

The *Perineal Body* is a small, wedge-shaped, fibromuscular mass which intervenes between the lower end of the vagina and the anal canal. Fibres from the sphincters of the vagina and anus, and from the levatores ani, enter into its constitution (*see also* p. 134).

The Perineal Membrane is not so strongly developed in the female subject, and it is interrupted by the passage through it of the vagina.

The **Greater Vestibular Glands** correspond to the bulbo-urethral glands, but they differ in position and in the mode of termination of their ducts. They lie under cover of the bulbospongiosus at the posterior extremity of the bulb of the vestibule, and are intimately related to the lateral walls of the vagina. The two ducts run down in the vaginal wall and open into the lower part of the vagina near the posterior part of each labium minus.

The **Urethra** is only 1½ inches long. It curves downwards and forwards to open into the vestibule an inch below the clitoris.

The vessels and nerves are very similar to those already described for the male subject. The clitoris is supplied by dorsal arteries and nerves in the same way as the penis.

THE ABDOMINAL WALL

(This title covers the structures forming the front and sides of the abdominal cavity. For the posterior part, v. p. 176.)

Cutaneous Nerves. The skin of the anterior abdominal wall is supplied by the lower six thoracic and the first lumbar nerves (anterior rami). The former give off anterior and lateral branches, but the lateral branch of the last thoracic nerve crosses the iliac crest to supply the skin of the buttock. The first lumbar nerve is represented by (1) the *anterior branch of the iliohypogastric nerve*, which pierces the external oblique aponeurosis about 1 inch above the superficial inguinal ring, and (2) the *ilioinguinal nerve*, which emerges through the superficial inguinal ring.

These nerves (T. 7–L. 1) supply successive and practically horizontal bands of skin, *T. 10 supplying the band which includes the umbilicus*. These segmental supplies overlays each other.

The **Superficial Veins** of the anterior abdominal wall form upper and lower groups on each side. The *upper group* returns the blood *via* the lateral thoracic and internal thoracic veins to the superior vena cava, and the *lower group* returns the blood *via* the femoral vein to the inferior vena cava. All four groups anastomose freely with one another, and their position amongst the soft, yielding fat of the abdominal wall allows the anastomosing channels to become widely dilated in obstruction of either the inferior or the superior vena cava, or in obstruction of the external or common iliac veins.

The radicles of the *para-umbilical veins* (p. 174) communicate with both groups, constituting an important connexion between the portal and the systemic venous systems.

The *Superficial Lymph Vessels* of the infra-umbilical region drain into the superficial inguinal lymph nodes (p. 51), and those of the supra-umbilical region into the pectoral lymph nodes (p. 10).

In the lower part of the wall the deepest layer of the superficial fascia is membranous in character. Its upper border is indefinite, but inferiorly it is firmly connected to the deep fascia on the front of the thigh just below the inguinal ligament. Medially, it is attached to the body of the pubis, but, instead of being attached to the pubes across the median plane, this portion of the sheet passes down into the perineum, where it forms the superficial boundary of the superficial perineal pouch (p. 132).

Muscles of the Anterior Abdominal Wall. The principal function of the abdominal muscles is to assist in respiration and defæcation, and, by their normal tonus, to exercise an important influence over the position of the abdominal viscera. They are also essential to other less common expulsive efforts, such as vomiting and childbirth.

The **External Oblique** is the most superficial of the three lateral abdominal muscles. Its fibres pass *from above* downwards, forwards and medially. It arises from the lower eight ribs, interdigitating with the serratus anterior and latissimus dorsi. Trace the fibres to their insertion consecutively. The lowermost fibres of origin descend vertically to be inserted into the anterior half of the iliac crest (outer lip). The remaining fibres end in a broad aponeurosis, so that *no fleshy fibres are found below the line joining the anterior superior spine to the umbilicus*. Between its attachments to the anterior superior spine and the pubic tubercle the lower border of the aponeurosis is folded backwards on itself, constituting the *inguinal ligament*, which is firmly attached to the deep fascia of the thigh. Above the pubic tubercle the aponeurosis is "pierced" by the spermatic cord, over which it is in reality continued as a thin covering, the *external spermatic fascia*. The artificial gap, created by severing the connexion of this fascia with the aponeurosis, constitutes the *superficial inguinal ring*. Medial to the ring the aponeurosis is attached to the pubic crest and symphysis, and then along the linea alba to the xiphoid process. The uppermost fibres, stretching from the fifth rib to the xiphoid, are therefore practically horizontal.

The *Pectineal Part of the Inguinal Ligament* occupies the small angular interval between the medial end of the inguinal ligament and the anterior end of the pectineal line. *Its lateral border is free and forms the medial boundary of the femoral ring as the lacunar ligament* (p. 53). Directly continuous with the inguinal ligament, it constitutes an additional insertion for the external oblique muscle.

The **Internal Oblique** lies deep to the external oblique, and its fibres run upwards, forwards and medially. Trace the fibres of origin consecutively. The lowest fibres arise from the lateral half, or more, of the grooved surface of the inguinal ligament. The next fibres arise from the intermediate area (middle lip) of the iliac crest, from the anterior superior spine backwards for two-thirds of its extent, where they meet the lateral edge of the lumbar fascia, up which the line of origin extends.

Trace the fibres to their insertion in the reverse order. The highest fibres of origin, fleshy throughout, are inserted into the lower borders of the twelfth, eleventh and tenth ribs and costal cartilages. The remaining fibres form a broad aponeurosis, the line of whose attachment extends upwards *along the costal margin* to the xiphoid process and then down the linea alba to the pubic symphysis. The lowest fibres arch medially above the spermatic cord and then descend behind it to reach the pubic crest and adjoining part of the pectineal line. Towards their insertion these fibres become tendinous and are joined, on their deep surface, by the lowest fibres of the transversus, to constitute the *conjoint tendon.*

The conjoint tendon has a free lateral border, but medially it is continuous with the rest of the aponeurosis of the internal oblique and, therefore, with the lowest part of the anterior wall of the sheath of the rectus abdominis muscle.

The **Transversus** is the deepest of the three lateral abdominal muscles. Its fibres run horizontally forwards. Trace the line of origin continuously, as in the case of the internal oblique. The highest fibres arise from the deep surfaces of the seventh to the twelfth costal cartilages, interdigitating with the diaphragm. The muscle gradually widens from above downwards, and the line of origin next descends along the lateral edge of the lumbar fascia to the iliac crest, and is then continued forwards along the anterior two-thirds of its inner lip to the anterior superior spine. Finally, the lowest fibres arise from the lateral third of the inguinal ligament.

Trace the insertion, which is entirely aponeurotic, in the same way. The highest fibres are short and pass medially to the xiphoid process, and the line of insertion then follows the linea alba to the pubic symphysis. The lowest fibres help to form the conjoint tendon (*vide supra*). In its upper part the aponeurosis is very narrow, and *fleshy fibres of transversus lie behind the rectus muscle.* As it is traced downwards, the aponeurosis widens out, but inferiorly it again becomes narrow.

The **Rectus Abdominis,** which is enclosed within a strong aponeurotic sheath, arises from the front of the pubis and the pubic crest, and, widening out as it ascends, crosses the costal margin to be inserted into the xiphoid process and the cartilages of the seventh, sixth, and fifth ribs. In the living subject its lateral margin corresponds to a conspicuous furrow, termed the *linea semilunaris,* which descends from the tip of the ninth costal cartilage and inclines medially at its lower end towards the pubic tubercle (Plate II, p. 16).

Its anterior surface is crossed by three *tendinous intersections,* one opposite the umbilicus, one opposite the xiphoid process, and a third midway between the other two. *The muscle is firmly adherent to the anterior wall of the sheath where these intersections occur, but, as the latter do not penetrate its whole depth, the muscle is nowhere adherent to the posterior wall of its sheath.* The rectus abdominis is developed from portions of the lower six thoracic myotomes and the tendinous intersections represent persistent intersegmental tissue.

The **Rectus Sheath** is in fact the aponeuroses of the three lateral abdominal muscles. Above the costal margin the posterior wall is absent and the anterior wall is formed by the external oblique aponeurosis. From the costal margin to a point, roughly midway between the umbilicus and the pubic symphysis, the internal oblique aponeurosis splits into two lamellæ, of which the anterior blends with the aponeurosis of the external oblique, and the posterior with that of the transversus muscle to form the corresponding walls of the sheath. It must be remembered, however, that *fleshy* fibres of the transversus muscle lie behind the upper part of the rectus. In its lower part the anterior wall of the sheath is formed by the aponeuroses of all three muscles, while the posterior wall, which possesses a free curved lower border termed the *arcuate (semicircular) line*, is entirely deficient, the rectus here coming into contact with the fascia transversalis.

The **Linea Alba,** which extends from the pubic symphysis to the xiphoid process, is a strong fibrous raphe formed by the interlacement of the aponeuroses of the lateral muscles of the two sides. Narrow below the umbilicus, it widens out superiorly. It contains no blood vessels of any size, and can therefore be incised freely without hæmorrhage. In the muscular young adult it can easily be identified in the interval between the two recti (Plate II, p. 16).

The **Pyramidalis,** which arises from the front of the pubis and is inserted into the lower part of the linea alba, is a small triangular muscle which lies between the rectus and the anterior wall of its sheath. It acts as a tensor of the linea alba, and is supplied by the last thoracic nerve. It is frequently absent.

The **Nerves of the Anterior Abdominal Wall** run at first in the interval between the internal oblique and the transversus muscle and then enter the rectus sheath. The *seventh* and *eighth* nerves pierce the posterior lamella of the internal oblique aponeurosis at the costal margin. They then run *upwards* and medially behind the rectus muscle before piercing it. The *ninth* nerve runs medially with a slight downward inclination, but the *tenth*, *eleventh* and *last thoracic nerves* descend appreciably as they pass medially. All four pierce the posterior layer of the internal oblique aponeurosis at the lateral edge of the rectus sheath, and continue medially behind the muscle before they pierce its substance. All these nerves supply the three lateral abdominal muscles and the rectus abdominis. In addition, the last thoracic nerve supplies the pyramidalis. Finally they pass out through the anterior wall of the sheath to end by supplying the skin.

Both the iliohypogastric and the ilioinguinal nerves supply branches to the lowest parts of the internal oblique and the transversus, and hence neither enters the rectus sheath (p. 134).

The **Transversalis Fascia** forms a complete fascial lining for the anterior and lateral abdominal walls, deep to the muscles and their aponeuroses. It may be regarded as a part of an abdominopelvic fascial envelope, which lies immediately outside the extra-peritoneal fat. The principal arterial trunks of the abdominal walls and pelvis lie, at first, inside this fascial envelope, and the femoral sheath may be regarded as a downward prolongation of the envelope behind the inguinal ligament. *The principal nerves, on the other hand, lie outside the fascial envelope*, and so it comes about that the femoral nerve is not enclosed inside the femoral sheath.

The fascia transversalis is attached to the inner lip of the iliac crest and the lateral half of the inguinal ligament, in both situations becoming continuous with the fascia iliaca. It is then drawn downwards to form the anterior part of the femoral sheath, and more medially is attached to the pectineal line and the pubic crest. Above the middle of the inguinal ligament it is pierced by the spermatic cord at the *deep inguinal ring*, and the edges of this opening are continued on to the cord as the *internal spermatic fascia*.

The **Inferior Epigastric Artery** arises from the external iliac just above the inguinal ligament. It runs upwards and medially in the extraperitoneal fat along the medial side of the deep inguinal ring. After piercing the transversalis fascia it comes into direct contact with the posterior surface of the rectus muscle, and runs upwards, passing in front of the arcuate line. Its terminal branches enter the rectus and anastomose with those of the superior epigastric artery.

It gives off (1) a *Cremasteric* branch to the spermatic cord, and (2) a *Pubic* branch, and other muscular and cutaneous branches. The pubic branch runs downwards and medially to the posterior surface of the pubis, where it anastomoses with the pubic branch of the obturator artery (p. 204). It would be of no importance were it not that this anastomosing channel is frequently enlarged and straightened out to form the main trunk of the obturator artery, which is therefore, in these cases, a branch of the inferior epigastric. It is then termed the *abnormal obturator artery*, and in its course to the obturator foramen it comes into close relationship with the femoral ring. It would, therefore, be intimately related to the neck of the sac of a femoral hernia, should one occur.

The *Superior Epigastric Artery* is one of the terminal branches of the internal thoracic. It passes downwards between the sternal and costal origins of the diaphragm, crosses the upper border of the transversus, and so enters the rectus sheath. It descends vertically, supplying the rectus muscle, and anastomoses with the inferior epigastric artery.

The **Deep Circumflex Iliac Artery** arises from the lateral side of the external iliac opposite the origin of the inferior epigastric. It runs laterally and upwards parallel to the inguinal ligament, pierces the fascia transversalis, and is continued along the iliac crest. It pierces the transversus muscle opposite the middle of the crest and terminates in the interval between the transversus and the internal oblique. In the region of the anterior superior spine of the ilium, branches of this artery anastomose with branches from the superior gluteal and the lateral circumflex femoral arteries.

Just behind the anterior superior iliac spine it gives off an *ascending branch*, which runs upwards between the transversus and the internal oblique muscles.

The **Inguinal Canal** commences at the *deep inguinal ring*, which is situated in the transversalis fascia about half an inch above the mid-inguinal point (*i.e.*, midway between the symphysis pubis and the anterior superior spine of the ilium). It passes, medially, forwards and downwards through the lower part of the anterior abdominal wall to the *superficial inguinal ring*, which lies in the external oblique aponeurosis above the lateral part of the pubic crest, the pubic tubercle and the medial end of the inguinal ligament. It is about $1\frac{1}{2}$ inches in length, and it is occupied by the spermatic cord in the male and by the round ligament of the uterus in the female.

The *Anterior Wall* of the canal is formed by the external oblique aponeurosis and also, in its lateral part, by the lowest fibres of origin of the internal oblique. *Consequently this wall is strongest where it lies opposite to the deep inguinal ring.*

The *Posterior Wall* of the canal is formed by the fascia transversalis and, in its medial part, by the conjoint tendon. *Consequently this wall is strongest where it lies opposite to the superficial inguinal ring.*

The *Floor* of the canal is formed by the grooved surface of the inguinal ligament and, at its medial end, by the pectineal part of that ligament.

The *Roof* of the canal is formed by the arched lower border of the internal oblique muscle.

Observe the threefold relationship which the lower fibres of the internal oblique bear to the spermatic cord. They arch obliquely across it in much the same way as a railway bridge obliquely may span a road.

Before the muscles of the abdominal wall become differentiated, the site of the inguinal canal is occupied by the *gubernaculum testis.* This is a bundle of unstriped muscle fibres connected at one end to the labioscrotal swelling and, at the other, to the lower pole of the testis or ovary, which pass the earlier stages of their development on the posterior abdominal wall and in the pelvis, close to the deep inguinal ring in the case of the testis. During the seventh month of fœtal life the testis passes through the inguinal canal into the scrotum, preceded by a peritoneal diverticulum, termed the *processus vaginalis*, and dragging its vessels, nerves, and duct after it. As these structures pass through the deep inguinal ring, they evaginate the transversalis fascia so as to obtain a tubular covering, termed the *internal spermatic fascia.* Having entered the canal through the deep inguinal ring, they have next to pass below the curved lower border of the internal oblique and, as they do so, they drag down the lowest fibres with them in a series of loops, thus gaining a second covering, named the *cremaster muscle* and *cremasteric fascia.* Finally, at the superficial inguinal ring, they evaginate the aponeurosis of the external oblique so as to form a superficial tubular covering, termed the *external spermatic fascia.* Thus the testis and the spermatic cord acquire three coverings as they traverse the canal, and do not, in fact, puncture the abdominal wall at all.

The *Processus Vaginalis,* in the normal case, becomes shut off from the general peritoneal cavity at, or shortly before, birth, and loses its lumen except in its lowest part, which becomes the tunica vaginalis of the testis. Sometimes the processus retains its connexion with the peritoneal cavity, and it is then a potential hernial sac. Should a hernia descend into this ready-made sac, it must lie within the identical coverings of the spermatic cord. Such a hernia can only enter the inguinal canal at the deep inguinal ring, and all such herniæ are known as *oblique inguinal herniæ.* The proximal part of the sac lies at the deep inguinal ring and is termed the neck of the sac. *The neck of the sac of an oblique inguinal hernia has the inferior epigastric artery to its medial side.*

A hernia may, however, push its way into the inguinal canal medial to the inferior epigastric artery, *i.e.*, at some point in the posterior wall other than the deep inguinal ring. Such a hernia is termed a *direct inguinal hernia* and, as it has no preformed sac, it has to form one for itself by thrusting the parietal peritoneum in front of it. *The neck of the sac of a direct inguinal hernia usually has the inferior epigastric artery to its lateral side.* The hernia, in its sac, pushes the transversalis fascia in front of it into the canal and so acquires a covering similar to the internal spermatic fascia of the spermatic cord but not identical with it. But, although herniæ may enter the canal at more points than one, they can leave the canal only by passing through the superficial inguinal ring. In this way a direct hernia descends inside the external spermatic fascia and so insinuates itself amongst the coverings of the spermatic cord.

It should be observed that although the inguinal canal necessarily constitutes a potential weakness in the anterior abdominal wall, that weakness is lessened by the fact that the two abdominal rings do not lie opposite to each other, *i.e.*, by the obliquity of the canal. Consequently, any force which would tend to thrust a hernia into the canal helps to counteract this effect by pressing the posterior wall against the anterior wall, and in normal health the weakness is trivial.

The **Spermatic Cord** commences at the deep inguinal ring. Within the abdomen its constituent parts are widely separated, but from the deep inguinal ring to the testis they are wrapped up together within the coverings already described (p. 140). Inside the inguinal canal the cord is related to the structures which form its walls, floor and roof (*vide supra*). From the superficial inguinal ring to the testis it is covered only by the skin, the superficial fascia (dartos muscle in the scrotum), and the membranous layer of the superficial fascia (p. 132), and is crossed by the superficial external pudendal artery from the femoral. As it leaves the inguinal canal it crosses the medial end of the inguinal ligament and the pubic tubercle, and then the origin of the adductor longus and the deep external pudendal vessels.

Constituents of the Spermatic Cord. (1) The *vas deferens* (p. 199) is easily identified in the spermatic cord of the living subject. On examination it feels like a piece of whipcord, this character being due to the thickness of the wall relative to the narrow lumen. (2) Three *arteries* run down in the spermatic cord: (*a*) The *testicular artery* from the abdominal aorta is the principal artery of supply to the testis and the epididymis. It anastomoses with (*b*) the *artery to the vas deferens*, which closely accompanies the duct and usually arises from the persistent proximal end of the umbilical artery (p. 200). (*c*) The *cremasteric artery*, which arises from the inferior epigastric close to the deep inguinal ring, supplies the coverings. (3) Numerous veins and lymph vessels ascend from the testis and epididymis. The former constitute the *pampiniform plexus*. (4) The genital branch of the genitofemoral nerve (L. 1 and 2) supplies the cremaster muscle and a sensory branch to the tunica vaginalis. Sympathetic fibres from the renal and aortic plexuses (carried by the testicular artery) and from the pelvic plexus (carried by the artery to the vas deferens) supply branches to the testis (T. 10) and to the epididymis (T. 11 and 12 and L. 1). (5) There are also remains of the processus vaginalis.

Though very mobile, the **Testis** usually lies in the scrotum with its long axis oblique, the upper pole of the gland being tilted forwards. The vas deferens and the epididymis are applied to its posterior border, the former to the medial side of the latter. Anteriorly and on each side the testis is enveloped by the tunica vaginalis, which, is usually a completely closed sac. The visceral layer of the tunica vaginalis is adherent to the testis and becomes continuous with the parietal layer at the upper and lower poles of the gland and along the posterior parts of both of its sides. On the lateral aspect of the gland it is reflected on to the medial side of the epididymis to line the small *sinus of the epididymis*, which partially separates the body of the epididymis from the testis.

Outside the tunica vaginalis the testis possesses coverings continuous with those of the spermatic cord (p. 145). The *tunica albuginea* is a complete fibrous covering of the testis, deep to the tunica vaginalis. Along the posterior border of the gland it is considerably thickened, constituting the *mediastinum testis*, from which incomplete fibrous septa pass forwards to subdivide the gland into lobes. The convoluted seminiferous tubules, which are the actively functioning structures, lie in the lobes and pass backwards into the mediastinum testis, where they unite with one another to form a network, termed the *rete testis*. From this network about twenty efferent ductules arise, which emerge from the *upper pole* of the testis to enter the head of the epididymis.

The testis is developed on the medial side of the mesonephric ridge as a patch of thickened cœlomic epithelium. The germinal cells lie at first deep to its free surface, but later they migrate into its substance, where they become incorporated in the germinal cords, which are formed by ingrowths from the covering cœlomic epithelium. The deeper parts of the germinal cords establish connexions with one another to form the *rete testis*, while their more superficial parts form the seminiferous tubules. The rete cords become canaliculised and connect up with some of the glomerular capsules. In this way they become connected to the mesonephric duct, which forms the canal of the epididymis and the vas deferens.

The **Epididymis** is an elongated structure applied to the lateral part of the posterior border of the testis. Its upper end, or *head*, is enlarged and sits like a cap on the upper pole of the testis, to which it is connected by the efferent ductules. The body and tail of the epididymis are attached to the gland only by connective tissue.

Within the head, the efferent ductules unite to form the canal of the epididymis, which is coiled up in a very remarkable manner within the body and the tail. When unravelled it is found to be nearly 20 feet in length. This duct emerges from the tail as the *vas deferens,* which ascends medial to the epididymis to enter the spermatic cord.

The *Lymph Vessels* of the testis and epididymis ascend in the spermatic cord, and terminate in the aortic lymph nodes, which are closely related to the abdominal aorta.

THE ABDOMINAL CAVITY

In order to facilitate the description of the topography of the abdominal viscera, the cavity can be subdivided into nine regions by means of two vertical and two horizontal planes. The two vertical planes pass through the mid-inguinal points and are termed the *right* and *left lateral planes.* The upper horizontal plane is drawn round the body at the level of the lowest points on the tenth costal cartilages, and is consequently termed the *subcostal plane.* The lower horizontal plane passes through the tubercles on the iliac crests, and is termed the *intertubercular plane* (Plate II, p. 16). In this way the abdominal cavity is subdivided into *hypochrondriac, lumbar* and *iliac regions* on each side, and into the *epigastric, umbilical* and *hypogastric regions* in the median area. It should be noted that the distance between the subcostal and the intertubercular planes is open to considerable variation and that the lumbar and umbilical regions may form a very narrow band.

The **Transpyloric Plane** (Plate II, p. 16) is also useful as a surface reference. *It is drawn round the body through the mid-point of the line joining the suprasternal notch to the upper border of the pubic symphysis. When the body is lying on its back*, this plane passes through the pylorus. It should be pointed out that the vertebral column is cut by the transpyloric plane near the lower border of the *first* lumbar vertebra, by the subcostal plane at the upper border of the *third* lumbar vertebra, and by the intertubercular plane at the upper border of the *fifth* lumbar vertebra.

The **Peritoneum,** in the male, forms a closed serous sac which lines the walls of the abdominal cavity (parietal layer), and is reflected so as to invest, more or less completely as the case may be, the various abdominal and pelvic viscera (visceral layer). In the female, however, the sac is not closed, for through the ostium pelvinum (p. 213) it communicates with the lumen of the uterine tube and so indirectly, through the uterus and vagina, with the exterior. Take the opportunity of examining the general arrangement of the peritoneum in a recently opened abdomen, for the softness of the viscera, unhardened by formalin, makes it far easier to trace out this arrangement—and its intricacies.

The *Greater Omentum* will be readily recognised, hanging down like an apron from the greater curvature of the stomach. It forms a natural but incidental separation between structures lying above and in front of it from those which lie below and behind. In this way the peritoneal cavity is naturally subdivided into *supra-* and *infra-colic compartments.* When the greater omentum is drawn up over the costal margin, the infracolic compartment will be seen to be partly divided into right and left parts by the mesentery, which connects the jejunum and ileum to the posterior abdominal wall. The left infracolic compartment communicates freely with the *pelvis,* which constitutes a fourth natural subdivision of the general peritoneal cavity. The right and left *paracolic grooves* lie lateral to the ascending colon and the descending colon, respectively.

The *Lesser Sac of the Peritoneum*, which lies behind the stomach and extends upwards and downwards beyond it, may be regarded as a diverticulum of the supracolic compartment.

The General Arrangement of the Abdominal Viscera. Revise the general arrangement of the viscera in an undisturbed abdomen if you can. In the following description the relations and positions of the viscera are described *as they are found when the body is lying on its back.* In the erect attitude most of the viscera tend to sink downwards in the abdominal cavity. This applies especially to those which are provided with a mesentery, and the levels at which the stomach and the transverse colon are found on X-ray examination carried out in the erect position are subject not only to variations as between different individuals but also to variations in the same individual examined at different times. These variations are usually quite independent of any pathological condition and are so great that it is impossible, for example, to state a normal level at which the transverse colon crosses the median plane.

The **Stomach** occupies the left hypochondriac and the epigastric regions. Its anterior surface can be seen and explored in the posterior wall of the supracolic compartment. The long axis of the viscus passes downwards, forwards, to the right, and finally backwards and slightly upwards, as it crosses the vertebral column.

The *Œsophageal* or *Cardiac End* of the stomach lies in the upper part of the epigastrium in contact with the left lobe of the liver and is difficult to examine at this stage, but the *pylorus*, where the stomach becomes continuous with the duodenum, can be identified easily. It lies in the transpyloric plane, $\frac{1}{2}$ inch to the right of the median plane, and its position is usually indicated by a slight constriction. Further, the circular muscular coat of the stomach is much thickened at the pylorus to form the pyloric sphincter, and this thickening can easily be recognised by the fingers. In the living subject it may be identified by a prepyloric vein, which crosses its anterior surface.

When the stomach is empty, or moderately distended, the pylorus is in contact with the quadrate lobe of the liver, but when it is greatly distended the pylorus may come into contact with the gall-bladder. Observe that the pylorus has a slight range of movement, in this respect contrasting markedly with the cardiac end of the stomach, which is fixed. (The full description of the stomach will be found on pp. 161–164.)

In the early embryo the stomach can be identified as a localised dilatation of the foregut. At first it is median in position with ventral and dorsal borders, and right and left surfaces. As it enlarges, it becomes rotated to the right, so that its right surface becomes postero-inferior and its left surface antero-superior. The ventral border becomes the lesser and the dorsal border the greater curvature. As a result of the rotation of the stomach the omental bursa, which appears first as a pocket on the right aspect of the dorsal mesogastrium, becomes enlarged to form the lesser sac.

The **Duodenum** can be traced upwards, backwards and to the right and then downwards until it is crossed by the transverse colon. This portion, which comprises the whole of the first and the upper half of the second part of the duodenum, lies in the supracolic compartment, related anteriorly to the quadrate lobe, the gall-bladder and the adjoining part of the right lobe of the liver.

In order to follow the duodenum it is necessary to turn the greater omentum upwards over the costal margin and displace the coils of the jejunum and ileum downwards and to the left. When this is done the duodenum can be traced downwards, and then horizontally to the left, on the upper part of the posterior wall of the right infracolic compartment. It then disappears behind the root of the mesentery. This segment of the duodenum is not easy to demonstrate, as it lies entirely behind the peritoneum on the posterior abdominal wall. Anteriorly, it is related to a coil of small intestine, which separates it from the transverse mesocolon. To its right side the lower pole of the kidney may intervene between it and the upper end of the ascending colon.

The rest of the duodenum lies in the left infracolic compartment and, in order that it may be exposed, the coils of jejunum and ileum must be drawn upwards and to the right (*i.e.*, at right angles to the line of attachment of the mesentery). This portion is always easy to identify and can be traced upwards, close to the root of the mesentery, to the duodenojejunal flexure, where it bends forwards and downwards to become continuous with the jejunum. The flexure usually lies on the left side of the body of the second lumbar vertebra.

The duodenum, therefore, is found in the supracolic compartment and in both infracolic compartments. It is plastered on to the posterior abdominal wall by the peritoneum and, except for its first inch or so, is relatively *fixed in position.* It is important to appreciate that since the vertebral bodies bulge markedly into the abdomen, the duodenum is much curved in the vertical plane.

The **Jejunum and Ileum,** together about 20 feet long, are found in both infracolic compartments and in the pelvis—it is usually the terminal coils of the ileum which are found in the latter position. If the coils of the gut are drawn forwards from the posterior abdominal wall, it will be seen that they are slung from it by the *mesentery*, which consists of two layers of peritoneum, with fat, vessels and lymph nodes between them. The whole mass can be swung upwards and to the right, and downwards and to the left, since the mesentery is attached to the posterior abdominal wall along a line which passes from the duodenojejunal flexure obliquely downwards and to the right into the right iliac fossa.

The **Cæcum** lies in the right iliac fossa and projects downwards as a blind diverticulum from the point where the ileum joins the large intestine. It is about 2½ inches long, and is completely invested by the peritoneum. From its anterior surface the peritoneum is continued upwards, covering the ascending colon, but from the upper part of its posterior surface the peritoneum is reflected backwards and downwards over the iliacus muscle. In this way a small cul-de-sac is formed behind the cæcum termed the *retrocæcal recess*. By reason of its complete peritoneal investment the cæcum possesses a certain degree of mobility, but it is anchored in place by its continuity with the ascending colon, which is fixed.

Anteriorly, the cæcum, when distended, may come into contact with the anterior abdominal wall in the right iliac region. As a rule either some coils of the small intestine or the lower part of the greater omentum, or both, are interposed. *Posteriorly*, it is related to the iliacus and psoas muscles and to the lateral cutaneous nerve of the thigh. *Medially*, the vermiform appendix springs from the cæcum about an inch below the ileal termination.

The *Tæniæ Coli* (p. 170) of the cæcum lie, one on its anterior, one on its posterior and one on its medial aspect. They converge on the base of the vermiform appendix, for which they provide a complete longitudinal muscle coat.

The **Vermiform Appendix** varies greatly in length, the average being about 3 inches. As a rule it has a complete peritoneal investment, and is anchored to the lower layer of the mesentery by a short mesentery of its own. It possesses a considerable range of movement, and may be found: (1) projecting upwards and medially from the cæcum, in close relationship with the mesentery; (2) hanging down over the pelvic brim; (3) coiled up in the retrocæcal recess; or (4) projecting towards the anterior abdominal wall. The pelvic and the retrocæcal positions are much commoner than the other two.

The *Appendicular Artery* is a small branch from the ileocolic (p. 172). It descends behind the root of the mesentery and, entering the mesentery of the vermiform appendix, runs in or near its free border to its tip.

The cæcum and vermiform appendix are first recognisable in the embryo as a diverticulum from the antimesenteric border of the distal limb of the U loop of gut, which is formed as the gut begins to grow in length more rapidly than the embryo. This diverticulum grows out into a finger-like process and later its proximal part enlarges to form the cæcum, while its distal part remains attenuated and forms the vermiform appendix. In the fœtus the appendix springs from the apex of a conical cæcum, but the more rapid growth of the right side of the cæcum produces the condition found in the normal adult.

The **Ileocæcal Valve** is placed at the orifice of the ileum into the colon. It consists of two horizontal crescentic folds of mucous membrane, which unite at the extremities of the opening, and are continued for a short distance round the gut as the *frenula* of the valve. This valve may be regarded as a vestigial structure, representing a cæcocolic sphincter. At the lower end of the ileum, however, the circular muscle coat is thickened to form a true sphincter, which regulates the flow of chyme from the ileum to the cæcum. It is normally in a state of tonic contraction as a result of impulses which reach it from the sympathetic system *via* the splanchnic nerves. Relaxation of the sphincter is due to vagal stimuli and is associated with the arrival of a peristaltic wave at the lower end of the ileum.

The **Ascending Colon** extends from the cæcum to the inferior surface of the right lobe of the liver, where it bends to the left, forming the *right colic flexure*. It is 4 or 5 inches long and lies in the right lumbar region, immediately lateral to the right lateral plane. Covered with peritoneum in front and on each side, but not behind, the ascending colon is *fixed in position.*

Anteriorly, it is related to coils of small intestine and the right edge of the greater omentum. *Posteriorly*, it lies successively in front of (1) the iliacus; (2) the quadratus lumborum, the lumbar fascia and the origin of the transversus; and (3) the lower pole of the right kidney. The right iliohypogastric and ilioinguinal nerves and the right fourth lumbar artery cross behind it.

At the **Right Colic Flexure,** which has the liver above and in front of it, the colon bends forwards, downwards and to the left, and becomes the transverse colon.

The **Transverse Colon** extends across the abdomen from the right to the left colic flexure, forming a wide U-shaped curve, the lowest part of which lies nearer to the anterior abdominal wall than either extremity. This part of the gut varies from 15 to 20 inches in length. In the supine position the intermediate part of the transverse colon lies in the lower part of the umbilical region or even higher, but when in erect attitude it commonly reaches the hypogastrium and may even enter the pelvis.

The transverse colon possesses a mesentery (p. 156), and so has a wide range of movement. It is related *anteriorly* to the anterior two layers of the greater omentum and the anterior abdominal wall. *Posteriorly*, it lies first in contact with the second part of the duodenum and the head of the pancreas. In the rest of its extent it is separated from the posterior abdominal wall by coils of the small intestine. The *upper border* of the transverse colon is separated from the greater curvature of the stomach by the anterior two layers of the greater omentum and the lesser sac behind them.

At the **Left Colic Flexure** the transverse colon bends downwards and backwards and becomes the descending colon. This flexure is in contact with the medial aspect of the spleen, and is higher and further back than the right colic flexure.

The **Descending Colon** is 10 or 11 inches long and extends from the left colic flexure above to the pelvic inlet below. The peritoneum covers this part of the colon in front and on each side, but not behind; it is consequently fixed in position. At first it descends in front of the lateral border of the kidney and curves medially round its lower pole. Then it runs vertically downwards in front of the quadratus lumborum and, crossing the iliac crest, continues downwards on the iliacus muscle almost to the inguinal ligament. It next turns medially across the left psoas muscle to become the pelvic colon in front of the external iliac artery. The left paracolic groove lies along its lateral side.

The left iliohypogastric and ilioinguinal nerves cross behind the upper end of the descending colon, separated from it by the fascia covering the quadratus lumborum. The lateral cutaneous nerve of the thigh and the femoral nerve are separated from it, below, by the fascia iliaca.

The **Pelvic Colon** and the **Rectum** are described on pp. 191 and 195.

The disposition of the large intestine, and the relationship of the transverse colon to the duodenum, are determined during the second and third months of intrauterine life. Owing to rapid growth of the liver, the U loop of the gut cannot be accommodated within the abdomen, and passes out into the proximal part of the umbilical cord, where it forms a normal umbilical hernia from the sixth to the tenth week. In the cord the distal (colic) limb of the U lies to the left and the proximal limb to the right. Normally, the hernia becomes reduced about the tenth week. The small intestine returns first, and the caudal part of the colon is thrust over to the left of the abdominal cavity. The cæcum is the last part of the hernia to be returned to the abdomen, and it lies at first in front of the other coils below the liver. As the gut lengthens the cæcum grows to the right and then downwards into the right iliac fossa. This series of changes is termed the "rotation of the gut," and a precisely similar condition would have resulted if the U loop had been rotated through three right angles, the distal limb passing first to the left, then headwards and, finally, to the right. As a result of the rotation, the transverse colon crosses in front of the second part of the duodenum and the superior mesenteric artery crosses in front of the third part.

The **Lymph Nodes and Vessels** of the colon are closely related to the colic blood vessels. The lymph nodes form three groups: (*a*) The *epicolic* lymph nodes are isolated nodes on the surface of the gut. (*b*) The *paracolic group* lies along the medial borders of the ascending and the descending colon, and along the mesenteric border of the transverse and the pelvic colon. They receive afferents from (*a*) and also direct from the gut. Their efferents pass to (*c*) the *intermediate group*. This group is associated with the ileocolic artery for the cæcum and ascending colon—*ileocolic lymph nodes*—and lies behind the peritoneum of the posterior wall of the right infracolic compartment. The intermediate lymph nodes for the right colic flexure are similarly situated in relation to the right colic artery. The intermediate nodes for the transverse colon—*middle colic lymph nodes*—lie in relation to the middle colic artery in the transverse mesocolon. Those for the descending colon are disposed around the left colic artery on the posterior wall of the left infracolic compartment—*left colic lymph nodes*.

The efferents from the intermediate nodes join the aortic group of lymph nodes in the neighbourhood of the origin of the superior mesenteric artery, in the case of the gut from the cæcum to the left colic flexure. They join those near the origin of the inferior mesenteric artery in the case of the rest of the large intestine.

The **Lesser Omentum** is a fold of peritoneum connecting the lesser curvature of the stomach to the liver. Below and to the left its two layers separate to enclose the stomach and the commencement of the duodenum. Above and to the right, it passes to the bottom of the fissure for the ligamentum venosum (ductus venosus) and to the edges of the porta hepatis where its layers separate on to the adjoining parts of the liver. Immediately to the right of the œsophagus the lesser omentum reaches the diaphragm in the interval between the œsophagus and the upper end of the fissure for the ligamentum venosum. At its other extremity (*i.e.*, between the duodenum and the porta hepatis) the lesser omentum possesses a *right free border*, around which its two layers are continuous.

This right free border is much the thickest part of the lesser omentum, for it contains between its layers three large and important structures, viz., the bile duct, the portal vein and the hepatic artery. The portal vein lies posteriorly, with the bile duct overlapping its right edge and the hepatic artery in front of its left edge. The whole thickened border forms the anterior boundary of a short tubular passage, *the aditus to the lesser sac*, which passes to the left into the sac. At the aditus the anterior layer of the lesser omentum passes downwards over the duodenum, but the posterior layer is reflected backwards on to the posterior abdominal wall, forming a gutter-like floor on which the finger rests inferiorly when it is introduced into the lesser sac.

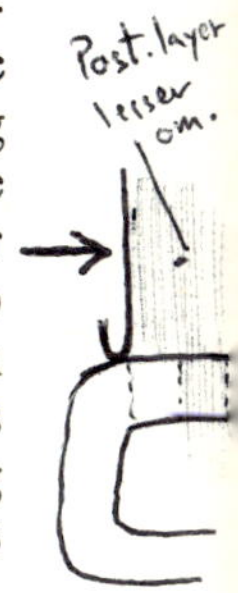

It is then continued upwards on the posterior abdominal wall, covering the inferior vena cava and forming the posterior boundary of the aditus, until it reaches the liver. There it passes forwards over the caudate process, which forms the roof of the aditus, and reaches the posterior edge of the porta hepatis.

Except at its right free border and along the lesser curvature of the stomach, where it contains gastric vessels and lymph nodes, the lesser omentum forms a thin, translucent sheet which is torn very easily in the cadaver. It forms the uppermost part of the anterior wall of the lesser sac.

The **Greater Omentum,** with variable fat content, hangs down from the greater curvature of the stomach. In its uppermost part it consists of two layers of peritoneum which are continued upwards to enclose the stomach, and so are continuous with the two layers of the lesser omentum. At its lower border these two layers are folded back on themselves and pass upwards until they reach the transverse colon, where they are adherent to the front and upper aspect of the gut and to the anterior layer of the transverse mesocolon. In the living subject at operation the transverse colon and the adjoining part of its mesentery can often be stripped away from the posterior aspect of the greater omentum over an area that is variable in extent. The part of the greater omentum which lies below the transverse colon consists, therefore, of four layers of peritoneum, but, as a rule, in the adult they are so fused that it is impossible to distinguish them. Accordingly, the lesser sac extends downwards for a variable distance between the anterior and the posterior layers.

The greater omentum is an incidental partition between the supracolic and the infracolic compartments and may act as a barrier to prevent the spread of infective processes.

The **Transverse Mesocolon** connects the transverse colon to the posterior abdominal wall. It is fused with the posterior layers of the greater omentum, so that when the latter is thrown upwards over the costal margin the transverse colon is also drawn upwards and its mesocolon is put on the stretch. The middle colic artery passes downwards between its two layers to reach the gut *well to the right of the middle of the transverse mesocolon.* To its left there is a wide area containing no blood vessels, and when this is incised the fingers can be introduced into the lesser sac through its postero-inferior wall. The posterior surface of the stomach, with the lesser omentum above and the anterior two layers of the greater omentum below, can then be explored in the anterior wall of the lesser sac.

The **Gastrosplenic Ligament** extends from the upper third of the greater curvature of the stomach to the hilum of the spleen. It is in direct continuity along the greater curvature with the greater omentum, of which it is merely an extension to the left. Its two layers, after the left, or anterior, one has invested the surfaces of the spleen, pass backwards to the posterior abdominal wall, where they meet the left kidney. This continuation of the layers of the gastrosplenic ligament constitutes the *Lienorenal "Ligament"*—a fold rather than a ligament. The splenic artery traverses the lienorenal ligament as it passes to the spleen, and its terminal branches traverse the gastrosplenic ligament on their way to the stomach. These two folds form the left boundary of the lesser sac.

The **Lesser Sac** of the peritoneum is a deep potential recess which lies behind the stomach, intervening between it and the "stomach bed." It extends upwards and to the right beyond the lesser curvature, and downwards beyond the greater curvature of the stomach into the greater omentum. Near the upper part of its right border it communicates with the rest of the peritoneal cavity through the aditus to the lesser sac.

The *Anterior Wall* of the lesser sac is formed by (1) the caudate lobe of the liver, (2) the lesser omentum, (3) the stomach, and (4) the anterior two layers of the greater omentum. The *Posterior Wall* is formed by (1) the stomach bed (p. 162), excluding the spleen, (2) the transverse mesocolon, (3) the transverse colon, and (4) the posterior two layers of the greater omentum. The upper limit, or roof, is formed by the reflection on to the diaphragm of the posterior layer of the lesser omentum in the area between the œsophagus and the upper end of the fissure for the ligamentum venosum (ductus venosus).

The *Lower Limit* is, theoretically, at the lower border of the greater omentum, but it is commonly situated in the neighbourhood of the transverse colon, as the anterior layers of the greater omentum become blended with the posterior layers before they reach its lower border.

The *Left Border* is formed above by the gastrosplenic and the lienorenal ligaments, and below by the left free border of the greater omentum.

The *Right Border* is rather complicated. It is formed (1) by the reflection of the peritoneum from the right edge of the caudate lobe backwards on to the diaphragm; (2) by the aditus to the lesser sac; (3) by the reflection of the peritoneum from the posterior surface of the duodenum on to the pancreas; (4) by the right free border of the greater omentum.

At the left end of the aditus its gutter-like floor becomes continuous with (3), and the two meet each other at a right angle. In this angle, extraperitoneally, the hepatic artery comes forwards from behind the posterior wall of the lesser sac to enter the lesser omentum. Pass the index finger, palmar surface downwards, through the aditus and hook it downwards into the lesser sac. Keeping the finger flexed, try to withdraw it. The hepatic artery can then be felt stretched across the palmar surface of the finger at the flexed joint.

Two other arteries, the splenic and left gastric, which at first lie behind the lesser sac, terminate in its anterior wall. The splenic artery passes round the left border of the sac in the lienorenal ligament and the gastrosplenic ligament; the left gastric artery circumvents the sac by hooking round the upper part of its left border in the immediate vicinity of the œsophagus.

The **Intestinal Mesentery** connects the coils of the jejunum and ileum to the posterior abdominal wall below the line of attachment of the transverse mesocolon. Its line of attachment to the abdominal wall is 6 or 7 inches long and begins above at the duodenojejunal flexure, in front of the terminal part of the duodenum. From there it runs downwards and to the right, crossing obliquely in front of (1) the third part of the duodenum; (2) the abdominal aorta; (3) the inferior vena cava; (4) the right psoas muscle and the ureter; and (5) the right iliacus muscle.

The intestinal branches of the superior mesenteric vessels, mesenteric lymph nodes and vessels, and a varying quantity of fat lie between the two layers of the mesentery, and the arrangement of the arteries and the disposition of fat should be examined in a freshly opened abdomen. At the upper end of the mesentery the fat is deposited near the root, and is very scanty, or entirely absent, near the gut; in this situation the arterial arcades are comparatively simple and easily seen, and the terminal branches to the gut are relatively long. At the lower end of the mesentery the fat is not only deposited near the root, but also extends as far as the gut, and sometimes encroaches on it. In this part of the mesentery the arterial arcades are more complex, the terminal branches to the gut are relatively short, and the "windows" between them are obscured by the fat. The transition from the one type to the other is not sudden, but occurs gradually, as will be seen on examination of the mesentery.

The **Falciform Ligament of the Liver** is a sickle-shaped fold of peritoneum which connects the anterior surface of the liver to the diaphragm and to the anterior abdominal wall above the umbilicus. The lower or posterior border, around which the two constituent layers of the ligament become continuous, is free and extends from the umbilicus to the anterior extremity of the fissure for the ligamentum teres on the under surface of the liver. It contains the obliterated umbilical vein or ligamentum teres (p. 167), and, when present, the para-umbilical veins (p. 174).

The **Spleen** lies partly in the epigastrium but chiefly in the left hypochondrium, occupying the left upper posterior part of the supracolic compartment. It is an elongated organ, and *its long axis corresponds to the posterior part of the shaft of the tenth rib.*

Its *Diaphragmatic Surface* is gently convex and lies opposite the posterior parts of the ninth, tenth and eleventh ribs, being separated from the left pleural sac and, in its upper half, from the base of the left lung by the diaphragm.

The *Visceral Surface* comes into relationship with the stomach, the left kidney, the left colic flexure and the tail of the pancreas. The *gastric area* is hollowed out to form the upper and left part of the stomach bed, and it is separated from the diaphragmatic surface by the notched anterior border of the gland. The *hilum* is situated posterior to this area.

The *Renal Area* is in contact with the upper and lateral part of the anterior surface of the left kidney. It is separated from the diaphragmatic surface by the thickened posterior border of the gland, and an irregular ridge separates it from the gastric area.

The *Colic Area* is in contact with the left colic flexure and is placed low down and in front of the hilum.

The *Pancreatic Area* is very variable. It is near the lower part of the hilum and intervenes between the renal and gastric areas.

The spleen is mapped out on the surface by an ellipse with its long axis corresponding to the tenth rib. The ellipse reaches the ninth and eleventh ribs, and it does not normally project forwards much beyond the mid-axillary line.

Peritoneal Relations. Except at its hilum, the spleen is completely invested with peritoneum, and projects into the supracolic compartment behind the upper part of the stomach. At the hilum the gastrosplenic ligament and the lienorenal ligament are attached, and the right layer of the one passes without interruption into the right layer of the other. On the other hand, the left layer of the gastrosplenic ligament passes round the spleen before it becomes continuous with the corresponding layer of the lienorenal ligament. On this account the spleen can be handled—and its diaphragmatic, renal, gastric and colic areas examined—from the greater sac.

The spleen is an accessory organ of the blood-vascular system. Its chief functions are the production of lymphocytes and the destruction of worn-out red blood corpuscles. In addition, it is able to store blood, as it is capable of distension owing to the amount of elastic tissue present in its capsule and trabeculæ. The spleen undergoes a slow, rhythmical contraction about once per minute in some animals, but the human spleen undergoes only small changes in volume. Bilirubin and certain antibodies are produced in the spleen, which also stores iron derived from the breakdown of haemoglobin.

The spleen arises as a number of localised thickenings in the cœlomic epithelium on the left side of the cephalic part of the dorsal mesogastrium. (The dorsal mesogastrium is the forerunner of greater and gastrosplenic omenta and the lienorenal "ligament".)

The notch or notches on the upper border of the organ are the only surface traces of lobulation in the adult spleen.

The *Splenic Lymph Nodes* lie at the hilum of the spleen. They receive afferents from the spleen and also direct from the fundus and adjoining portion of the stomach. Their efferents pass to the lymph nodes which lie along the upper border of the pancreas, and these in turn become continuous with the cœliac group of the aortic lymph nodes.

The **Cœliac Artery** arises from the ventral surface of the commencement of the abdominal aorta. It therefore lies between the two crura of the diaphragm and behind the peritoneum on the posterior wall of the lesser sac and it is surrounded by the cœliac plexus, which connects the two cœliac ganglia (p. 190). The upper border of the pancreas crosses the abdominal aorta immediately below the origin of the artery. It is very short, and breaks up almost at once into its three terminal branches, viz.: the left gastric, the splenic, and the hepatic arteries.

1. The **Left Gastric Artery** passes upwards to the left to the œsophageal opening of the diaphragm. It is closely related to the left cœliac ganglion, the left inferior phrenic artery and the medial border of the left adrenal gland. On reaching the œsophagus it gives off an ascending œsophageal branch, and then turns downwards and to the right round the upper end of the left border of the lesser sac (p. 155). It then follows the lesser curvature of the stomach, giving off gastric branches, and anastomoses with the right gastric artery.

2. The **Splenic Artery** runs to the left behind the lesser sac. It follows a wavy course, the troughs of the waves lying behind the pancreas and their crests emerging above it, so forming a posterior relation of the stomach. In its course the artery lies above its corresponding vein, and crosses in front of the left psoas muscle, the lower end of the left adrenal gland and the gastric area of the left kidney. It then turns forwards between the two layers of the lienorenal ligament to reach the hilum of the spleen.

The short gastric arteries and the left gastro-epiploic branch are continued onwards to the stomach between the two layers of the gastrosplenic ligament, thus reaching their destination by passing round the left border of the lesser sac.

Branches. (1) Pancreatic, to the body and tail of the pancreas; (2) splenic; (3) gastric.

The gastric branches include the *short gastric arteries* which supply the fundus of the stomach, and the *left gastro-epiploic*, which follows the greater curvature from left to right, giving off numerous branches to both surfaces of the stomach and to the greater omentum, and finally anastomosing with the right gastro-epiploic between the anterior two layers of the greater omentum.

3. The **Hepatic Artery** runs forwards below the medial end of the aditus to the lesser sac (p. 157), and reaches the upper border of the duodenum. There it turns upwards between the two layers of the lesser omentum, in front of the portal vein and to the left of the bile duct, and ascends in front of the aditus to reach the porta hepatis.

Branches. (*a*) The *Right Gastric Artery* arises at the upper border of the duodenum and runs to the left along the lesser curvature. It anastomoses with the trunk of the left gastric artery.

(*b*) The *Gastroduodenal Artery* arises close to the last-named artery. It runs downwards behind the first part of the duodenum and immediately to the right of the right border of the lesser sac. It divides into the *superior pancreaticoduodenal*, which runs to the right in the groove between the head of the pancreas and the duodenum, supplying both structures, and the *right gastro-epiploic*, which follows the greater curvature of the stomach and anastomoses with the left gastro-epiploic.

(*c*) The *Cystic Artery* arises from the right terminal branch, and passes posterior to the common hepatic and cystic ducts to be distributed to the gall-bladder.

(*d*) Nearing the liver, the hepatic artery divides into right and left terminal branches, which enter the corresponding extremities of the porta hepatis behind the hepatic ducts but in front of the right and left branches of the portal vein.

Each of the numerous branches derived from the cœliac artery carries off a mixed plexus of autonomic nerves from the cœliac plexus, and these are distributed to the viscera which the artery supplies.

The Stomach. The position of the stomach and its two orifices has already been indicated (p. 149).

The fact that the stomach is a localised dilatation of a simple tube is well brought out by radiograms taken in the upright posture, following a barium meal (Plate XVIII, p. 172). When the viscus is in a normal condition it commonly presents a J-shape, the longer limb lying to the left of the median plane.

When the stomach is filled, its borders, which are known as "curvatures," disappear as such, and are only indicated by the lines of attachment of the omenta. When, however, the stomach is empty and flattened, as is usually the case in the cadaver, the borders are apparent as such.

The *Lesser Curvature* extends from the right side of the cardiac orifice to the upper border of the pylorus, and the lesser omentum extends from it to the liver. In the erect attitude it forms a J-shaped curve, and its concavity curves below the omental tuberosity of the pancreas. The lowest part of the curve is often represented by a notch, termed the *incisura angularis*, and this indicates the subdivision of the stomach into a *body*, proximal to the notch, and a *pyloric portion*, distal to it. The pyloric portion shows a further subdivision into a proximal and a distal part. The proximal part shows a slight dilatation and is termed the *pyloric antrum*; the distal part is more tubular and is called the *pyloric canal*. The *Greater Curvature*, from which the greater omentum passes downwards into the abdominal cavity, forms the lower and left border of the stomach.

When the peritoneal cavity is opened, the stomach sinks backwards so that peritoneal recesses are found between it and the diaphragm, and also between it and the liver, if the latter has been hardened *in situ*. These recesses are only potential spaces during life. Try to restore the stomach to its natural position relative to the diaphragm and the liver. When this is done it will be seen that the left lobe of the liver is in direct contact with the stomach over a narrow area adjoining the lesser curvature. Of the rest of the antero-superior surface of the stomach, the lower and right portion lies in direct contact with the anterior abdominal wall in the region of the upper part of the left rectus muscle and linea alba, while the upper and left portion lies under cover of the left costal margin and in contact with the left half of the diaphragm. To the left of the cardiac orifice the *fundus* of the stomach bulges upwards as high as the level of the fifth costal cartilage, and becomes related to the heart and pericardium. It can easily be identified in X-ray photographs taken in the erect attitude (Plate XVIII, p. 172), since it usually contains a large bubble of gas. It will be remembered that the pleura extends downwards below the lower border of the lung (p. 103), and therefore a larger part of the antero-superior surface of the stomach is related to the pleura than to the lung.

The *Posterior Surface* of the stomach takes a large share in the formation of the anterior wall of the lesser sac, which intervenes between it and the structures forming the so-called "stomach bed."

The greater curvature of the stomach is related, below and behind, to the transverse colon, and the adjoining part of the posterior surface rests on the transverse mesocolon. Above the latter structure the stomach is in contact with the anterior surface of the pancreas. These structures form a gently sloping shelf, over which the stomach may slide downwards or upwards, as the position of the body

Coeliac art — (L) gastric 1.
— Splenic 2
— Hepatic 3

(L) gastric - 1. ascending oesophageal *
2. Gastric - lesser curvature of [illegible]. *

Splenic - 1. Pancreatic *
2. Splenic *
3. Gastric — short gastric *
— (L) gastro-epiploic *
gt. curvature.

Hepatic
1. (R) gastric *
2. Gastroduodenal → sup. pancreatico * duodenal.
→ (R) gastro-epiploic *.
supraduod.
3. Cystic art *
terminates — R hepatic *
— L — " — *.

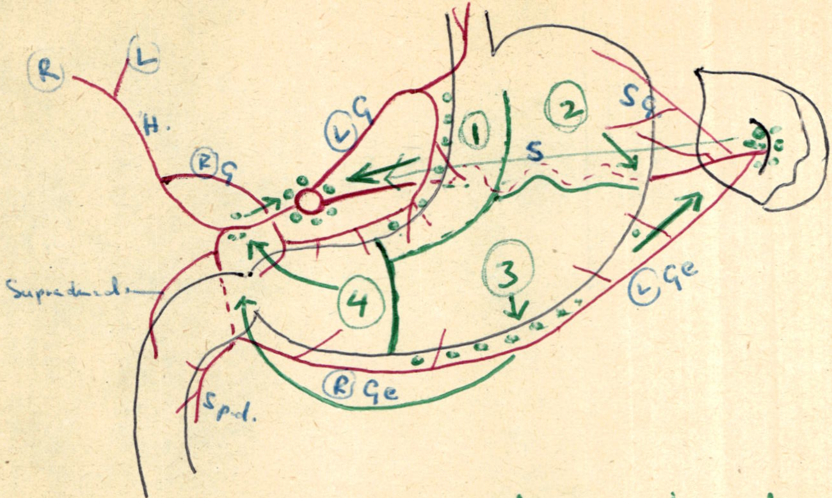

All drain to celiac lymph n.

is altered from time to time, with each contraction of the diaphragm, and as it fills or empties.

Above the pancreas the stomach lies entirely to the left of the median plane, and adjoins the left adrenal gland and the upper part of the anterior surface of the left kidney. At a still higher level, *i.e.*, in the region of the fundus, the stomach produces the concave gastric area of the spleen, and touches the left half of the diaphragm.

The Arteries which supply the stomach are derived from the branches of the cœliac artery (p. 160). Their main trunks run along the curvatures and their branches run at right angles to the long axis of the viscus. The veins of the stomach join the portal circulation. The right and left gastric veins end in the portal vein itself, while the left gastro-epiploic and the short gastric veins join the splenic vein, and the right gastro-epiploic is a tributary of the superior mesenteric vein.

The *Lymph Vessels* of the stomach are arranged in four principal groups: 1. The lymph vessels from both surfaces in the neighbourhood of the lesser curvature end in a chain of lymph nodes which lies along the lesser curvature in close relationship with the left gastric vessels. The efferents from these nodes pass to the cœliac lymph nodes, which surround the cœliac artery at its origin.

2. The lymph vessels from the region adjoining the upper third of the greater curvature accompany the left gastro-epiploic vein to the lymph nodes in the hilum of the spleen, and thence to the pancreaticosplenic lymph nodes, which, in turn, are drained by the cœliac lymph nodes.

3. The lymph vessels from the regions adjoining the lower two-thirds of the greater curvature join the right gastro-epiploic lymph nodes, which lie along that part of the greater curvature. Their efferents join the pyloric lymph nodes, which are associated with the gastroduodenal artery, and thence reach the cœliac lymph nodes.

4. The lymph vessels from the pyloric region end in two or three lymph nodes which lie along the hepatic artery, and thence they drain into the cœliac group.

It will be observed that the cœliac lymph nodes constitute the central group for all the gastric lymph vessels.

The *Nerves* of the stomach come from the cœliac plexus of the sympathetic system and from both vagus nerves. The vagal fibres are secretomotor to the gastric glands, motor to its muscular wall but inhibitory to the pyloric sphincter, which receives its motor supply from the sympathetic. The sympathetic fibres arise from the fifth, sixth, seventh and eighth thoracic segments of the spinal cord, and it is consequently in the cutaneous areas supplied by the corresponding intercostal nerves that referred pains may occur in gastric disorders.

The *Muscular Wall* of the stomach contains: (1) longitudinal fibres; (2) circular fibres; and (3) oblique fibres. The *longitudinal layer* is best developed in the neighbourhood of the curvatures, and is the most superficial. It is continuous with the longitudinal layer of the œsophagus on the one hand, and of the duodenum on the other. The *circular fibres* are deep to the preceding. Practically absent at the fundus, they encircle the body of the stomach, and are specially thickened at the pylorus to form the pyloric sphincter. A fibrous septum intervenes between the pyloric sphincter and the circular fibres of the duodenum. The *oblique fibres* constitute the deepest layer; they are most numerous over the body, and are absent in the pyloric region and along the lesser curvature. Near the greater curvature they blend with the circular fibres.

The **Liver** occupies nearly the whole of the right hypochondrium and extends into the upper and anterior part of the epigastrium, while its lower border usually descends for a short distance into the right lumbar region. It is imperfectly divided into a large right and a much smaller left lobe, and the line of division on the anterior and superior surfaces corresponds to the attachment of the falciform ligament. (The "surfaces" of the liver are not all clearly separable, and are largely a descriptive convenience.)

The *Superior Surface* is related to the central tendon and the adjoining muscular parts of the diaphragm, and is separated by the diaphragm from the basal surfaces of the right and left lungs. The intermediate depressed area is related to the heart and pericardium.

The *Right Surface*, which merges into the superior and anterior surfaces, lies opposite the seventh to the eleventh ribs inclusive, but is separated from them by the diaphragm. The upper two-thirds of this surface is related to the lowest part of the costodiaphragmatic recess of the right pleural sac, and its upper third to the lower border of the right lung.

The *Anterior Surface* is limited inferiorly by the sharp lower border of the liver, which slopes upwards and to the left. It is in contact with the right half of the diaphragm, the anterior abdominal wall in the infrasternal angle, and also, but to a lesser extent, with the left half of the diaphragm. The upper part of this surface is related, on the right side, to the lower limit of the pleura. The falciform ligament is attached to this surface of the liver, a little to the right of the median plane.

The *Inferior* and *Posterior Surfaces* are not separated sharply from each other. The inferior surface is set very obliquely and looks backwards and to the left. The *porta hepatis*, through which the hepatic artery, portal vein, etc., enter and the bile duct, lymph vessels, etc., emerge from the liver, is situated on this surface. Its left extremity is joined by (*a*) the *fissure* for the *ligamentum teres*, which crosses the inferior surface from the inferior border, and (*b*) the *fissure* for the *ligamentum venosum*, which cuts into the posterior surface. These two fissures mark the subdivision into right and left lobes on the inferior and posterior surfaces.

The right lobe is further subdivided into a quadrate lobe, a caudate lobe, with a caudate process, and a large unnamed area. The *Quadrate lobe* lies on the inferior surface, and is bounded behind by the porta hepatis, in front by the inferior border, on its left side by the fissure for the ligamentum teres, and on its right side by a shallow fossa which lodges the gall-bladder. The *Caudate lobe* lies on the posterior surface, and is bounded on the right by the inferior vena cava. It projects inwards from the upper part of the right border of the lesser sac, and has a free left margin, which forms the lateral lip of the fissure for the ligamentum venosum. Its anterior surface forms the posterior wall of the fissure and is in contact with the hepatic part of the lesser omentum. The *caudate process* is a narrow ridge of liver substance which connects the lower end of the caudate lobe to the unnamed area of the right lobe. It forms the upper boundary of the aditus to the lesser sac, and lies in front of the inferior vena cava.

The quadrate lobe is related to the pyloric part of the stomach and the first part of the duodenum, below, and to the right portion of the lesser omentum, above. The gall-bladder lies in front of the first and second parts of the duodenum, but the latter extends beyond it and comes into relationship with the adjoining part of the right lobe. Immediately to the right of the duodenal area the right colic flexure leaves its imprint on the formalin-hardened liver, and above and behind this area the under surface of the right lobe is extensively related to the right kidney.

The *Posterior Surface* is triangular in shape, with its apex tailing off to the left. The right extremity of this surface—which is known as the *bare area*, because it is devoid of peritoneal covering—is in direct contact with the diaphragm, but its lower and medial corner shows a small triangular impression on the formalin-hardened organ. This impression is produced by the right adrenal gland, and it abuts on the one hand on the inferior vena cava, and on the other on the upper end of the renal area. The left border of the *bare area* is occupied by the inferior vena cava, which is always lodged in a deep groove and is often bridged over by liver substance.

To the left of the inferior vena cava lies the caudate lobe, which forms the uppermost part of the anterior wall of the lesser sac. It is related posteriorly to the diaphragm, which separates it from the descending *thoracic* aorta and the lower thoracic vertebræ. On its left side the caudate lobe is limited by the fissure for the ligamentum venosum, which cuts deeply into the substance of the liver. The under surface of the left lobe is related to the stomach (p. 163) and the lesser omentum. Near the left extremity of the porta hepatis it presents a rounded elevation termed the *omental tuberosity* (p. 185).

The posterior surface of the left lobe is very narrow, and may be notched by the intra-abdominal portion of the œsophagus.

Blood Vessels. Both the hepatic artery and the portal vein bring blood to the liver, and their principal branches are included, along with branches of the biliary ducts, in a fibrous capsule. The blood conveyed by the portal vein has already passed through one set of capillaries in the submucosa of the small intestine and has there absorbed products of digestion from the alimentary canal. The smallest branches of the portal vein form venous plexuses between the lobules of the liver and from the plexuses the hepatic sinusoids penetrate into the lobules between the columns of liver cells, converging on the central vein. The walls of the sinusoids are lined in part by Kuppfer's cells and are elsewhere incomplete. As a result substances such as glucose in the blood readily pass into the liver cells, for conversion into glycogen, etc. The central veins drain ultimately into the right and left *hepatic veins*, which issue from the posterior aspect of the liver and open directly into the inferior vena cava, having no extra hepatic course on account of the intimate relationship of the vena cava to the liver.

The *Lymph vessels* of the liver terminate for the most part in a small group of lymph nodes in and below the porta hepatis. The efferents from these nodes pass direct to the cœliac lymph nodes (p. 190). Some of the superficial lymph vessels from the anterior surface ascend to the diaphragm in the falciform ligament and ultimately reach the mediastinal lymph nodes. Others accompany the inferior vena cava into the thorax and end in one or two small lymph nodes related to the intrathoracic part of the vessel.

The *Nerves* of the liver are derived from the two vagi and from the hepatic plexus of the sympathetic. The latter are connected with the seventh, eighth and ninth segments of the spinal cord.

The liver arises from a hollow endodermal outgrowth from the ventral border of the duodenum. This diverticulum grows into the septum transversum, bifurcates and from the two extremities solid buds of epithelial cells grow out to form the liver cells. Mesenchymal cells of the septum transversum are incorporated in the growing mass to form the stroma of the organ. The gall-bladder and cystic duct arise from the stalk of the diverticulum as a solid outgrowth, which later acquires a lumen. The duodenal end of the stalk forms the bile duct (*see also* p. 168).

Fœtal Circulation and the Liver. In the fœtus the umbilical vein brings fresh blood direct from the placenta to the fœtal circulation. Entering at the umbilicus, it runs upwards and backwards in the falciform ligament to the liver, where it joins the left branch of the portal vein. Its union with the *left* branch of the portal vein is explained by the fact that the umbilical vein was originally a paired structure, the left one alone persisting. Only a small part of the blood brought by the umbilical vein circulates through the left lobe of the liver before reaching the heart, for the greater proportion passes along the *ductus venosus*. This large vessel runs upwards from the left branch of the portal vein, in its fissure on the left side of the caudate lobe, and joins the inferior vena cava just below the diaphragm. After ligature of the umbilical cord at birth the umbilical vein becomes converted into a fibrous cord, termed the *ligamentum teres*, which can be recognised in the free border of the falciform ligament and in the bottom of the corresponding fissure. The remains of the ductus venosus can also be identified in the adult liver as a fibrous strand—the ligamentum venosum—attached by one end to the left branch of the portal vein, and by the other to the left side of the inferior vena cava. It runs up along the bottom of the fissure for the ligamentum venosum, at the upper end of which it curves to the right to reach the inferior vena cava.

Peritoneal Connexions of the Liver. The liver is completely invested with peritoneum except over the "bare area," and along the lines of attachment of the various folds.

The lines of peritoneal reflection along the upper and lower borders of the bare area are termed the upper and lower layers of the *coronary ligament*. The former connects the liver to the diaphragm, and the latter connects it either to the diaphragm or to the anterior surface of the right kidney. At their right extremities the two layers become continuous, forming the *right triangular ligament* of the liver.

The *falciform ligament* (p. 158) connects the anterior surface of the liver to the diaphragm and the anterior abdominal wall. Its right layer becomes continuous with the superior layer of the coronary ligament, and its left layer is continued to the left on the upper surface of the left lobe. It is folded backwards on itself to form the *left triangular ligament*, which connects the upper surface of the left lobe with the under surface of the diaphragm.

The *lesser omentum* is attached to the margins of the porta hepatis and around its right extremity. The two layers are continued from the left extremity of the porta hepatis up the fissure for the ligamentum venosum, at the upper end of which they separate. The anterior, or left, layer becomes continuous with the posterior layer of the left triangular ligament, while the posterior layer skirts the upper end of the caudate lobe and descends along its right border to become continuous with the lower layer of the coronary ligament. This layer is reflected from the caudate lobe on to the diaphragm and forms the right boundary of the uppermost recess of the lesser sac.

These "ligaments" must not be regarded as supporting the weight of the organ. The liver, like all the other abdominal and pelvic organs, is retained in place by the intra-abdominal pressure, which is attributable, mainly, to the tonus of the muscles of the anterior and lateral abdominal walls.

The **Gall-bladder** is a pear-shaped sac (Plate XIX, p. 172) which is closely connected to the inferior surface of the right lobe of the liver and forms the right boundary of its quadrate lobe. The fundus of the gall-bladder projects from the lower margin of the liver, opposite the angle formed by the right costal margin and the right linea semilunaris (Plate II), *i.e.*, opposite the tip of the ninth costal cartilage. Its neck becomes continuous with the cystic duct.

The *postero-inferior* surface of the gall-bladder is covered with peritoneum, and is related to the first and second parts of the duodenum. The *antero-superior surface* is in direct contact with the liver, no peritoneum usually intervening though the gall-bladder sometimes has a short mesentery.

The **Cystic Duct,** about 1 inch long, runs from the neck of the gall-bladder to the porta hepatis, where it joins the common hepatic duct to form the bile duct; but it may descend for a variable distance in the right free margin of the lesser omentum before doing so. In its course it makes an S-shaped bend (Plate XIX), and the mucous membrane in its interior is folded to constitute a *spiral valve.*

The *Right* and *Left Hepatic Ducts* issue from the right and left lobes of the liver, and unite in the porta hepatis to form the common hepatic duct, which is joined by the cystic duct to form the bile duct.

The **Bile Duct,** so formed, begins in or just below the porta hepatis. In the first part of its course it lies in the right free border of the lesser omentum; in the second part of its course it crosses behind the first part of the duodenum; in the third part of its course it is associated with the head of the pancreas. Altogether the duct is about 3 inches long.

Relations. (*a*) In the first part of its course the bile duct lies in the right free border of the lesser omentum, to the right of the hepatic artery, and in front of the portal vein. When the index finger is passed into the aditus to the lesser sac, the right border of the lesser omentum can be gripped between the finger and thumb, and the whole of this part of the bile duct can be palpated.

(*b*) In the second part of its course the bile duct lies behind the first part of the duodenum, with the right edge of the portal vein behind it, and the gastroduodenal artery to its medial or left side.

(*c*) The terminal part of the bile duct is embedded in a groove on the upper and lateral part of the posterior surface of the head of the pancreas. It is thus separated from the portal vein, which inclines to the left behind the neck of the pancreas, but it is closely related to the right edge of the inferior vena cava, which lies behind it.

At its lower end the bile duct pierces the medial wall of the second part of the duodenum in an oblique manner and, in common with the duct of the pancreas, opens into a small ampulla in the duodenal wall (pp. 182, 184). The terminal portions of both ducts and the duodenal ampulla are surrounded by circular muscle fibres, known clinically as the *sphincter of Oddi*, though there is little evidence of sphincteric control here.

The Structure of the Small Intestine. Throughout its whole length, from the pylorus to the ileocolic valve, the small intestine is provided with a complete external muscular coat of longitudinal fibres, and a complete internal muscular coat of circular fibres.

The characters of the mucous membrane differ in the different parts of the gut. The mucous membrane of the first part of the duodenum is smooth and the branched tubular duodenal glands are numerous, especially near the pylorus. The *plicæ circulares*, which are permanent infoldings of the mucous membrane, set at right angles to the long axis of the gut, begin in the second part of the duodenum and become very closely set below the duodenal papilla. They are equally close in the upper part of the jejunum, but towards its lower end they are not so numerous. In the ileum they become more widely separated, and in the lower part of the ileum they are entirely absent. The plicæ circulares serve to increase the extent of the absorptive surface without increasing the length of the gut.

Minute projections of the mucous membrane, termed *villi*, are characteristic of the whole length of the small intestine. The simple tubular glands of the intestine open on the surface between the bases of the villi.

Small collections of lymphoid tissue form rounded or oval elevations in the mucous membrane. They are known as *solitary lymphatic nodules.* Much larger collections of lymphoid tissue constitute the *aggregated lymphatic nodules.* They are most numerous towards the lower end of the ileum, where they form elongated oval areas on the anti-mesenteric aspect of the gut. They do not occur in the upper two-thirds of the jejunum. Best marked in the young subject, they tend to disappear as age advances.

If an empty coil of the upper end of the jejunum be compared with an empty coil from the lower end of the ileum, it will be found that, owing to the presence of the numerous plicæ circulares, the former feels much thicker to the touch.

The jejunum (approximately upper two-fifths of the intestine) is not distinctly identifiable. No characteristics change gradually into those of the ileum.

Differences between the Small Intestine and the Large Intestine. *External Appearances.* (1) The wall of the large intestine is sacculated. (2) The longitudinal muscle coat of the large intestine is not equally distributed throughout the wall of the gut, but is collected into three distinct bundles, termed the *tæniæ coli,* which can be seen through the serous coat. In the intervals between the tæniæ coli, the longitudinal muscle coat forms a very thin layer. (3) When occupied the large intestine is greater in calibre than that of the small intestine. (4) Little fatty tags project from the serous coat of the large intestine. They are little peritoneal bags of fat, termed *appendices epiploicæ.*

In contrast to the large intestine the wall of the small intestine shows no localised constrictions. The longitudinal muscle coat is spread out evenly so as to cover the wall completely. True appendices epiploicæ are not found in the small intestine, although in a fat subject the mesenteric fat at the lower end of thc ileum overlaps the intestinal wall and gives it a somewhat similar appearance.

Internal Appearances. (1) The mucous membrane of the large intestine is devoid of villi; villi are found in the mucous membrane throughout the whole extent of the small intestine. (2) The mucous membrane of the large intestine is thrown into folds opposite the constrictions between sacculations. These folds can be smoothed out when the longitudinal muscle band which causes the puckering relaxes. The plicæ circulares of the small intestine are permanent folds. (3) Aggregated lymph nodules are found in the ileum, particularly in its lower part; they are not found in the large intestine.

The **Superior Mesenteric Artery** arises from the front of the abdominal aorta behind the neck of the pancreas and, therefore, a little below the origin of the cœliac artery. It runs downwards and to the right, at first behind the neck of the pancreas and then in front of the uncinate process. In this way it reaches the third part of the duodenum, in front of which it passes to enter the root of the mesentery. In the latter it is continued downwards in front of the inferior vena cava and the right psoas muscle and the ureter, and ends by anastomosing with the ileal terminals of its own ileocolic branch.

Branches. 1. The *Jejunal* and *Ileal Branches* arise from its left side and run between the layers of the mesentery to reach the gut. They anastomose very freely with one another and form a series of arterial arcades prior to giving off the terminal branches, which run at right angles to the long axis of the intestine. The termination of the main trunk constitutes the lowest of these branches.

2. The *Inferior Pancreaticoduodenal Artery* arises from the superior mesenteric as it crosses the uncinate process of the head of the pancreas. It passes to the right in the groove between the head of the pancreas and the duodenum, where it ends, after supplying both these structures, by anastomosing with the superior pancreaticoduodenal artery.

3. The *Middle Colic* arises from the right side of the artery close to the origin of the last-named branch. It passes downwards, between the two layers of the transverse mesocolon and nearer to its right than to its left border. Reaching the transverse colon, which it supplies, it divides into right and left branches, which anastomose respectively with the right colic and the superior left colic arteries.

4. The *Right Colic Artery* arises a little below (3) and runs to the right behind the peritoneum on the posterior wall of the right infracolic compartment. It crosses in front of the inferior vena cava, the right testicular (or ovarian) vessels and the right ureter and, on reaching the upper part of the ascending colon, it divides into a superior branch, which anastomoses with the middle colic, and an inferior branch, which anastomoses with the ileocolic artery. Not infrequently it fails to arise as an independent branch and springs instead from the ileocolic or from the middle colic artery.

5. The *Ileocolic Artery* arises from the right side of the superior mesenteric at a lower level and runs downwards and to the right, behind the peritoneum on the posterior wall of the right infracolic compartment. It crosses in front of the inferior vena cava and the right ureter and testicular vessels.

Its terminal branches are: (*a*) an ascending branch to the ascending colon, which anastomoses with the right colic; (*b*) an anterior cæcal artery; (*c*) a posterior cæcal artery, which gives off the *appendicular artery* (p. 152); (*d*) a descending branch, which enters the root of the mesentery and anastomoses with the terminal part of the superior mesenteric artery, both vessels giving off branches to supply the lowest part of the ileum.

The **Inferior Mesenteric Artery** arises from the front of the abdominal aorta about 1½ inches above its bifurcation. Closely applied to the parietal peritoneum, the artery runs downwards, inclining to the left, leaves the anterior surface of the aorta and crosses the left common iliac artery. It then passes into the pelvis as the *superior rectal artery*.

Branches. 1. The *Superior Left Colic Artery* is the first branch to arise. It runs *upwards* and to the left, immediately behind the peritoneum of the posterior wall of the left infracolic compartment, crossing in front of the left psoas muscle, testicular vessels and ureter. It then ascends in front of the jejunal area of the left kidney (p. 178), and reaches the left colic flexure. It divides into branches which anastomose with the middle colic in the transverse mesocolon, and the uppermost of the inferior left colic arteries.

2. The *Inferior Left Colic Branches*, usually three or four in number, supply the descending and the pelvic colon. They anastomose freely with each other and with the superior left colic, *but the anastomosing channel connecting the lowest and the superior rectal is very small or absent*.

3. The *Superior Rectal Artery* is the terminal part of the inferior mesenteric artery. It enters the pelvic mesocolon and continues downwards behind the rectum, where it divides into right and left branches. These vessels subsequently anastomose with the middle and inferior rectal vessels in the submucous tissue of the anal canal.

It should be noted that prior to the reduction of the embryonic umbilical hernia (p. 154) the greater part of the colon shares a common mesentery with the small intestine, and this mesentery contains the colic vessels. Subsequently the mesentery of the ascending and descending portions of the large intestine comes into contact with the posterior abdominal wall, the opposed peritoneal layers fuse and the colic vessels therefore cross anterior to those structures which develop *in situ* on the posterior body wall, *e.g.*, inferior vena cava, ureter, etc.

The **Inferior Mesenteric Vein** is a tributary of the portal circulation. It begins at the lower end of the rectum as the superior rectal vein, and runs up on the posterior abdominal wall to the left side of the inferior mesenteric artery. After receiving tributaries which correspond to the branches of the artery, it curves to the right above

Plate XVIII. Radiograph of the Stomach Taken in the Upright Position after a Barium Meal.

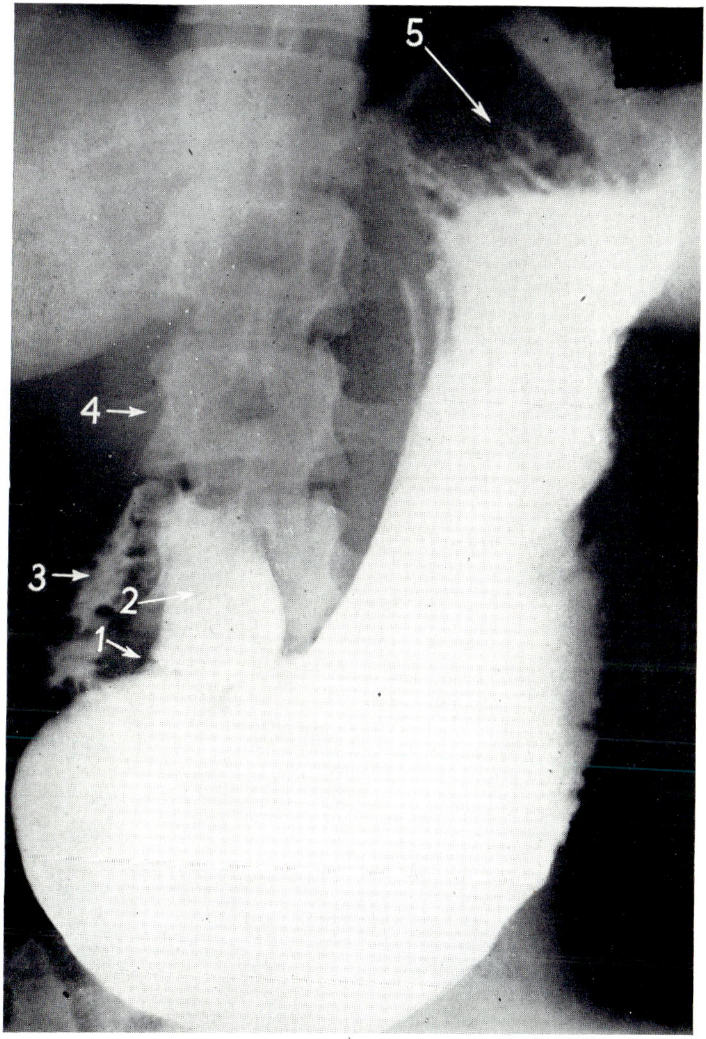

1. Pyloric constriction.
2. Duodenal cap.
3. Barium in the second part of the duodenum.
4. Second lumbar vertebra.
5. Bubble of gas in fundus of stomach.

Note that the pylorus lies below the lower border of the body of L.3. This is a little lower than its average position.

To face p. 172

PLATE XIX. RADIOGRAPH OF THE GALL-BLADDER AND BILE DUCTS TAKEN AFTER THE ORAL ADMINISTRATION OF SODIUM TETRAIODOPHENOLPHTHALEINE.

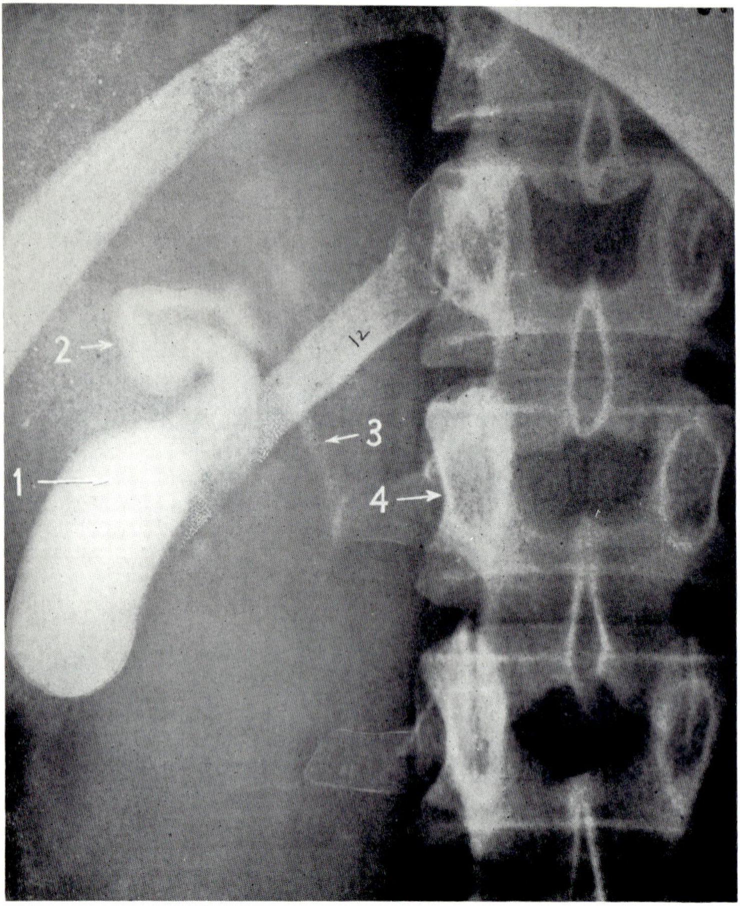

1. Gall bladder
2. Cystic duct. Note the S-shaped bend.
3. Bile duct, at its upper end.
4. First lumbar vertebra.

The irregularly shaped dark area, *apparently* in the bodies of the vertebræ, corresponds to the interspinous and interlaminar intervals.

Note the relationship of the gall-bladder to the twelfth rib.

Plate XX. The Lumbar Region, after an Intravenous Injection of Uroselectan B.

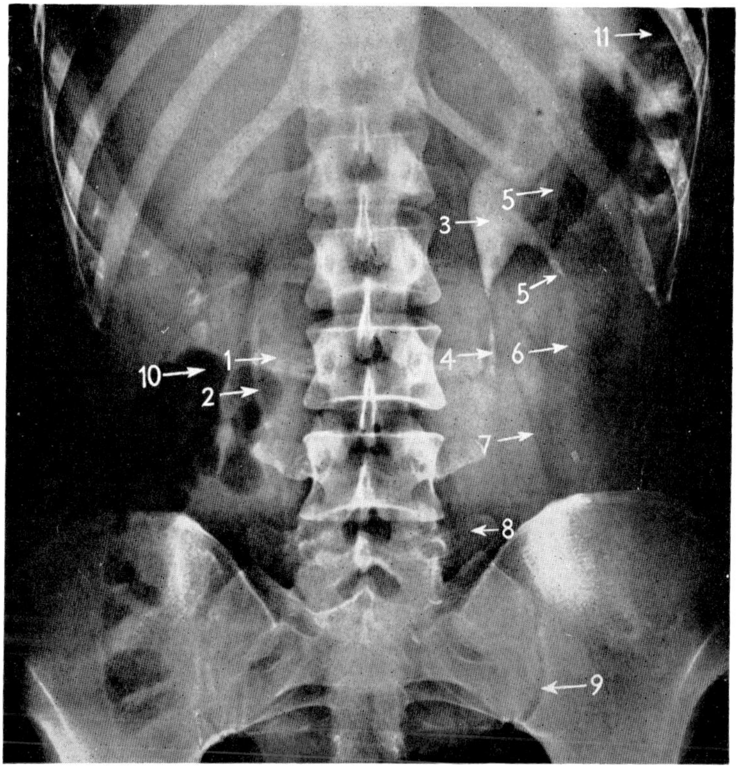

1. Transverse process of L.3.
2. Right ureter.
3. Pelvis of left kidney.
4. Left ureter.
5. Minor calyces of left kidney.
6. Lower pole of left kidney.
7. Lateral edge of left psoas major m.
8. Transverse process of L.5.
9. Line of left sacro-iliac joint.
10. Gas in right colic flexure.
11. Gas in left colic flexure.

Note that, although on the left side (right side of figure) the renal pelvis is well shown, on the right side it cannot be identified, although some of the minor calyces of the right kidney are conspicuous.

Much gas is present in the ascending colon, and the right colic flexure (10) lies at a much lower level than the left colic flexure (11).

The irregular dark areas, visible through the bodies of the vertebræ, represent the interlaminar intervals, which are partially obscured by the shadows of the vertebral spines.

Distortion, caused by divergence of the rays, accounts for the appearances of T.11 and L.5.

PLATE XXI. ARTERIOGRAM OF LEFT INTERNAL CAROTID ARTERY.

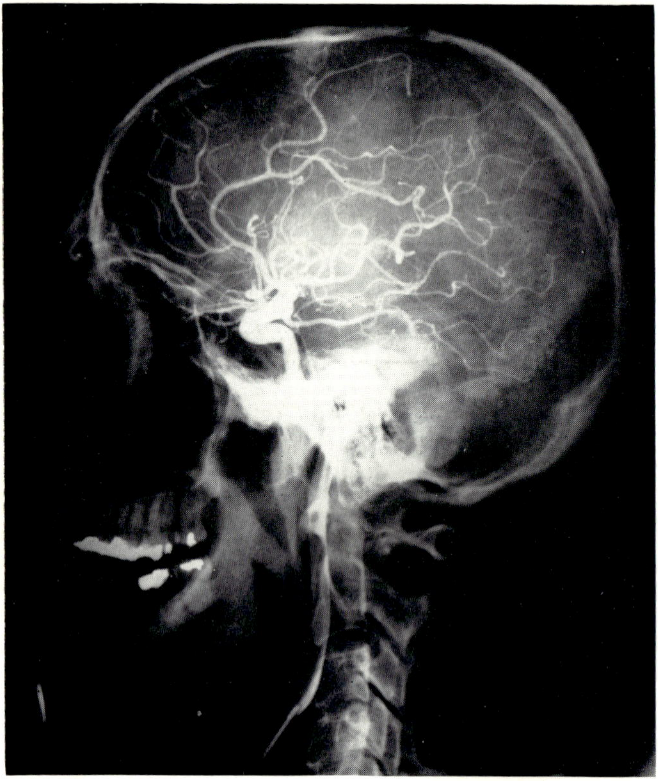

Radio-opaque material, introduced into the left internal carotid artery, has entered its branches, which can be readliy identified.

the duodenojejunal flexure, passes behind the body of the pancreas, and joins the splenic vein.

The **Superior Mesenteric Vein** begins at the lower end of the root of the mesentery, and runs upwards and to the left, receiving tributaries which correspond to the branches of the superior mesenteric artery and, in addition, the right gastro-epiploic vein from the greater curvature of the stomach. It emerges from the root of the mesentery and crosses in front of the third part of the duodenum and the uncinate process of the pancreas, lying to the right side of its artery. It ends behind the neck of the pancreas by joining the splenic vein to form the portal vein.

The **Splenic Vein** is formed at the hilum of the spleen, where the veins issuing from the gland are joined by the left gastro-epiploic and other veins from the greater curvature of the stomach. It traverses the lienorenal ligament and then passes to the right behind the body of the pancreas, crossing in front of the left kidney, adrenal gland, psoas muscle, and the abdominal aorta. In its course it lies below the splenic artery. Behind the neck of the pancreas it joins the superior mesenteric vein to form the portal vein.

In its course it receives the inferior mesenteric vein and additional tributaries from the body of the pancreas.

The **Portal Vein** is formed behind the neck of the pancreas by the union of the superior mesenteric and the splenic veins. It runs upwards and to the right, overlapping the head of the pancreas and behind the first part of the duodenum. At the upper border of the duodenum it enters the lesser omentum near its right free margin and ascends, in front of the aditus to the lesser sac, to the porta hepatis, where it divides into right and left branches.

As it lies in the lesser omentum the portal vein has (1) the hepatic artery, in front and to its left side; (2) the bile duct, in front and to its right side; and (3) the inferior vena cava, behind it and separated from it by the aditus to the lesser sac.

As it lies behind the first part of the duodenum the portal vein has (1) the gastroduodenal artery in front; (2) the bile duct, in front and to its right side; and (3) the inferior vena cava, behind it. [*Cf.* the relations of the bile duct (p. 168).]

In its course the portal vein receives the left and right gastric veins from the lesser curvature of the stomach and a pancreaticoduodenal vein.

The portal vein brings to the liver blood which has already circulated (1) *through the whole length of the abdominal part of the alimentary canal, from the lower end of the œsophagus to the upper end of the anal canal;* (2) *through the spleen; and* (3) *through the pancreas.*

The connections of the portal vein or its tributaries with the systemic veins are of importance, because obstruction of the portal circulation is by no means an uncommon occurrence.

1. In the submucous tissue at the lower end of the œsophagus the radicles of the left gastric vein anastomose with the radicles of the thoracic œsophageal veins. These vessels may become greatly dilated in portal obstruction and may rupture, causing hæmatemesis (vomiting of blood).

2. In the submucous tissue of the anal canal the radicles of the superior rectal vein anastomose with those of the middle and inferior rectal veins. Varicosity of these vessels occurs in the condition known as internal hæmorrhoids.

3. The para-umbilical veins, not always present, commence at the umbilicus, where they communicate with the superficial abdominal veins, and run up along the ligamentum teres to terminate in the left branch of the portal vein. (When this connexion is greatly enlarged, as happens occasionally in portal obstruction, the appearance of the dilated veins, which radiate from the umbilicus, has been likened to the head of Medusa, with her radiating crown of snakes!)

4. The lumbar veins are stated to be connected to the colic and intestinal veins.

The **Diaphragm** is a muscular and tendinous curved sheet between pleuræ and pericardium above and peritoneal cavity below. When it is relaxed, it is shaped like a dome, above it the abdomen, as viewed from below. Its attachments are extensive and must be studied in detail.

(*a*) The *Crura* of the *Diaphragm* arise, on the right side, from the sides of the bodies of the upper three lumbar vertebræ, on the left side the upper two, and on both sides from the intervertebral discs. The medial fibres of the two crura decussate in front of the commencement of the abdominal aorta, and the medial fibres of the right crus surround the lower end of the œsophagus. Both crura ascend and curve forwards to reach the posterior border of the central tendon.

(*b*) Lateral to the crura the diaphragm arises from the *Medial* and *Lateral Arcuate Ligaments*. The former is the thickened upper border of the fascia covering the psoas muscle, and it stretches from the side of the body of the second to the tip of the transverse process of the first lumbar vertebra. The *lateral arcuate ligament* is a thickening in the anterior lamella of the lumbar fascia, and extends from the tip of the first lumbar transverse process to the lower border of the last rib. From this origin the fibres arch upwards to reach the postero-lateral aspect of the central tendon.

(*c*) The *Costal Origin* of the diaphragm consists of six fleshy slips, which arise from the deep surfaces of the lower six costal cartilages, interdigitating with the costal origin of the transversus. These fibres are inserted into the antero-lateral aspect of the central tendon.

(*d*) The *Sternal Origin* consists of right and left slips from the posterior surface of the xiphoid process. These fibres are relatively short, and pass upwards and backwards to the anterior margin of the central tendon.

The central tendon of the diaphragm is the highest part of the muscle. In shape it resembles a trefoil leaf, with a median part, projecting forwards, and right and left lateral parts, curving laterally and backwards. Above, the tendon is inseparably blended with the fibrous layer of the pericardium.

The *Nerve Supply* of the diaphragm is derived from the right and left phrenic nerves (C. 3, 4 and 5).

Action. When the muscle of the diaphragm contracts it tends to straighten, so that its peripheral part becomes flattened, losing its dome-like appearance. At the same time the central tendon descends for a short distance.

The aorta, œsophagus, inferior vena cava and other smaller structures pierce the diaphragm in passing from the thorax to the abdomen, or *vice versâ*.

The *Aortic Opening* lies in front of the first lumbar vertebra, between the two crura, and is bounded anteriorly by a tendinous band which connects the medial borders of the crura to each other. Through this opening pass the aorta, the thoracic duct and the vena azygos. The two latter lie deeply under cover of the right crus. Note that the aortic "opening" is in fact a *notch*. The aorta really passes *behind* the diaphragm, not *through* it.

The *Œsophageal Opening* lies level with the tenth thoracic vertebra in the fleshy part of the diaphragm, in front and to the left of the aortic notch and behind the central tendon. It transmits the œsophagus and the two vagus nerves.

The *Vena Caval Opening* is at the level of the ninth thoracic vertebra. It is situated to the right of the median plane and pierces the central tendon near its posterior border, where the right and median portions of the tendon join each other. Owing to the position of the opening, the inferior vena cava is not constricted by each diaphragmatic contraction. A few twigs from the right phrenic nerve accompany the inferior vena cava through the opening.

In addition, the splanchnic nerves pierce the crura, and the sympathetic trunk passes behind the medial arcuate ligament on each side.

The central part of the diaphragm is derived from the septum transversum, which originally lies in the cervical region and is then invaded by cells from the fourth cervical myotome accompanied by the phrenic nerve. The crura are formed in the dorsal mesentery of the gastric end of the œsophagus. In the early embryo the postero-lateral parts of the diaphragm are deficient, and at this time the pleural and peritoneal cavities communicate on each side. These openings are closed by the pleuroperitoneal membranes.

The **Muscles of the Posterior Abdominal Wall** comprise the crura and adjoining parts of the diaphragm above, and the psoas, the quadratus lumborum and the transversus below.

The **Psoas** occupies the angle between the bodies and the transverse processes of the lumbar vertebræ. It arises from the sides of the vertebral bodies and from the intervertebral discs (from the lower border of the twelfth thoracic to the upper border of the fifth lumbar), from the roots of the transverse processes, and from tendinous arches which are thrown over the lumbar arteries as they pass backwards round the vertebral bodies.

The fibres run downwards and laterally, converging to end in a strong tendon, which passes behind the inguinal ligament to gain the thigh, where it is inserted into the lesser trochanter of the femur (p. 55).

Its *Nerve Supply* is derived from L. 2, 3 and 4.

Action. The psoas is a flexor of the thigh and is often said to be also a medial rotator. It may also flex the trunk on the lower limbs, when these are fixed.

The **Quadratus Lumborum** is a flat muscle which lies lateral to the psoas. It arises from the iliolumbar ligament—which extends from the fifth lumbar transverse process to the posterior part of the iliac crest—from the adjoining part of the crest, and from the tips of the lower two or three lumbar transverse processes. It runs upwards and medially, so that its lateral border is oblique, and is inserted into the lower border of the last rib.

Its *Nerve Supply* is derived from L. 1, 2, 3 and 4.

Action. It probably fixes the last rib to assist the diaphragm in inspiration, and may bend the vertebral column to the same side.

The anterior surface of the quadratus lumborum is covered by the anterior lamella of the lumbar fascia, and the main part of the latter structure lies along its lateral border, giving origin to the intermediate fibres of the transversus.

The **Iliacus** arises from the fossa of the ilium, and its fibres converge to leave the pelvis on the lateral side of the psoas tendon (p. 56).

The iliac fascia covers the muscle and is continuous with the thinner layer of connective tissue over the psoas. It is attached to the inner lip of the crest and to the lateral half of the inguinal ligament, and in both of these situations it is continuous above with the fascia transversalis. Opposite the medial half of the inguinal ligament the fascia is carried down into the thigh behind the femoral vessels, as the posterior wall of the femoral sheath (p. 52).

The arrangement will be better understood if the iliac fascia is regarded as part of an abdominopelvic connective tissue, which encloses the extraperitoneal fat. The nerves of the lumbar plexus lie outside this fascial envelope, and so the femoral and the lateral cutaneous nerves need not pierce it as they pass behind the inguinal ligament. On the other hand, the external iliac artery lies within the fascial envelope, and so, when it reaches the inguinal ligament, it has the fascia transversalis in front of it and the fascia iliaca behind it. These structures are therefore carried down into the thigh as the femoral sheath.

Superiorly, the abdominopelvic fascial envelope is completed by the fascia on the under surface of the diaphragm. On the posterior abdominal wall it can be distinguished, laterally, covering transversus, and medially, the psoas; but between these two muscles it blends with the anterior lamella of the lumbar fascia.

The **Kidneys** lie behind the peritoneum, on the posterior abdominal wall opposite the bodies of the last thoracic and the upper three lumbar vertebræ. The left kidney is on a slightly higher level than the right, and is usually restricted to the epigastric and hypochondriac regions, but the right kidney extends into the upper and adjoining portions of the lumbar and umbilical regions as well. (N.B. Most radiologists consider that this difference in level is exaggerated in cadaveric anatomy.)

The average kidney measures $4\frac{1}{2}$ inches long by 2 inches wide, and its long axis is inclined downwards and slightly laterally. The hilum of the right kidney lies about 2 inches from the midline, while that of the left kidney is nearer by $\frac{1}{2}$ inch. The transpyloric plane passes through the hila of both kidneys, a little above the middle of the right and a little below the middle of the left. With this information it is not difficult to refer the outline of the two kidneys to the anterior abdominal wall.

The *Posterior Relations* of the kidneys are very similar. The upper pole rests on the diaphragm [the lateral edge of the crus, the arcuate ligaments and the fibres arising from them]. The kidney is separated from the lower limit of the pleural sac by the diaphragm. The left kidney extends upwards as high as the vertebral end of the eleventh rib, but the right kidney is rarely higher than the upper border of the twelfth. Below the arcuate ligaments the flattened posterior surface of the kidney rests on the quadratus lumborum, but the more rounded lateral and medial parts of this surface are related to the origin of the transversus from the lumbar fascia, and to the lateral border of the psoas, respectively.

The subcostal, the iliohypogastric and the ilio-inguinal nerves run downwards and laterally behind the kidneys and in front of the quadratus lumborum. In the angle between the lateral border of the psoas and the quadratus lumborum, the tips of the transverse processes of the upper three lumbar vertebræ indent the posterior surface of the kidney, so as to leave impressions on the organ when it is hardened *in situ*.

The *Anterior Relations* of the two kidneys are very different from each other. *On the right side:* (1) the adrenal is related to a strip at the upper pole. (2) The second part of the duodenum lies in front of the area immediately adjoining the hilum. (3) The upper end of the ascending colon lies on the lower and lateral part of this surface. Each of these three structures lifts the peritoneum away from the anterior surface of the kidney. (4) Between the duodenum and the ascending colon there is frequently a small interval. Here the lower part of the anterior surface is directly covered by peritoneum and occupies the right upper corner of the posterior wall of the right infracolic compartment. It thus comes into relationship with a coil of small intestine. (5) The rest of the anterior surface—roughly, its upper and lateral two-thirds—is directly covered by peritoneum and is related to the inferior surface of the right lobe of the liver.

The anterior relations of the *left kidney* are quite different. (1) The pancreas forms a broad band across the anterior surface, usually situated nearer to the upper than to the lower pole. (2) The left adrenal occupies a strip along the medial border, from the upper pole to the hilum. (3) The spleen is related to the upper third or more of the lateral border and the adjoining part of the anterior surface. (4) The stomach comes into contact with a somewhat triangular area, bounded below by the pancreatic area, medially by the suprarenal area, and laterally by the splenic area. (5) The descending colon is related to the lower two-thirds or less of the lateral border and slightly overlaps the anterior surface. (6) The first coils of the jejunum lie in contact with the lower part of the anterior surface. This area is frequently extensive; it is limited above by the pancreas, and laterally by the descending colon.

The pancreas, adrenal, and descending colon, being fixed or "retroperitoneal" viscera, lift the peritoneum away from the kidney, but the rest of the anterior surface is covered by peritoneum, being in contact with mobile viscera peritoneum. The gastric area lies in the posterior wall of the lesser sac and is separated from the splenic area by the attachment of the root of the lienorenal ligament. The splenic area lies in the greater sac, and is separated from the upper end of the left paracolic groove by the phrenicocolic ligament. Finally, the jejunal area occupies the left upper corner of the posterior wall of the left infracolic compartment.

In addition to these viscera, certain vessels are related to the anterior surface of the left kidney. (1) The splenic vein is interposed between pancreas and kidney. (2) The splenic artery crosses the lower part of the gastric area. (3) The superior left colic vessels cross the jejunal area as they make for the left colic flexure.

The *Hilum* of the *Kidney*, which is a vertical slit leading into the *renal sinus*, is on the medial border and is bounded, in front and behind, by thick lips of renal substance. Through it the branches of the renal artery enter the gland, and the veins and ureter emerge.

On coronal section of the kidney it will be seen that, within the renal sinus, the ureter expands to form the *ureteral pelvis*, which divides into 2 or 3 *major calyces*. These divide into *minor calyces*, into which the striated pyramids of the renal medulla project, forming the *renal papillæ*. Hence, in radiographs of the kidneys (Plate XX, p. 172) the ends of the minor calyces are cupped.

The *fibrous capsule* of the kidney is closely applied to the cortex, but in a healthy organ it can be stripped off readily. A variable amount of fat is packed round the kidney—perinephric fat—outside its capsule, but within a condensation of the subperitoneal areolar tissue, which forms a subsidiary sheath termed the *perinephric fascia*.

The emerging veins usually lie in front of the entering arteries, and most of the vessels lie in front of the pelvis of the ureter, but there is always at least one artery which enters the hilum behind the ureter.

The **Ureter** emerges from the hilum of the kidney and runs vertically downwards on the psoas muscle in line, more or less, with the tips of the lumbar transverse processes and about $1\frac{1}{2}$ inches from the median plane (Plate XX). At the pelvic brim it crosses the bifurcation of the common iliac artery. It shows three slight constrictions, one at its upper end, one at the pelvic brim and one as it pierces the bladder wall.

On both sides it is immediately behind the posterior parietal peritoneum, the colic and testicular (or ovarian) vessels alone intervening. *On the right side*, close to its commencement, it is placed behind the duodenum, at the junction of the second and third parts, and before it enters the pelvis it is crossed by the root of the mesentery. *On the left side* the inferior mesenteric vein lies to its medial side, and as the ureter enters the pelvis it is crossed by the pelvic mesocolon.

The *nerves* of the ureter are derived from the renal, the testicular (or ovarian) and, in the pelvis, from the hypogastric plexuses (T. 11, 12, and L. 1 and 2).

The kidney, or metanephros, has a twofold origin. A *ureteric outgrowth* arises from the caudal end of the mesonephric duct and extends cranially into the caudal end of the mesonephric ridge. Around its expanding blind end the mesoderm of the ridge condenses to form a *metanephrogenic cap*. The ureter and its pelvis, the calyces and the collecting tubules of the kidney are all developed from the ureteric outgrowth, but the renal corpuscles and the convoluted and secreting tubules all take origin from the metanephrogenic cap. It will be clear, therefore, that before the kidney can function, connexions must be established between the collecting tubules on the one hand and the secreting tubules on the other. Congenital cysts occur in the kidney, when the connexions fail.

As the kidney enlarges, it grows in a headward direction, and relative to the growing vertebral column it ascends from its original position in the pelvis to its adult position opposite the upper lumbar vertebræ; the ureter lengthens correspondingly. As the lower end of the mesonephric duct is absorbed into the growing bladder (p. 198), the ureter acquires an independent opening into the latter.

The **Suprarenal (Adrenal) Glands** are closely related to the upper poles of the kidneys, and both lie in the epigastrium.

The *Right Suprarenal* is triangular in shape. *Below*, it is related to the upper pole of the right kidney. *Posteriorly* it rests on the upper lateral part of the right crus of the diaphragm. *Anteriorly*, it is related to the inferior vena cava medially, and to the bare area of the liver laterally. The cœliac ganglion lies close to its infero-medial extremity.

The *Left Suprarenal* is semilunar in outline, and the concavity is applied to the medial border of the left kidney from the hilum to the upper pole. *Posteriorly*, it rests upon the left crus of the diaphragm. *Anteriorly*, it is covered by peritoneum and lies in the posterior wall of the lesser sac, forming a part of the stomach bed. Its lower part is crossed by the splenic vessels and the pancreas, which separate it from the peritoneum.

Each gland receives three *arteries*, viz., a superior suprarenal from the (inferior) phrenic, a middle suprarenal from the aorta, and an inferior suprarenal from the renal artery. A single *vein* emerges from the hilum on the anterior surface. The right vein is very short, and joins the *inferior vena cava*; the left vein runs downwards and medially, and ends in the *left renal vein*.

The cortex of the suprarenal gland is developed from the cœlomic epithelium close to the root of the dorsal mesentery. The medulla is developed from groups of sympatho-chromaffin cells, derived from the primitive spinal ganglia (neural crest tissue).

Adrenalin is secreted actively by the medulla under the influence of its sympathetic nerve-supply, which consists of preganglionic fibres from the splanchnic nerves, the cells of the medulla representing the ganglionic neurones.

The **Duodenum** has already been referred to as it lies *in situ* before the viscera are disturbed (p. 150). For descriptive purposes it is divided into four parts, but these do not correspond to the subdivision which is brought about by the peritoneal arrangements. Taken as a whole, the duodenum forms an irregular C-shaped curve around the head of the pancreas—the lower part of the C being disproportionately long. Except for its first half-inch, which is covered by peritoneum both in front and behind, the duodenum is fixed on to the posterior abdominal wall and is covered by peritoneum only in front where it is related to mobile organs. It is situated in the epigastric and umbilical regions, but its second part approaches very near the right lateral plane.

The *First Part of the Duodenum*, about 2 inches long, begins at the pylorus and runs backwards and upwards round the right side of the first lumbar vertebral body. It can easily be identified in X-ray photographs as the "duodenal cap," which is separated from the stomach by the pyloric constriction (Plate XVIII, p. 172). It is related *anteriorly* to the quadrate lobe of the liver and to the gall-bladder. *Posteriorly*, at its commencement, the duodenum is related to the pancreas, and (more to the right) the gastroduodenal artery, the portal vein and the bile duct run downwards behind it and separate it from the inferior vena cava. *Below* lies the head of the pancreas, and *above*, the hepatic artery, the portal vein and the bile duct intervene between the duodenum and the floor of the aditus to the lesser sac.

The *Second Part of the Duodenum* is about 3 inches long. It runs vertically downwards in front of the hilum and adjoining part of the anterior surface of the right kidney. Its *anterior surface* is crossed by the commencement of the transverse colon. Above the transverse colon the second part of the duodenum lies in the supracolic compartment, and is related anteriorly to the gall-bladder and right lobe of the liver; below the transverse colon it lies in the posterior wall of the right infracolic compartment, and is related anteriorly to a coil of small intestine. The head of the pancreas lies to its *medial side*, and the ascending colon, the right colic flexure and the right lobe of the liver, to its *lateral side*, in that order from below upwards.

The *Third Part of the Duodenum* is about 3 inches long. It runs horizontally to the left just below the subcostal plane, and being crossed by the root of the mesentery, it is found in both the right and left infracolic compartments. Its *upper border* is related to the head of the pancreas, and its *lower border* to coils of jejunum. From right to left it crosses in front of the right psoas muscle and the ureter, the inferior vena cava, the abdominal aorta and the left side of the body of the third lumbar vertebra. *Anteriorly* the third part of the duodenum is related to coils of jejunum and is crossed about its middle by the superior mesenteric vessels as they pass to enter the root of the mesentery, and by the root of the mesentery itself.

The *Fourth Part of the Duodenum*, about 2 inches long, runs upwards on the left side of the vertebral bodies and terminates by turning forwards to form the duodenojejunal flexure on the left side of the body of the second lumbar vertebra. *Posteriorly*, it is related to the medial border of the left psoas muscle. *Anteriorly*, it is related to the root of the mesentery and coils of jejunum. On its *right side* it is related to the vertebral column, and on its left side to the initial coils of the jejunum.

The *Duodenojejunal Flexure* lies in front of the left psoas muscle and medial to the lower part of the hilum of the left kidney. *Above*, it is related to the transverse mesocolon and the body of the pancreas.

Peritoneal Relations. The first half-inch of the duodenum is covered, in front and behind, by the anterior and posterior layers of the lesser omentum, so that its peritoneal relations are identical with those of the stomach. It consequently lies in the anterior wall of the lesser sac. Half-an-inch beyond the pylorus the peritoneum is reflected from its posterior surface backwards on to the pancreas, so forming the right border of the lesser sac immediately below the aditus (*see* pp. 155 and 157).

The rest of the duodenum is covered by peritoneum only on its anterior surface, and the transverse colon and the superior mesenteric vessels lift the peritoneum from its surface.

The *Mucous Membrane* of the duodenum is smooth for the first inch or two. The plicæ circulares begin in the second part, and are very numerous in the third and fourth parts. The whole of the interior of the duodenum is covered with villi. The *duodenal papilla* is a small rounded elevation on the medial wall of the second part. A small orifice on its summit leads into the *ampulla of the bile duct*—a dilatation in the duodenal wall into which both the bile duct and the duct of the pancreas open. The minute orifice of the accessory pancreatic duct lies a little above the duodenal papilla. In the fresh specimen the *duodenal glands* can just be felt, especially near the pylorus, where they are most numerous.

When the stomach becomes rotated to the right in the embryo, the duodenum is necessarily affected in a similar manner and comes to lie in contact with the posterior abdominal wall. Later it loses its mesentery and becomes fixed. That the growth of the duodenal wall proceeds in an unequal manner is indicated clearly by the fact that the liver grows out from its *ventral* aspect in the first instance, whereas the bile duct opens on its *medial* wall at a later stage.

The **Pancreas** stretches obliquely across the posterior abdominal wall in the lower part of the epigastric region, but its left extremity, or tail, comes into relationship with the spleen in the left hypochondriac region.

The *Head* of the pancreas occupies the concavity of the curve of the duodenum, and lies on the right side of the vertebral column. Its lower and medial part is drawn out to the left, forming the *uncinate process*. *Posteriorly*, the head is in contact with the inferior vena cava and the terminal portions of the two renal veins, and the uncinate process encroaches on to the aorta. The upper and lateral part of this surface has the bile duct embedded in it (p. 168). *Anteriorly*, the head of the pancreas is related to the pylorus and to the transverse colon, while the uncinate process is crossed by the superior mesenteric vessels. The *margins* of the head are related to the duodenum.

The *Neck* of the pancreas emerges from the upper and medial part of the anterior surface of the head. (The "neck" is hardly distinguishable from the "body," except by its relations—or the "tail" from the body; but for descriptive purposes the terms have some slight use.) *Posteriorly*, the neck is related to the commencement of the portal vein. *Anteriorly*, it is covered with peritoneum and lies in the posterior wall of the lesser sac, which intervenes between it and the stomach. To its *lower border* the root of the transverse mesocolon is attached.

The *Body* of the pancreas runs upwards and to the left, crossing the median plane in front of the first lumbar vertebra. *Posteriorly*, it is related to (1) the aorta and the origin of the superior mesenteric artery; (2) the left psoas muscle; (3) the lower pole of the left adrenal gland, and the hilum and anterior surface of the left kidney; (4) the splenic vein is closely applied to the posterior aspect of the gland and is connected to it by the short pancreatic veins.

The *Anterior Surface* of the body lies in the posterior wall of the lesser sac, and is covered with peritoneum. It forms a part of the bed of the stomach (p. 162).

The *Lower Border* receives the attachment of the transverse mesocolon, and the narrow *Inferior Surface* is related to the duodenojejunal flexure and the first coil of jejunum.

The *Upper Border*, as it leaves the neck, is raised up to form the *omental tuberosity*, which projects above the lower end of the lesser curvature of the stomach, and is separated from the omental tuberosity of the liver (p. 165) by the lesser sac and the lesser omentum. The rest of this border is associated with the splenic artery (p. 160).

The *Tail* of the pancreas passes forwards in the lienorenal ligament, and comes into contact with the spleen just above and medial to the left colic flexure. Like the body, it is intimately related to the splenic vessels.

The *Duct* of the pancreas begins in the tail and runs to the right and downwards through the body and neck to the head. It is joined by numerous tributaries *en route*, and it pierces the postero-medial wall of the second part of the duodenum about its middle. It ends in the ampulla of the bile duct (pp. 169, 182). The *accessory duct* drains the uncinate process and the lower part of the head, and runs upwards to open into the duodenum above the duodenal papilla. The two ducts frequently communicate.

Blood Supply. The arteries of the pancreas are derived from the superior and inferior pancreaticoduodenal and the splenic arteries. The two former supply the head. The veins of the tail and body join the splenic vein; those from the head and neck pass directly into the portal vein.

The *Lymph Vessels* join the pancreaticosplenic lymph nodes, and efferents from these glands join the cœliac lymph nodes.

The pancreas is developed from a ventral rudiment, which arises as an endodermal outgrowth from the ventral aspect of the duodenum just caudal to the outgrowth of the liver, and a dorsal rudiment, which arises from the dorsal aspect of the duodenum. Both rudiments grow dorsally in the meso-duodenum and the caudal part of the dorsal mesogastrium. The two rudiments become fused. The dorsal diverticulum forms the body, neck and a part of the head of the gland. The ducts of the two rudiments become connected and eventually the duct of the pancreas is derived, at its duodenal end, from the ventral rudiment and in the rest of its extent from the dorsal rudiment. The accessory duct represents the duodenal end of the dorsal rudiment.

The **Abdominal Aorta** commences in front of the first lumbar vertebra, where it comes through the aortic opening of the diaphragm. It descends in front of the bodies of the lumbar vertebræ and ends opposite the fourth lumbar vertebra, a little to the left of the median plane, by dividing into the two common iliac arteries.

Its *Anterior Relations* are numerous and important: (1) The cœliac artery and the cœliac plexus intervene between the aorta and the peritoneal posterior wall of the lesser sac. More anteriorly lie the lesser sac, the lesser omentum and the liver. (2) Immediately below the origin of the cœliac artery, the aorta is crossed by the pancreas. Situated more anteriorly are the lesser sac and the stomach. (3) It is next crossed by the third part of the duodenum, which separates the aorta from coils of the jejunum. (4) Below the duodenum, the aorta is covered with the peritoneum of the posterior wall of the left infracolic compartment, and is related anteriorly to coils of the small intestine, which intervene between the vessel and the transverse colon and the greater omentum.

Posteriorly, the aorta is related (1) to the bodies of the lumbar vertebræ and the corresponding intervertebral discs; (2) to the anterior longitudinal ligament; and (3) to the left lumbar veins, as they cross the median plane to reach the inferior vena cava, and to the origins of its own dorsal branches, viz., the lumbar arteries.

To its *Right Side* lie the inferior vena cava with the sympathetic trunk behind it and, at a higher level, the right crus of the diaphragm, the cisterna chyli and the vena azygos.

To its *Left Side*, from above downwards, the aorta is related to (1) the left crus of the diaphragm, (2) the pancreas, (3) the duodeno-jejunal flexure, (4) the fourth part of the duodenum, (5) the posterior parietal peritoneum and coils of the small intestine, and (6) the left sympathetic trunk.

Branches. The three ventral branches, viz., the cœliac (p. 160), the superior mesenteric (p. 170), and the inferior mesenteric (p. 172), have already been described. They are distributed entirely to the gut, its outgrowths (the liver and the pancreas), and the spleen. In the early stages of development these arteries pass directly into the dorsal mesentery, and when the spleen develops in the upper part of the dorsal mesogastrium it receives its blood supply from one of the branches to the stomach.

The lateral branches of the aorta are persistent mesonephric arteries.

The **Phrenic Arteries** arise from the aorta near the origin of the cœliac artery. They run upwards and laterally, skirting the supra-renal gland, to which a superior suprarenal artery is given. The right artery passes behind the inferior vena cava, and the left behind the œsophagus. The two arteries supply the diaphragm and anastomose with each other.

The **Middle Suprarenal Arteries** arise at a slightly lower level, and run laterally, the right passing behind the inferior vena cava, to reach the suprarenal gland.

The **Renal Arteries** arise from the lateral aspect of the aorta a little below the level of the transpyloric plane. The *right renal artery* passes laterally behind the inferior vena cava and the head of the pancreas to reach the hilum of the right kidney. The *left renal artery* runs to the left, behind its accompanying vein, the splenic vein and the body of the pancreas, and, usually, the duodenojejunal flexure. On each side, the renal artery gives off inferior suprarenal and ureteral branches, and on each side one of the terminal branches enters the hilum behind the pelvis of the ureter.

The **Testicular Arteries** arise from the anterior aspect of the aorta a little below the origin of the renals. The *Right Testicular Artery* runs downwards and to the right, crossing obliquely in front of the inferior vena cava. It is then continued downwards in front of the psoas muscle, crossing in front of the ureter, and ultimately reaches the deep inguinal ring, where it enters the spermatic cord (p. 146). Anteriorly, it is separated from the posterior parietal peritoneum by the third part of the duodenum and the ileo colic vessels, and is crossed by the terminal part of the ileum.

The *Left Testicular Artery* has a corresponding course on the left side of the body, but it crosses behind the lower part of the descending colon.

In the intra-abdominal part of its course each testicular artery gives off branches to the ureter.

The **Ovarian Artery** in the female has a similar origin and course, but it crosses the external iliac vessels at the pelvic inlet and enters the infundibulopelvic ligament of the ovary (p. 208).

The dorsal branches of the abdominal aorta are persistent intersegmental arteries and are distributed on the same plan as the posterior intercostal arteries (p. 125).

Four Pairs of Lumbar Arteries arise from the dorsal aspect of the aorta and pass backwards round the bodies of the upper four lumbar vertebræ. The lower arteries run behind the sympathetic trunk and the psoas muscle; the upper arteries, in addition, pass behind the crus of the diaphragm. On reaching the interval between the transverse processes, each lumbar artery gives off a posterior branch and then runs laterally into the anterior abdominal wall. As a general rule the upper three pass behind the quadratus lumborum muscle, and the lowest passes in front of it. They terminate in the interval between the transversus abdominis and the internal oblique muscle.

The *Posterior Branch* corresponds exactly to the posterior branch of an intercostal artery (p. 125).

The **Median Sacral Artery** arises from the posterior aspect of the aorta just above its bifurcation and runs down behind the left common iliac vein and in front of the sacral promontory into the pelvis, where it anastomoses with the lateral sacral arteries.

The **Cisterna Chyli** is an elongated lymph sac which lies on the right side of the bodies of the first and second lumbar vertebræ, under cover of the right crus of the diaphragm. It receives the intestinal and both lumbar lymph trunks (p. 191). The thoracic duct arises from its upper end and enters the thorax on the right side of the aorta (p. 175).

The **Inferior Vena Cava** is formed on the right side of the body of the fifth lumbar vertebra by the union of the two common iliac veins. It ascends on the posterior abdominal wall to the vena caval opening in the diaphragm, where, on a level with the upper part of the ninth thoracic vertebra, it passes through the central tendon and ends in the right atrium.

Posteriorly, the vena cava is related below to the right sympathetic trunk and the medial border of the right psoas, and above to the right crus of the diaphragm. Several structures are interposed between the vessel and the crus. These include the right renal, middle suprarenal and the phrenic arteries, the right cœliac ganglion and the medial part of the right suprarenal gland.

Anteriorly, from above downwards, the vessel is related to (1) the posterior aspect of the liver; (2) the aditus to the lesser sac; (3) the first part of the duodenum and the portal vein; (4) *the head of the pancreas*, with the terminal part of the bile duct embedded in it; (5) the third part of the duodenum and the right testicular artery; (6) the posterior parietal peritoneum, the root of the mesentery and its contents; (7) the right common iliac artery.

The abdominal aorta lies to its left side, and the right ureter lies half-an-inch from its right border.

Tributaries. In its course the inferior vena cava is joined by numerous tributaries.

1. The *Lumbar Veins*, which run with the corresponding arteries, open into its posterior aspect, the veins of the left side crossing behind the abdominal aorta. The first and second lumbar veins do not open directly into the vena cava. They may turn downwards and join the third lumbar vein, or they may end in the ascending lumbar vein or the vena azygos on the right side, or the vena hemiazygos inferior on the left side.

2. The *Right Testicular* (or *Ovarian*) *Vein*, frequently duplicated, opens into the anterior surface of the inferior vena cava just below the entrance of the renal veins. It is formed near the deep inguinal

ring by the union of the veins of the pampiniform plexus (p. 146). The left testicular (or ovarian) vein ends in the left renal vein behind the duodenojejunal flexure. Both veins are closely related to their accompanying arteries.

3. The *Renal Veins* join the vena cava just below the transpyloric plane and each lies in front of the corresponding artery. *The right vein is very short* and lies behind the second part of the duodenum. The *left vein* crosses in front of the left psoas and the aorta and lies behind the pancreas and splenic vein. It receives the left suprarenal and testicular (or ovarian) veins.

4. The *Right Suprarenal Vein* is extremely short, owing to the proximity of the hilum of the right suprarenal to the trunk of the inferior vena cava. The left suprarenal vein runs downwards and medially to join the left renal vein.

5. The *Hepatic Veins* open directly into the anterior surface of the vena cava just before it pierces the diaphragm. They have no extrahepatic course.

The peculiar behaviour of the upper lumbar veins and of the left suprarenal and testicular veins can be explained in the light of the developmental history of the inferior vena cava. Above the renal veins the vessel represents the persistent right subcardinal vein and its headward continuation to the vena hepatis communis; below the renal veins it represents the right supracardinal vein, which replaces the primitive posterior cardinal vein. The subcardinal vein lies in the ventral part of the mesonephric ridge, whereas the supracardinal vein lies in its dorsal part. The two are therefore on different planes. On this account the third and fourth lumbar veins pass direct to the inferior vena cava (supracardinal segment), but the first and second, which lie opposite its subcardinal segment have to take a different course (p. 187). For the same reason the mesonephric arteries which persist as the phrenic, middle suprarenal and renal arteries cross dorsal to the vena cava (subcardinal segment) but the testicular artery crosses ventral to its supracardinal segment.

Further, as the supracardinal and subcardinal veins of the left side disappear, the left suprarenal, renal and testicular veins are forced to send their blood over to the right side. This they are able to do owing to the presence of a previously established intersubcardinal anastomosis, which becomes incorporated in the terminal part of the left renal vein.

The **Lumbar Plexus** is formed in the substance of the psoas muscle by the ventral rami of the upper four lumbar nerves.

The first lumbar nerve gives origin to (1) the iliohypogastric, (2) the ilio-inguinal, and (3) one root of the genitofemoral nerve.

The **Iliohypogastric** and **Ilio-inguinal Nerves** frequently arise by a common trunk. They emerge at the lateral border of the psoas and run downwards and laterally in front of the quadratus lumborum and behind the kidney and colon (ascending or descending, as the case may be). They pierce the transversus and are continued onwards between that muscle and the internal oblique (p. 139).

The **Genitofemoral Nerve** arises from the first and second lumbar nerves and emerges on the *anterior* surface of the psoas muscle near its medial border. It runs downwards in front of the muscle, being crossed by the root of the mesentery and the ureter on the right side, and by the ureter and the lower part of the descending colon on the left side. Near the deep inguinal ring it lies in front of the external iliac artery and divides into (*a*) a genital branch, which enters the spermatic cord (p. 146), and (*b*) a femoral branch, which is distributed to the skin of the thigh (p. 50).

The second lumbar nerve gives origin to (1) one root of the genitofemoral nerve; (2) one root of the lateral cutaneous nerve of the thigh; (3) one root of the femoral nerve; and (4) one root of the obturator nerve.

The **Lateral Cutaneous Nerve** of the thigh arises from L. 2 and L. 3. It emerges at the lateral border of the psoas and runs downwards and laterally across the right iliac fossa, in front of the iliacus muscle and behind the iliac fascia, to pass behind the lateral end of the inguinal ligament (p. 50).

The **Femoral Nerve** arises from the *posterior* branches of L. 2, L. 3 and L. 4 (being an "extensor" nerve), and emerges at the lateral border of the psoas, running downwards and slightly laterally, situated deeply in the furrow between the psoas and the iliacus. It lies under cover of the iliac fascia and passes behind the inguinal ligament on the lateral side of the femoral artery and femoral sheath. Before it enters the thigh it supplies the iliacus muscle.

The **Obturator Nerve** arises from the *anterior* branches of L. 2, L. 3 and L. 4 (the adductors being "flexor" or ventral musculature in origin). It emerges on the medial side of the psoas muscle and runs forwards and downwards on the pelvic wall, below the pelvic brim. Near its commencement it is crossed by the internal iliac vessels and the ureter (p. 202).

The third lumbar nerve gives origin to (1) one root of the lateral cutaneous nerve of the thigh; (2) one root of the femoral nerve; and (3) one root of the obturator nerve.

The fourth lumbar nerve gives origin to (1) one root of the femoral nerve; (2) one root of the obturator; and (3) one root of the lumbosacral trunk (p. 205), which takes part in the formation of the sacral plexus.

The **Sympathetic System (Abdominal Part)** consists of the two ganglionated trunks and their subsidiary ganglia and plexuses.

The *Sympathetic Trunk* enters the abdomen by passing downwards behind the medial arcuate ligament, and descends along the medial border of the psoas muscle, lying on the bodies of the lumbar vertebræ. On the *right* side it lies behind the inferior vena cava, and on the *left* side it lies close to the left side of the aorta. In the lower part of the abdomen it passes behind the common iliac artery and crosses the sacral promontory to gain the pelvis. Throughout its course the lumbar vessels alone intervene between the trunk and the vertebral bodies. There are usually four lumbar ganglia, the first and second being fused to each other.

Branches: 1. *Lateral.* Each ganglion is connected to the anterior primary ramus of the corresponding lumbar nerve by a *grey ramus communicans.* The upper two, sometimes three, ganglia are also connected to the corresponding lumbar nerves by *white rami communicantes* (p. 238). These branches pass backwards across the sides of the bodies of the vertebræ in company with the lumbar vessels and deep to the psoas muscle.

2. *Medial.* Numerous branches run medially to join the aortic plexus, while others descend, in front of the common iliac artery, to the anterior surface of the body of the fifth lumbar vertebra, where they form the hypogastric plexus (p. 206).

Each **Cœliac Ganglion** is a large, irregularly shaped mass, which lies on the crus of the diaphragm medial to the lower pole of the adrenal gland. It is joined on its deep surface by the greater and lesser splanchnic nerves (pre-ganglionic fibres), which are derived from the fifth to the tenth or eleventh thoracic ganglia, inclusive. The two cœliac ganglia are connected to each other by a large network of fibres, which surrounds the origin of the cœliac artery. From the nerve cells of the ganglia post-ganglionic branches arise, which accompany the cœliac artery and its branches, forming the cœliac plexus. Other branches accompany the renal, the middle suprarenal, superior mesenteric, and testicular (or ovarian) arteries, while others are associated with the aorta. These constitute the renal, suprarenal, superior mesenteric, spermatic and aortic plexuses, which are, of course, merely regional parts of the same great abdominal peri-vascular plexus. In this way sympathetic fibres connected with thoracic segments of the spinal cord are carried to the abdominal viscera. Branches from the aortic plexus continue as the inferior mesenteric plexus, while others join the hypogastric plexus.

In addition to their vasomotor functions, the branches of the cœliac plexus are inhibitory to the muscle and glands of the stomach and intestines, but supply motor fibres to the pyloric and ileocolic sphincters.

The *Aortic Lymph Nodes* are closely associated with the abdominal aorta, forming a pre-aortic and right and left lateral aortic chains. The *Pre-aortic Lymph Nodes* comprise the cœliac, the superior and the inferior mesenteric lymph nodes, and therefore drain practically the whole of the abdominal and pelvic portions of the alimentary canal, the spleen, the pancreas and the greater part of the liver. Their efferents form a large *intestinal trunk*, which joins the cisterna chyli.

The *Lateral Aortic Lymph Nodes* receive efferents (1) from the common iliac nodes, (2) from the kidneys and suprarenals, (3) from the testes in the male, and from the ovary, uterine tube, and body of the uterus in the female, and they receive the deep lymph vessels of the abdominal parietes. Their efferents form the right and left lumbar trunks, which join the cisterna chyli (p. 187).

THE PELVIS IN THE MALE

The **Peritoneum** sweeps down from the anterior abdominal wall on to the superior surface of the urinary bladder, but instead of descending on the sides of that viscus it passes laterally on to the pelvic wall. Towards the back of the upper surface of the bladder, the peritoneum dips down for a short distance on its posterior surface, and is then carried backwards on to the anterior aspect of the rectum, forming the *rectovesical fossa.* On each side of the rectum the peritoneum is closely applied to the sacrum and the lateral walls of the pelvis, and the various vessels, etc., are thus excluded from the pelvic peritoneal cavity. On the left side, however, it is drawn off from the wall to form a mesentery for the pelvic colon.

In natural circumstances, the pelvis contains the pelvic colon and the terminal coils of the ileum both mobile organs.

The **Pelvic Colon** begins in front of the external iliac artery about 2 inches above the inguinal ligament. It is usually 12 to 15 inches long, but its length is subject to great variation. It is provided with a mesentery by which it is attached to the upper part of the posterior wall of the pelvis. As it lies in the pelvis, this part of the colon is related to the urinary bladder below and anteriorly, to the rectum and sacrum posteriorly, and to the terminal coils of the ileum on its right side.

The *Blood Supply* is obtained from the inferior left colic branches of the inferior mesenteric artery. They form a series of arterial arcades in the mesocolon before supplying the gut. The *nerves* are derived from the pelvic plexuses (p. 206). The lymph vessels are described on p. 154.

The **Pelvic Mesocolon** varies in extent with the length of the pelvic colon, but the attachment of its root is fairly constant. Beginning on the medial side of the left external iliac artery, 2 inches from its termination, it runs upwards and medially to the artery's bifurcation. There it blends sharply downwards and medially and it ends in front of the third sacral vertebra, where the pelvic colon gives place to the rectum. Thus the root of the mesocolon is attached along a line which resembles an inverted V. At the apex of the V there is a small peritoneal recess which opens downwards. This is termed the *recess of the pelvic mesocolon*, and when the peritoneum of its floor is divided, the left ureter is exposed. In addition to the inferior left colic vessels, nerves, lymph nodes (p. 154), etc., the superior rectal artery runs downwards and medially to the rectum in the descending limb of the pelvic mesocolon.

The Muscles and Fasciæ of the Pelvis. Before the pelvic viscera and blood vessels are described, it will be found more satisfactory to revise the arrangement of the pelvic muscles and their associated fasciæ. They form two groups, viz., one associated with the pelvic walls, and one associated with the pelvic floor.

The Parietal Pelvic Muscles. The **Piriformis,** which lies on the posterior wall of the pelvis, arises from the second, third and fourth sacral vertebrae and leaves the pelvis by passing through the greater sciatic foramen (p. 62).

The **Obturator Internus** lies on the side wall of the pelvis. It arises from the pelvic surface of the obturator membrane and from the pelvic surface of the hip bone behind the obturator foramen. In its posterior part the muscle extends up to the arcuate line (pelvic brim), but as it is traced forwards its upper border falls short of the upper margin of the obturator foramen, so that the obturator vessels and nerves pass out from the pelvis without piercing the muscle. The fibres of the muscle converge on the lesser sciatic foramen, and its tendon turns laterally, grooving the ischium, to be inserted into the greater trochanter (p. 62).

The **Sphincter Urethræ** lies in the triangular gap of the pubic arch. Its fibres arise on each side from the margin of the arch at the junction of the pubic and ischial rami, and they meet each other in a median raphe. The muscle surrounds the membranous urethra (p. 134).

The **Parietal Pelvic Fascia** covers the pelvic surfaces of the parietal muscles. Posteriorly, it covers the piriformis, and it sweeps forwards as a continuous sheet on to the obturator internus, so that it closes the greater sciatic foramen from the pelvic aspect. Its upper attachment follows the upper border of the obturator internus. Consequently, in the posterior part of the pelvis it is attached to the iliac part of the arcuate line, and is there continuous above with the psoas fascia, but as it is traced forwards it sinks below the line. In front the parietal pelvic fascia is carried medially to cover the pelvic surface of the sphincter urethræ, and its upper border, in this situation, reaches no higher than the lower margin of the symphysis pubis.

The lower limit of the parietal pelvic fascia is attached posteriorly to the falciform edge of the sacrotuberous ligament, and in front stretches across between the two ischial tuberosities, blending with the perineal membrane (p. 134).

The **Muscles of the Pelvic Floor** comprise the two coccygei and the two levator ani muscles, which together constitute the *pelvic diaphragm.*

The *Coccygeus* arises from the ischial spine, and is inserted into the lateral border of the fifth sacral and first coccygeal vertebrae. It covers the pelvic surface of the sacrospinous ligament. It is supplied by S. 4.

Action. The coccygeus assists the levator ani to sustain the pressure of the abdominopelvic viscera. It can also flex the coccyx.

The **Levator Ani** has a linear origin, which begins on the ischial spine and runs forwards across the parietal pelvic fascia, usually coinciding with a linear thickening of the fascia termed the *tendinous arch* (*white line*). Owing to the tilt of the pelvis, the horizontal linear origin of the levator ani crosses the upper border of the parietal pelvic fascia just in front of the obturator internus muscle, and anteriorly the muscle arises from the pubic bone. It does not extend medially as far as the symphysis, and on this account there is a gap between the two levatores ani anteriorly, in which the apex of the prostate is situated.

The levator ani is really a compound muscle consisting of two parts, the iliococcygeus and the pubococcygeus, and the separation is often indicated by a gap in the origin of the muscle.

The *iliococcygeus* arises from the ischial spine and the adjoining part of the parietal pelvic fascia wall, and its fibres run medially to be inserted into the side of the coccyx, and into a median raphe which extends from the tip of the coccyx to the anal canal. At their insertion they are overlapped by the posterior fibres of the pubococcygeus.

The *pubococcygeus* arises from the back of the body of the pubis and the adjoining part of the obturator fascia. Its anterior fibres, which constitute the *levator prostatæ* muscle, run backwards and slightly downwards, across the lateral aspect of the prostate to be inserted into the perineal body.

The succeeding fibres pass backwards across the lateral aspect of the prostate and the upper part of the anal canal, round which they sweep to become continuous with the corresponding fibres of the opposite side. They act as an additional sphincter for the anal canal and are often referred to as the *puborectalis* muscle.

The posterior fibres of the pubococcygeus run backwards and medially. Behind the anal canal they reach the median raphe and the side of the coccyx, overlapping the iliococcygeus, which they assist in supporting the horizontal part of the rectum.

The levator ani plays an important part in resisting the intrapelvic pressure and in maintaining the pelvic viscera in position (*vide infra*). It is called into action during all straining or expulsive efforts, to resist the downward thrust which the muscles of the abdominal wall exert on the abdominal and pelvic viscera.

The *Nerve Supply* is derived from the perineal branch of the pudendal nerve and from the perineal branch of S. 4.

The *Perineal Body* is a substantial fibromuscular node, which is the confluence of muscles important in maintaining the integrity of the pelvic floor.

In the male it lies behind the apex of the prostate and in front of the anal canal, and is intimately connected to the base of the perineal membrane. The external sphincter and the bulbospongiosus take origin from it, and the superficial transverse perineal muscles and the levatores ani (levatores prostatæ) are inserted into it. In addition it is intimately connected to the longitudinal fibres of the lower end of the rectum and the upper part of the anal canal.

In the female the pelvic floor is pierced by the vagina in addition to the urethra and the rectum, and the perineal body is of greater importance than it is in the male. It lies between the anal canal and the lower end of the vagina and receives the insertion of those fibres of the levatores ani which correspond to the levatores prostatæ. The latter sweep backwards across the sides of the vagina to reach the perineal body, and so act as an additional vaginal sphincter. Lacerations of the perineum may occur during delivery. When they rupture the posterior vaginal wall and the perineal body, they greatly diminish the efficiency of the pelvic floor. Unless adequately repaired, they lead subsequently to prolapse of the pelvic viscera.

The **Visceral Pelvic Fascia** is a layer of connective tissue which envelops the pelvic viscera. On each side it is continuous with the fascia on the pelvic surface of the levator ani muscle, and so indirectly becomes continuous with the parietal pelvic fascia along the origin of that muscle. The only portions which merit special description are the rectovesical fascia and the sheath of the prostate. Elsewhere the visceral pelvic fascia need not be regarded as anything more definite than the layer of connective tissue which is found on the outer wall of any viscus in the abdomen.

The *rectovesical fascia* is a non-vascular membranous sheet which is connected below to the perineal body. It extends upwards behind, and often firmly adherent to, the prostate, the seminal vesicles and the terminal portions of the vasa deferentia, and in front of the rectum, from which it is separated by some loose areolar tissue. Above, the rectovesical fascia is attached to the peritoneal floor of the rectovesical fossa, and it represents the fused walls of the obliterated lower part of the fossa. On each side, it is connected to the sheath which surrounds the prostatic and vesical venous plexuses.

The *sheath of the prostate* is formed in front and on each side by the fibroareolar tissue in which the veins of the prostatic plexus are embedded. Posteriorly, the sheath is non-vascular and is formed by the rectovesical fascia. The upper and anterior part of the sheath is connected to the posterior aspect of the pubic bones by the *puboprostatic ligaments*, which lie close together, one on each side of the median plane. These ligaments are included under the term "visceral pelvic fascia," and they consist partly of fibrous tissue and partly of unstriped muscle. They occupy the anterior part of the interval between the anterior fibres of the levatores ani, and on each side are continuous with the fascia covering the muscle.

The **Rectum** occupies the posterior part of the pelvis. It begins opposite the middle of the third sacral segment and, following the curve of the sacrum and coccyx, ends 1 inch in front of the tip of the latter by bending sharply downwards and backwards into the anal canal. In addition to the curve imposed upon it by the vertebral column, the rectum shows lateral flexures. A little below its commencement the rectum deviates to the left, but it soon returns to the median plane, and retains that position throughout the remainder of its extent. The sum total of the lateral flexures results in the rectum bulging over to the left of the median plane in its upper part.

The *Peritoneum* at first covers the rectum anteriorly and on each side, but it gradually leaves the sides, and 1 inch above the base of the prostate it is reflected from the anterior surface forwards to the bladder, forming the floor of the rectovesical fossa. The lower part of the rectum is thus devoid of peritoneal covering, and when the finger is introduced through the anal canal it is this portion which can be explored.

The lower portion of the rectum is dilated to form the *rectal ampulla*.

Posteriorly, the rectum is related to the median sacral artery and the sacrum, the coccyx and the median raphe of the levatores ani, although the last-named is, strictly speaking, an inferior relation.

On each side of the median plane the rectum is related to the piriformis muscle, the sympathetic trunk, the lateral sacral artery, and the lower sacral nerves as they issue from the anterior sacral foramina; but, owing to the lateral flexures of the gut, these relations are closer on the left than on the right side. In its last part the rectum rests on the coccygei and levatores ani.

Anteriorly, so long as it is covered with the peritoneum, the rectum is related to the terminal part of the pelvic colon. Below the reflection of the peritoneum the rectum is related to the posterior surface of the bladder in the median plane, and to the termination of the vas deferens and the seminal vesicle on each side of the median plane. The anterior wall of the rectal ampulla is related to the posterior aspect of the prostate. It is separated from all these structures by some loose cellular tissue and the rectovesical fascia (*vide supra*).

The **Anal Canal,** which is 1½ inches long, runs downwards and backwards through the posterior part of the gap between the two levatores ani muscles to reach the anus. *Posteriorly*, it is related to the anococcygeal body—a collection of dense fibrous tissue which lies between the anal canal and the coccyx, and which is blended above with the median raphe of the levatores ani. *Anteriorly*, it is related to the perineal body and the base of the perineal membrane, which separate it from the membranous urethra and the bulb of the penis. *On each side*, the puborectalis separates the anal canal from the ischiorectal fossa.

The *Blood Supply* of the rectum and anal canal is derived from the median sacral, and from the superior, middle and inferior rectal vessels (pp. 172, 204 and 131).

The *Lymph Vessels* of the rectum and the upper half of the anal canal end in (1) the anorectal lymph nodes, which lie in or on the wall of the rectal ampulla, and (2) the internal iliac lymph nodes. The efferents from these lymph nodes pass to the lower aortic lymph nodes.

From the lower half of the anal canal the lymphatics pass to the medial lymph nodes of the superficial inguinal group (p. 51).

The *Nerves* of the rectum and the upper half of the anal canal are derived from the pelvic splanchnics (p. 206). The lower half of the anal canal receives branches from the inferior rectal nerve (p. 131).

The Structure of the Rectum and Anal Canal. The muscular coat of the rectum differs from that found in the rest of the large intestine in that the longitudinal fibres form only two broad bands, of which one is placed on the anterior and the other on the posterior aspect of the gut. The circular coat is thickened at the upper end of the anal canal to form the *internal sphincter.* Fibres of the levator ani (puborectalis) lie outside the internal sphincter, but within the muscular ring of the external sphincter, which is developed in association with the other superficial perineal muscles.

The *Mucous Membrane* of the rectum is infolded at the site of each lateral flexure. These infoldings pass half-way round the gut-wall, and are termed the *transverse folds* of the rectum. Two are placed on the left and one on the right wall. The lowest horizontal fold can just be reached with the tip of the finger on digital examination. The folds are variable in number, but they are true infoldings of the rectal wall, and they involve the circular muscle coat as well as the mucous membrane.

The mucous membrane of the anal canal in its upper half displays a number of longitudinal ridges, termed the *anal columns*, which are connected to one another at their lower ends by short semilunar folds, named the *anal valves*. The lining membrane of the lower half of the anal canal is modified skin.

The rectum and the upper half of the anal canal are endodermal in origin and are derived from the dorsal part of the cloaca. After they have been separated off from the bladder and urogenital sinus, they remain closed below by the anal membrane.

The perineal aspect of the anal membrane lies at first at the bottom of a small depression, termed the *proctodeum*, which forms the lower half of the anal canal. The membrane, which later breaks down, lies at the level of the anal valves. The upper part of the anal canal is derived from the cloaca and is endodermal in origin, but the lower part is ectodermal in origin and is therefore lined with modified skin, supplied by the neighbouring cutaneous nerves. On this account, although extensive lesions of the upper half of the anal canal may be almost entirely painless, even a small tear of the wall of the lower half is exquisitely painful.

The **Common Iliac Artery** arises at the bifurcation of the abdominal aorta and runs downwards and laterally, along the medial border of the psoas, to end opposite the sacro-iliac joint at the level of the lumbosacral disc by dividing into the external and the internal iliac arteries. *Posteriorly*, the artery crosses the bodies of the fourth and fifth lumbar vertebræ, the sympathetic trunk, the obturator nerve and the lumbosacral trunk. On the right side the commencement of the inferior vena cava forms an additional posterior relation. *Anteriorly*, it is covered with peritoneum and is crossed by sympathetic branches on their way to the hypogastric plexus and, at its termination, by the ureter. On the left side, the vessel is also crossed by the superior rectal artery and, at its termination, by the pelvic mesocolon (p. 191).

The **Common Iliac Vein,** formed by the union of the internal and external veins, lies medial to its companion artery on the left side, but is postero-medial on the right side. The two veins unite behind the right common iliac artery to form the inferior vena cava. With the exception of the ureter, the relations are similar to those of the artery.

The **Urinary Bladder** occupies the anterior part of the pelvic cavity. When empty, it is flattened from above downwards by the pressure of the neighbouring viscera, but as it fills with urine it becomes ovoid in shape.

The *Peritoneal Relations* of the bladder are of great importance. The empty bladder lies below the peritoneal floor of the pelvis, and is consequently covered only on its superior surface by the peritoneum. As the bladder fills, it rises up into the hypogastric region. Its superior surface becomes larger, and as the peritoneum does not stretch, the additional peritoneal covering is obtained by peeling the peritoneum off the lower part of the anterior abdominal wall and from the side walls of the pelvis. *Thus the anterior part of the bladder comes into direct contact with the lower part of the anterior abdominal wall,* a fact which is important to the surgeon. It must be remembered, however, that the point where the urachus is attached does not remain the highest point on the bladder when it is distended. As a result the area left uncovered by the peritoneum is considerably smaller than is sometimes stated, and in approaching the distended bladder extraperitoneally the surgeon is careful to keep in the median plane until the viscus has been opened.

In the young child, the bladder projects further above the pubes than in adults and is, to a large extent, an abdominal organ.

The *Superior Surface* is related to the coils of the pelvic colon and the terminal coils of the ileum. The anterior part of this surface is somewhat pointed, and forms the *apex* of the bladder. From it a fibrous cord, termed the *urachus*, runs upwards in the extraperitoneal fat to the umbilicus.

The *Inferolateral Surfaces* are in contact, in front, with the retropubic pad of fat and the pubic bones. More posteriorly they are related to the obturator internus and the lateral umbilical ligament above, and to the levator ani muscle below. Numerous veins of the vesical venous plexus course backwards in intimate relationship with this surface.

The *Posterior Surface* of the bladder, which looks as much downwards as backwards, is related to the anterior surface of the rectum.

No peritoneum intervenes between the two viscera except to a very slight extent above, but they are separated from one another by the vasa deferentia, the seminal vesicles and the rectovesical fascia (p. 195). The two vasa deferentia lie side by side on the posterior surface of the bladder, and they intervene between the seminal vesicles, which are related to the lateral portions of this surface. The supero-lateral angles of the posterior surface are the site of entry of the ureters.

Inferiorly, the conical neck of the bladder is related to the prostate. The relationship is more than topographical, for *the muscular fibres of the bladder are uninterruptedly continuous with those of the prostate.* On the outside the union is marked by a groove in which lie the backwardly running veins of the prostatic and vesical plexuses, but the veins extend above the groove on to the infero-lateral surface of the bladder, and below it on to the lateral surface of the prostate.

The *Mucous Membrane* of the empty bladder is rugose, but the irregularities disappear when the bladder is full. Over the *trigone*, which corresponds to the posterior surface, the mucous membrane is always smooth. This area is limited above by a muscular ridge, termed the *interureteric ridge*, which runs from the opening of one ureter to that of the other. Below, it is limited by the orifice of the urethra. The *uvula vesicæ* is a small rounded elevation which lies immediately behind the urethral orifice. It is caused by the underlying *median lobe* of the prostate. A small degree of enlargement of this lobe easily causes obstruction to the urinary outflow.

Blood Supply. The superior and inferior vesical arteries (p. 204) supply the bladder. The *veins* constitute the vesical venous plexus (p. 201).

The *Nerves* of the bladder are derived from the hypogastric plexus of the sympathetic (L. 1 and 2) and the pelvic splanchnics (S. 2 and 3). The sympathetic is motor to the sphincter and inhibitory to the muscular wall of the bladder. The parasympathetic fibres of the pelvic splanchnics are visceromotor to the muscular wall of the bladder and inhibitory to its sphincter.

The bladder is derived from the ventral part of the cloaca. The allantois plays no part in its formation, although it may contribute to the formation of the urachus. The trigone, however, is formed from the incorporated caudal ends of the mesonephric ducts, and as a result the ureters (p. 179) are able to open into the bladder.

The **Vas Deferens** (p. 148) leaves the spermatic cord at the deep inguinal ring and, hooking round the origin of the inferior epigastric artery, runs backwards with a slight downward inclination on the side wall of the pelvis till it reaches the ischial spine. Although in this part of its course the vas is running almost horizontally, it becomes placed more and more deeply in the pelvis as it passes backwards, on account of the normal inclination of the pelvis. At the ischial spine it makes a right-angled bend, which carries it medially, forwards and downwards across the terminal part of the ureter and down the posterior surface of the bladder.

Until the vas reaches the posterior surface of the bladder, it is in direct contact on its medial side with the peritoneum, and thereafter it lies below the level of the peritoneal floor of the pelvis. After hooking round the inferior epigastric artery the vas deferens crosses the external iliac artery and vein, the superior ramus of the pubis and the obturator internus muscle, but it is separated from the latter by the lateral umbilical ligament and the obturator artery, the obturator nerve and the obturator vein.

On turning medially at the ischial spine, the vas crosses in front of the ureter, and then runs downwards on the posterior aspect of the bladder. In this part of its course the vas lies behind the bladder and in front of the rectum, with the seminal vesicle on its infero-lateral side and the vas of the opposite side in close contact.

The lower end of the vas deferens is dilated and constitutes the *ampulla*. Inferiorly, the ampulla narrows down in a very striking manner before it joins the duct of the seminal vesicle to form the *ejaculatory duct*. It commonly contains spermatozoa.

The *Artery to the Vas deferens* arises either from the umbilical (p. 204) or from one of the vesical arteries, and runs in close relationship with its wall from the base of the bladder to the epididymis, where it anastomoses with the testicular artery.

The **Seminal Vesicles** are two puckered, loculated sacs, each 2 inches in length, which lie between the rectum *behind* and the bladder *in front*. The blind upper end of the seminal vesicle lies below the terminal part of the ureter, and the long axis of the sac is directed forwards, medially, and slightly downwards, when the bladder is empty. On the *medial side* lies the terminal part of the vas deferens, with its ampulla; on the *lateral side* the prostatic and vesical plexuses of veins stream backwards to join the internal iliac vein, and the superior and inferior vesical arteries pass forwards to reach the bladder.

Inferiorly, the seminal vesicle becomes much narrowed, and joins the vas deferens to form the *ejaculatory duct*, which pierces the prostate to open into the prostatic urethra.

The seminal vesicle does not act as a reservoir for spermatozoa; its function is to produce a secretion which forms a large part of the seminal fluid.

The vas deferens is the persistent mesonephric duct (p. 180) and the seminal vesicle arises as an outgrowth from its caudal end.

The **Prostate** is a solid organ, consisting of fibrous tissue, plain muscle and glandular tissue. It lies between the neck of the bladder above and the perineal membrane below, and is traversed by the beginning of the urethra.

The *Superior Surface* of the prostate is structurally continuous with the superimposed bladder, neither the fibrous nor the muscular constituents showing any interruption as they pass from the one organ to the other. *Posteriorly*, the prostate is in contact with the anterior aspect of the rectal ampulla, the rectovesical fascia alone intervening. This surface can readily be palpated on digital examination through the rectum. It is pierced on each side of the median plane by the ejaculatory duct. The *infero-lateral surfaces* are related to the anterior fibres of the levator ani as they run backwards from the pubis. These two surfaces meet the posterior surface at the *apex* of the prostate, which lies just below the emerging urethra and is separated from the anal canal by the perineal body. The infero-lateral surfaces are separated from each other by the rounded *anterior surface*, which is pierced by the urethra immediately above the apex.

The prostate possesses a strong fibrous sheath, which is continuous above with the fascial covering of the bladder, and in front with the puboprostatic ligaments (p. 195). Posteriorly, the sheath is formed by the rectovesical fascia, and on each side it is little more than the fibro-areolar tissue in which the prostatic plexus of veins is embedded.

Blood Supply. The prostate is supplied by the inferior vesical and middle rectal arteries. The prostatic veins are joined in front by the deep dorsal vein of the penis (p. 134) and as they pass backwards in the lateral wall of the sheath of the prostate they are joined by numerous vesical veins. Finally they run backwards, lateral to the seminal vesicle and below the ureter, to join the internal iliac vein.

The *Lymph Vessels*, for the most part, end in the internal iliac and sacral lymph nodes.

The median lobe of the prostate roughly corresponds to the portion of the gland which lies between the two ejaculatory ducts and the urethra. It not uncommonly produces a slight elevation in the floor of the bladder immediately behind the internal urethral orifice. This elevation has already been mentioned as the *uvula vesicæ* (p. 199).

The **Prostatic Part of the Urethra** begins at the neck of the bladder and runs downwards and slightly forwards through the prostate, to emerge a little above its apex, where it becomes continuous with the second, or membranous, part of the urethra. One and a quarter inches long, the prostatic is the *widest and most dilatable part of the urethra.* Its floor, or posterior wall, is marked by a longitudinal elevation named the *urethral crest.* On each side of the crest is a groove, *the prostatic sinus,* into which the numerous minute ducts of the prostate open. The *prostatic utricle* is a small blind diverticulum which opens into the floor of the urethra near the lower end of the urethral crest. At the lateral margins of its orifice the ejaculatory ducts open into the urethra.

The **Ureter** (p. 179) enters the pelvis by crossing the pelvic brim in front of the bifurcation of the common iliac artery, and runs downwards and slightly backwards in front of the internal iliac artery until it reaches the level of the ischial spine. It then bends forwards and medially to reach the posterior aspect of the bladder at its upper and lateral angle.

Throughout its course in the pelvis the ureter is in intimate relation, on its *anterior* and *medial* aspects, with the peritoneum, except near its termination, where the vas deferens and the superior vesical artery intervene. The internal iliac artery lies immediately *behind* the ureter, and its obturator and obliterated umbilical branches and the obturator nerve run forwards *lateral* to the ureter and separate it from the posterior part of the obturator internus muscle (see also p. 204).

The **External Iliac Artery** commences opposite the sacro-iliac joint as one of the terminal branches of the common iliac artery. It runs downwards along the medial border of the psoas muscle, following the pelvic brim, until, at a point about half-an-inch above the inguinal ligament, it passes in front of the muscle and then runs downwards into the thigh.

On its *anterior* and *medial* aspects the artery is closely related to the peritoneum, except near its termination, where the testicular (or ovarian) artery crosses in front of it and the vas deferens crosses its medial side. On its *lateral* side the artery is related to the psoas muscle above, and to the femoral nerve below. Its companion vein lies *medial* to the artery below, but is posterior above. On the *right* the artery is related to the terminal coil of the ileum. On the *left* it is related to the pelvic colon and the root of the pelvic mesocolon (p. 191).

In the *female,* the external iliac artery is crossed near its commencement by the ovarian vessels, as they pass from the pelvic wall to enter the infundibulopelvic ligament of the ovary. Just above the inguinal ligament it is related anteriorly to the round ligament of the uterus before this structure enters the inguinal canal.

The *External Iliac Lymph Nodes* surround the artery near its termination. They draw their afferents from the deep inguinal lymph nodes (p. 51), and send their efferents upwards to the common iliac and aortic lymph nodes.

Branches. The inferior epigastric and the deep circumflex iliac arteries are the only branches worthy of note. They have been described in connexion with the anterior abdominal wall (p. 143).

The **External Iliac Vein** begins behind the inguinal ligament, where it is related to the medial side of its accompanying artery. As it passes up through the pelvis it lies on a plane postero-medial to the artery, and is in contact laterally with the upper part of the side walls of the pelvis, and medially with the peritoneum.

Near its commencement it receives the inferior epigastric and deep circumflex iliac veins, and it ends by joining the internal iliac to constitute the common iliac vein. On the right side, at its upper end, it lies directly behind the corresponding artery.

The **Internal Iliac Artery** is the other terminal branch of the common iliac trunk. Beginning on a level with the lumbosacral disc it runs downwards on the posterior pelvic wall in front of the sacro-iliac joint. At the upper border of the greater sciatic foramen the artery breaks up into anterior and posterior divisions, but the precise manner in which the terminal branches arise from these divisions is open to considerable variation.

Relations. Anteriorly, the artery is related to the ureter, and *medially*, to the peritoneum. On its *lateral side* it is separated from the obturator internus muscle by the external iliac vein and the obturator nerve. *Posteriorly*, it is related to the sacrum and the sacro-iliac joint, whilst the companion vein and the lumbosacral trunk lie to its postero-medial side.

Branches. The following branches usually arise from the *posterior division:*

1. The *Iliolumbar Artery*, which often arises from the main trunk, ascends along the pelvic inlet posterior to the external iliac vessels and passes deep to the psoas and iliacus muscles, supplying branches to both.

2. The *Lateral Sacral Artery* runs downwards and medially in front of the sacral plexus, and, therefore, lateral to the anterior sacral foramina. It gives off spinal branches, which enter the foramina and terminate inferiorly by anastomosing with the median sacral artery and its fellow of the opposite side. It is usually represented by two arteries on each side.

3. The *Superior Gluteal Artery* runs backwards and downwards between the lumbosacral trunk and the first sacral nerve and, piercing the parietal pelvic fascia, enters the gluteal region by passing

through the upper part of the greater sciatic foramen above the piriformis muscle (p. 62).

The following branches usually arise from the *anterior division* of the internal iliac artery:—

1. The *Umbilical Artery* is a large vessel in the fœtus. It is then the main continuation of the internal iliac, but in the adult it is only pervious in its first inch or two, and is thereafter a fibrous cord, which is termed the *lateral umbilical ligament.* It runs downwards on the pelvic wall below the external iliac vein, and is crossed by the ureter. After giving off the *artery to the vas deferens* and the *superior vesical artery*, it becomes fibrous and runs downwards and forwards on the lateral wall of the pelvis, just above the obturator nerve. Near the pubic tubercle it leaves the pelvis and ascends in the extra-peritoneal fat to the umbilicus.

2. The *Superior Vesical Artery* is usually a branch of the umbilical, which is, therefore, pervious until it has been given off. It supplies the superior surface of the bladder and may give off the *artery to the vas deferens.*

3. The *Obturator Artery* runs downwards and forwards on the pelvic wall, below and behind the obturator nerve, which separates it from the lateral umbilical ligament. Converging on the nerve, it passes through the upper part of the obturator foramen and divides into lateral and medial branches, which encircle the outer surface of the obturator membrane, supplying the obturator externus muscle and giving off an acetabular branch to the hip joint.

Before leaving the pelvis the obturator artery gives off a pubic branch, which anastomoses with a similar branch from the inferior epigastric artery. This anastomosis may be enlarged and form an abnormal obturator artery (p. 143).

4. The *Inferior Vesical Artery* runs forwards and medially on the levator ani, crosses the lateral aspect of the seminal vesicle, and is distributed to the infero-lateral surface of the bladder. It supplies the seminal vesicle and often gives off the *artery to the vas deferens.*

5. The *Middle Rectal Artery*, small and variable, pierces the muscular coat of the rectum and gains the submucous level, where it anastomoses with the superior and inferior rectal arteries.

A similar communication exists between the corresponding veins, and constitutes a link between the systemic veins and the veins of the portal system (p. 174).

6. The *Internal Pudendal Artery* and (7) the *Inferior Gluteal Artery* run downwards in front of the sacral plexus, which separates them from the piriformis muscle. At the lower border of the muscle they pierce the parietal pelvic fascia and pass through the lower part

of the greater sciatic foramen into the gluteal region (p. 62). The internal pudendal lies anterior to the inferior gluteal, and is usually the smaller artery.

The **Internal Iliac Vein** lies postero-medial to its companion artery, and ascends in front of the sacro-iliac joint. It receives tributaries which correspond to the branches of the artery save that the ilio-lumbar vein joins the common iliac. The tributaries from the viscera form venous plexuses from which one or more trunks finally emerge.

The **Sacral Plexus** is formed by the anterior primary rami of L. 4 and 5, S. 1, 2, 3 and 4. The portion of L. 4 which does not join the lumbar plexus runs downwards, medial to the psoas muscle, and joins L. 5 to form the *lumbrosacral trunk*. This nerve is joined by S. 1, and the resulting broad nerve band is joined by S. 2 and a part of S. 3, and lies in front of the piriformis muscle and behind the parietal pelvic fascia.

The sacral plexus is placed in front of the piriformis muscle, which separates it from the lateral part of the sacrum. *Anteriorly*, it is covered by the parietal pelvic fascia, which separates the plexus from the internal iliac vessels above, and from their lateral sacral, inferior gluteal and internal pudendal branches below. Still more anteriorly the rectum, especially when it is distended, is related to the lower part of the plexus.

Branches of the Plexus. 1. The *Superior Gluteal Nerve* (L. 4, 5 and S. 1) arises from the dorsal aspect of the plexus and passes backwards above the piriformis into the gluteal region. It is distributed to the gluteus medius and minimus and the tensor fasciæ latæ muscles.

2. The *Inferior Gluteal Nerve* (L. 5, S. 1 and 2) also arises from the posterior aspect of the plexus. It passes backwards below the piriformis and, gaining the buttock, to the supply of the gluteus maximus muscle.

3. The *Nerve to the Quadratus Femoris* (L. 4, 5 and S. 1) arises from the ventral surface of the plexus and enters the gluteal region below the piriformis (p. 62).

4. The *Nerve to the Obturator Internus* (L. 5, S. 1 and 2), like the preceding nerve, arises from the ventral aspect of the plexus, and in company with the internal pudendal vessels enters the gluteal region below the piriformis muscle.

5. The *Posterior Cutaneous Nerve of the thigh* (S. 1, 2 and 3) arises from the posterior aspect of the plexus, and passes below the piriformis muscle to enter the gluteal region behind the sciatic nerve (p. 63). It is a purely sensory nerve.

6. The *Sciatic Nerve* (L. 4, 5, S. 1, 2 and 3) is the main continuation of the broad nerve band within the pelvis. Like the preceding nerve it leaves the pelvis through the lower part of the greater sciatic foramen. Its subsequent course is described on pp. 63 and 66.

7. The *Pudendal Nerve* (S. 2, 3 and 4) runs in company with the internal pudendal vessels and the nerve to the obturator internus. It passes into the gluteal region through the greater sciatic foramen below the piriformis muscle, and, after crossing the sacrospinous ligament, gains the ischiorectal fossa (p. 130).

8. Branches from S. 2 and S. 3 supply the piriformis.

9. The *Pelvic Splanchnics*, which arise from S. 2 and 3 or S. 3 and 4, form a leash of small nerves which run forwards on the levator ani muscle, and join the branches of the pelvic plexus (*infra*), on the walls of the pelvic viscera. Small ganglia are situated at the points of junction. These nerves are distributed to the pelvic viscera, and they constitute the sacral part of the parasympathetic system (*infra*). They supply visceromotor fibres to the bladder wall and inhibitory fibres to its sphincter, visceromotor fibres to the rectum, vasodilator fibres to the erectile tissue of the penis or clitoris, and visceromotor fibres to the uterus.

10. The *Perforating Cutaneous Nerve* (S. 2 and 3) pierces the sacrotuberous ligament and the lower border of the gluteus maximus to supply the skin of the lower and medial part of the buttock.

The **Coccygeal Plexus** is formed by the remainder of S. 4 and the whole of S. 5 and the coccygeal nerve. It lies on the pelvic surface of the coccygeus muscle, and gives *muscular branches* to the levator ani, the coccygeus and the sphincter ani externus.

The coccygeal nerve, after being joined by S. 5, pierces the coccygeus and supplies the skin in the immediate neighbourhood of the coccyx.

The **Pelvic Portion of the Sympathetic Trunk** is directly continuous with the abdominal portion. It lies on the front of the sacrum, medial to the anterior sacral foramina. There are usually four ganglia on each side, and the two trunks unite in the *ganglion impar* in front of the coccyx.

Branches. A Grey Ramus Communicans connects each sympathetic ganglion to a sacral nerve, carrying post-ganglionic fibres into it. Numerous *visceral branches* leave the sacral ganglia and join the various offsets of the pelvic plexuses.

The **Superior Hypogastric Plexus (Hypogastric Plexus)** is formed in front of the fifth lumbar vertebra by branches from the aortic plexus and the lumbar ganglia of both sides and breaks up at once into the *right* and *left interior hypogastric* (*pelvic*) *plexuses.* These plexuses run downwards and forwards on the lateral wall of the pelvis to the pelvic viscera, where they join branches from the pelvic splanchnics.

Fibres of the pelvic splanchnic nerves pass back from the inferior to the superior hypogastric plexuses, ascending thence to the aortic plexus to reach the inferior mesenteric plexus. By this route that part of the colon which is not innervated by vagus fibres receives its parasympathetic supply. The junction between the two zones innervated by the cranial and sacral outflows is near the left colic flexure.

THE FEMALE PELVIS

The **Peritoneum** of the female pelvis is complicated by the presence of the uterus and vagina, which are interposed between the bladder and the rectum.

The peritoneal relations of the bladder are very similar to those already described for the male (p. 198). On leaving the posterior part of the upper surface of the bladder, the peritoneum passes directly on to the anterior surface of the uterus, which it meets on a level with the internal os uteri. It is carried upwards on the anterior surface, backwards over the fundus, and then downwards on the posterior surface. It covers the whole of this aspect of the uterus, *and is continued downwards over the upper part of the posterior wall of the vagina* before it is reflected backwards on to the rectum.

Along the right and left borders of the uterus the two layers which cover the anterior and posterior surfaces of the viscus do not become continuous with each other, but are carried laterally, in close apposition, to the pelvic wall, where they become continuous with the parietal peritoneum. In this way a loose fold of peritoneum connects the uterus to the side wall of the pelvis: it is known as the *broad ligament of the uterus.*

On account of the projection of the uterus into the pelvic cavity, two peritoneal fossæ are produced: (1) a shallow uterovesical fossa placed between the uterus and the bladder; and (2) a deep recto-uterine fossa, placed between the uterus and vagina in front, and the rectum behind. The first of these is usually obliterated by the close apposition of the uterus to the superior surface of the bladder, but the second is normally open and contains coils of ileum or pelvic colon.

The peritoneal relations of the rectum are the same in the female as in the male pelvis.

The **Broad Ligament of the Uterus** is a structure of great importance on account of the relationship which it bears to the uterine tube, the uterine and ovarian vessels, the ovary, etc. Formed like all other peritoneal ligaments as a two-layered fold, the broad ligament is somewhat triangular in shape. Medially the two layers separate to enclose the uterus. Inferiorly and laterally they separate to clothe the floor and side wall of the pelvis. Superiorly the two layers are continuous, so forming a free upper border for the ligament—it is really anterior in the standing position. Within this free border the uterine tube is situated, just as the ligamentum teres of the liver is situated in the free edge of the falciform ligament. The portion of the broad ligament which lies immediately below the uterine tube is usually termed the *mesosalpinx*.

The ovary lies behind the broad ligament, but it is connected to its posterior layer by a short peritoneal fold, known as the *mesovarium*. The upper and lateral part of the broad ligament constitutes the *infundibulopelvic ligament of the ovary*. It contains the ovarian vessels, etc., as they pass between the pelvic wall and the mesovarium.

In addition to the uterine tube, the following structures are found between the two layers of the broad ligament:—

1. The *Round Ligament of the Uterus*, a fibro-muscular cord which passes from the supero-lateral angle (*cornu*) of the uterus to the deep inguinal ring, raising a ridge on the anterior aspect of the broad ligament (p. 211).

2. The *Ovarian Ligament*, a fibromuscular cord which connects the uterine (lower) pole of the ovary to the supero-lateral angle of the uterus.

3. The *Epöophoron*, a vestigial tubular structure which lies in the mesosalpinx above the attachment of the mesovarium (p. 213).

4. The *Uterine Vessels*, which lie along the border of the uterus.

5. The *Ovarian Vessels*, which, after supplying the ovary, run medially to the uterus to anastomose with the uterine vessels.

The muscles and fasciæ of the pelvis do not require much further explanation (p. 192). The gap between the two levatores ani in the anterior part of the pelvic floor is occupied by the neck of the bladder—the prostate being absent in the female—the vagina and the anal canal. Consequently, the vagina and the uterus become clothed in visceral pelvic fascia. Pubovesical ligaments replace the puboprostatic ligaments (p. 195), but are not so strongly developed. The perineal body (p. 194) lies between the anal canal and the lower end of the vagina. As in the male, it receives the insertion of the anterior fibres of the levatores ani, and the importance of this fact has already been emphasised (see p. 194).

The **Bladder** presents certain differences in relations which are of importance. *Superiorly*, it is related to the body of the uterus and the uterovesical fossa. *Posteriorly*, it is separated from the rectum by the vagina. *Inferiorly*, the neck of the bladder is related to the sphincter urethræ. The infero-lateral relations are as already described (p. 198).

Owing to the absence of the prostate the bladder occupies a rather lower level in the pelvis. As it becomes filled and rises up into the abdomen, it thrusts the uterus upwards and backwards, decreasing the angle of anteversion.

The **Uterus** is a hollow viscus with thick muscular walls. In the adult, during the child-bearing period, it is 3 inches long, 2 inches wide, and 1 inch thick, but it is capable of enormous growth during pregnancy. The lowest part of the uterus is somewhat narrowed and is termed the *cervix*. It projects into the upper part of the vagina, with which it communicates by means of the *external os uteri*. The lumen of the cervical canal is spindle-shaped, and opens above into the uterine cavity proper through the *internal os uteri*.

The portion of the uterus which lies above the cervix is termed the *body*, and its convex upper extremity is the *fundus*.

Under normal conditions the long axis of the uterus is bent forwards on the long axis of the vagina; this position is termed *anteversion*. Further, the uterus is itself curved forwards, a condition known as *anteflexion*.

Relations of the Uterus. *Anteriorly*, the body of the uterus is separated from the superior surface of the bladder only by the potential uterovesical fossa. The cervix, in its upper part, is in direct relationship with the bladder; in its lower part it forms the posterior wall of the anterior part of the fornix of the vagina. *Posteriorly*, both the body and cervix lie in the anterior wall of the recto-uterine fossa, and are therefore related to coils of ileum or pelvic colon. *On each side*, the body is related to the broad ligament and the uterine vessels. The cervix is related to the vaginal branch of the uterine artery and, *half-an-inch to its lateral side, the ureter passes forwards to the bladder*.

The supero-lateral angle of the uterus is traversed by the uterine tube, and has the round ligament connected to its anterior aspect and the ovarian ligament to its posterior aspect.

Blood Supply. The **Uterine Artery** arises from the anterior division of the internal iliac artery, and runs forwards on the pelvic floor to reach the lateral aspect of the cervix, making a wide spiral turn round the ureter. *Half-an-inch from the cervix the artery crosses above and in front of the ureter*. On reaching the cervix the vessel gives off a small vaginal branch and then turns upwards in the medial part of the broad ligament along the border of the uterus.

Near the supero-lateral angle of the uterus it meets and anastomoses with the terminal branch of the ovarian artery, which also helps to supply the organ (p. 208).

The *Uterine Vein* accompanies the artery and ends in the internal iliac vein.

The *Lymph vessels* of the body and fundus pass to the aortic lymph nodes for the most part, but some run along the round ligament and join the external iliac and the superficial inguinal lymph nodes (pp. 51 and 203). The lymph vessels of the cervix join the internal iliac and sacral lymph nodes.

The *Mucous Membrane* of the body of the uterus, the *endometrium*, is smooth and featureless, but in the canal of the cervix, median ridges are found on both the anterior and posterior walls of the cervix, and from them smaller ridges radiate upwards and laterally in a very regular manner (the *arbor vitæ* appearance).

In the vagina are similar median ridges of the mucous membrane, the *columnæ rugarum.* Transverse ridges run laterally from the columns, and the ridges of the anterior wall fit into the grooves of the posterior wall and *vice versâ.* This condition is seen best in the lower part of the vagina; in the upper part, particularly in the fornix, the mucous membrane tends to be smooth and featureless.

From puberty to menopause the endometrium undergoes a series of cyclical changes which recur every twenty-eight days. Following the rupture of a ripe vesicular ovarian follicle and the discharge of an ovum, the endometrium becomes swollen, softer and more vascular. These changes are associated with the presence in the blood-stream of progesterone, secreted by the fresh corpus luteum, and of œstrogen, secreted by the interstitial cells of the ovary. They ensure that, if the ovum is fertilised during its passage along the uterine tube, the endometrium will be prepared to receive it. On the other hand, if the ovum does not become fertilised, the corpus luteum degenerates and progesterone disappears from the bloodstream. As a result the endometrium becomes unstable, some of the dilated vessels rupture, portions of the epithelium necrose and are shed together with the ovum, blood and blood-clot. This constitutes the menstrual flow, which begins 14 ($\pm$2) days after the discharge of an ovum and usually lasts for five to seven days. It is followed by a period of about seven days, during which active repair is effected under the influence of œstrogen. A short quiescent interval follows, and then the series of changes recommences with the rupture of another vesicular ovarian follicle.

Prior to puberty the endometrium is lined with ciliated columnar epithelium, but owing to the repeated destructive changes, it is lined with non-ciliated cylindrical epithelium in the adult.

The groove which surrounds the vaginal portion of the cervix is termed the *fornix.* The deepest part of the fornix is placed posteriorly and through it, on vaginal examination, the promontory of the sacrum can be reached with the finger.

The *External Os* of the Uterus is situated on the vaginal portion of the cervix, and it is directed backwards against the posterior wall of the vagina. In the virgin the opening is small and circular, but after childbirth it is a transverse slit, with thick rounded anterior and posterior lips.

The mucous membrane of the cervix is lined with ciliated, low columnar epithelium in its upper part, but in its lower third there are no cilia and, just above the external os, the epithelium changes to the stratified squamous variety which covers the vaginal surface of the cervix and lines the vagina.

The **Round Ligament of the Uterus** is a fibro-muscular cord attached by one extremity to the supero-lateral angle of the uterus in front of the isthmus of the uterine tube, and by the other extremity to the subcutaneous tissue and skin of the labium majus. It passes forwards and laterally between the two layers of the broad ligament, and crosses the pelvic brim and the external iliac vessels to reach the deep inguinal ring (*cf.* the vas deferens, p. 199). Having traversed the inguinal canal, it terminates in the skin and fascia of the labium majus. Together with the ovarian ligament (p. 208), the round ligament of the uterus is homologous with the gubernaculum testis (p. 145).

The *Uterosacral Ligaments* are two short fibro-muscular cords, which pass from the posterior aspect of the upper end of the cervix backwards to the sacrum on each side of the rectum. They lie immediately in contact with the peritoneum and form ridges in the lateral walls of the recto-uterine fossa, which are termed the *recto-uterine folds*. (Shortening of these ligaments following inflammation may over-accentuate anteflexion of the uterus.)

The Vagina passes upwards and backwards for 3 inches from the pudendal cleft. Owing to the anteversion of the uterus, the posterior wall of the vagina is longer than the anterior wall, being $3\frac{1}{2}$ inches long. At its upper end the vagina is firmly attached to the outside of the cervix.

Relations. Anteriorly, the vagina is intimately related to the *posterior wall of the bladder above, and to the urethra below. Posteriorly*, the upper part is *covered with peritoneum* and lies in the anterior wall of the recto-uterine fossa, being related to coils of ileum or pelvic colon. The succeeding part is closely related to the anterior aspect of the rectum, while the lowest part is separated from the anal canal by the perineal body (p. 194). *Laterally*, the vagina is related to the ureter above, and to the anterior fibres of the levator ani, as they pass backwards to reach the perineal body and to sweep round the anorectal flexure. Below, the vagina pierces the perineal membrane, and in the perineum it is related on each side to the bulb of the vestibule (p. 138) and the bulbospongiosus muscle.

Blood Supply. The *Vaginal Artery* replaces the inferior vesical artery of the male. It arises from the anterior division of the internal iliac artery, and runs forwards and medially on the levator ani to reach the vagina. In addition it usually sends branches forwards to supply the bladder.

The *Lymph Vessels* of the upper part of the vagina join the internal and external iliac lymph nodes; *those from the lower part join the medial lymph nodes of the superficial inguinal group.*

The **Ovary** of the virgin lies in contact with the lateral pelvic wall in a small depression, termed the *ovarian fossa,* which is bounded behind by the ureter, and in front by the lateral umbilical ligament. Its peritoneal floor separates the ovary from the obturator nerve, artery and vein. The ovary is about 1 inch long by $\frac{1}{2}$ inch wide, and it lies with its long axis nearly vertical.

Covered by germinal epithelium, which is cubical in character, the ovary is connected to the posterior layer of the broad ligament by the mesovarium, which is attached to its *anterior border.*

The *Medial Surface* of the ovary is covered by the uterine tube and the mesosalpinx. The tube passes upwards along the anterior border of this surface and downwards along its posterior border.

The ovarian fimbria is attached to the *tubal (upper) pole*; the ovarian ligament, which connects the ovary to the supero-lateral angle of the uterus, is attached to the *uterine (lower) pole.*

During pregnancy the ovary is carried upwards with the enlarging uterus into the abdomen, and subsequently its position in the pelvis is open to considerable variation, although it always remains attached by the ovarian ligament, the infundibulopelvic ligament and the mesovarium.

Within its covering of germinal epithelium the ovary is surrounded by a thin *tunica albuginea.* The fibro-areolar stroma of the gland contains oöcytes in all stages of development and patches of interstitial epithelial cells, which are responsible for the secretion of œstrin.

Blood Supply. The *ovarian artery* arises from the aorta just below the origin of the renal artery, and runs downwards and laterally on the posterior abdominal wall (p. 186). Unlike the corresponding artery in the male, the ovarian artery does not pass to the deep inguinal ring but turns medially over the pelvic brim, leaving the psoas muscle and crossing the external iliac vessels to enter the infundibulo-pelvic ligament of the ovary. The ovarian branches reach the hilum by way of the mesovarium, but the terminal branches are continued medially in the broad ligament to supply the uterine tube and the upper part of the uterus. They anastomose with branches of the uterine artery.

Several *veins* issue from the hilum of the gland, but they soon unite to form a double or single ovarian vein. The right ovarian vein ends in the inferior vena cava; the left ovarian joins the left renal vein.

The *Lymph Vessels* of the ovary follow the ovarian veins and end in the aortic lymph nodes.

The **Uterine (Fallopian) Tube** lies in the upper border of the broad ligament. It is 4 inches long. The medial end opens into the supero-lateral angle of the uterus; *the lateral end communicates with the general peritoneal cavity through the ostium pelvinum.* Near the uterus the tube is narrow, but near the mesovarium it becomes distinctly dilated. The narrow portion is termed the *isthmus*, and the expanded portion the *ampulla.* The lateral extremity of the tube projects freely from the broad ligament. It is enlarged and funnel-shaped, but the surface of the funnel is broken up into a number of finger-like processes which are known as the *fimbriæ.* Of these one is constantly found attached to the tubal pole of the ovary, and is consequently termed the *ovarian fimbria.* The outer surfaces of the fimbriæ are covered with peritoneum but their inner surfaces are lined with ciliated columnar epithelium. These cilia provide the mechanism which enables an ovum to reach the ostium pelvinum and gain the interior of the tube.

In the virgin the tube runs backwards and laterally from the uterus to the pelvic wall, and then comes into relationship with the ovary in the manner already described (p. 212). In the whole of its course it is related to the coils of intestine which occupy the pelvis. After the first pregnancy the relationship of the tube to the ovary is not so constant, though the two remain attached to each other by the ovarian fimbria.

The *Blood Supply* of the uterine tube is derived from the uterine and ovarian arteries, while its nerves are branches from the pelvic plexus (T. 11 and 12 and L. 1).

A *paramesonephric* (*Mullerian*) *duct* develops on the lateral aspect of the mesonephric ridge as a small surface depression of the cœlomic epithelium, which burrows tailwards in the substance of the ridge. The right and left ducts approach each other in the pelvis and descend side by side to the urogenital sinus. The caudal portions of the two ducts fuse to form the uterus and the vagina, but their cephalic portions remain separate and constitute the uterine tubes. The original invagination persists as the pelvic ostium of the tube. The *Epoöphoron* is a vestigial structure which lies between the two layers of the broad ligament, below the ampulla of the tube. It represents a few persistent tubules of the mesonephros, and may give rise to cysts of the broad ligament. A portion of the mesonephric duct persists as the duct of the epoöphoron. It may end blindly, or it may pass medially in the broad ligament and open through the vaginal wall.

The **Rectum** in the female shows few differences from the description given for the male subject on p. 195. Below the peritoneal reflection, however, the anterior surface of the rectum is related to the posterior wall of the vagina.

THE JOINTS OF THE PELVIS

The **Sacro-iliac Joint** is a synovial joint of the plane variety, formed by the auricular surfaces of the ilium and of the sacrum.

Despite the fact that the sacrum is broader in front than it is behind, the anterior sacro-iliac ligaments are comparatively weak. On the other hand, the posterior and interosseous sacro-iliac ligaments, which pass between the roughened areas on the bones behind the auricular surfaces, are of unusual strength. They serve to suspend the weight of the trunk from the hip bones.

The **Symphysis Pubis** is a cartilaginous joint placed between the opposed bodies of the pubic bones. Weak anterior and posterior ligaments pass across the joint, but the real uniting medium is a disc of fibrocartilage, very similar to an intervertebral disc, but possessing a very small cavity instead of a nucleus pulposus.

The **Sacrotuberous Ligament** is a strong band which extends from the medial border of the ischial tuberosity to the lateral part of the sacrum and coccyx, and to the posterior inferior iliac spine. From the ischial tuberosity its attachment extends forwards along the ischial ramus, and in this situation the free edge of its *falciform process* blends with the parietal pelvic fascia covering the obturator internus muscle.

The posterior surface of the ligament gives origin to the lower fibres of the gluteus maximus, and the ligament is exposed in the buttock when that muscle is reflected.

In addition to forming the postero-lateral boundary of the outlet of the pelvis, the sacrotuberous ligament also forms the lower boundary of the lesser sciatic foramen.

The **Sacrospinous Ligament** is a short fan-shaped sheet which extends from the spine of the ischium to the side of the sacrum and coccyx. Its pelvic or anterior surface is partially blended with the coccygeus muscle, of which it is considered to be a degenerate part, and its gluteal or dorsal surface is crossed by the pudendal nerve. Situated between the greater and the lesser sciatic foramina, the ligament takes part in the formation of the boundaries of both of these openings.

Owing to the backward inclination of the long axis of the sacrum, the weight of the body tends to thrust the upper end of the bone downwards and forwards and to rotate it around a transverse axis. Such a rotation would be accompanied by an upward movement of the lower end of the bone, but this is effectively prevented by the tension of the sacrotuberous and the sacrospinous ligaments.

The *Iliolumbar Ligament* stretches from the tip of the fifth lumbar transverse process to the iliac crest. Anteriorly, it is continuous with the anterior layer of the lumbar fascia (p. 224), and, superiorly, it gives origin to the quadratus lumborum muscle.

Section V

THE HEAD AND NECK

THE FRONT AND SIDE OF THE NECK

For the satisfactory revision of the neck, the student must take advantage of dissections. Prepared dissections are very helpful, but they are not so valuable as dissections which can be handled and explored.

The **Platysma** muscle lies in the superficial connective tissue of the neck. It starts from the deep fascia covering the pectoralis major and the deltoid, and its fibres run upwards and medially to be attached to the lower border of the mandible. Some fibres reach the face and mingle with the muscles of the lower lip. The two muscles may blend for a short distance below the chin. When the angles of the mouth are actively drawn downwards and laterally, the muscle fibres can be made to stand out prominently.

Its *Nerve Supply* is the cervical branch of the facial nerve.

Superficial Veins. The **External Jugular Vein,** which varies greatly in size, is formed by the union of the posterior auricular vein with a branch of the posterior facial vein. It begins at the lower part of the parotid gland and runs almost vertically downwards, superficial to the sternomastoid muscle. In the angle between the clavicle and the posterior border of that muscle it pierces the deep fascia, which is strongly adherent to its wall, and joins the subclavian vein.

The **Anterior Jugular** vein commences in the submental region by the union of a few small radicles, and runs downwards in the superficial fascia a short distance from the median plane. Just above the sternum it pierces the investing layer of the deep cervical fascia and makes a sharp bend laterally. At this point it is connected to the corresponding vein of the opposite side by a transverse branch, termed the *jugular arch*, which lies in the suprasternal space. It then runs laterally deep to the sternomastoid, and ends in the external jugular or subclavian vein.

It is not uncommon to find the anterior jugular a large vein, and in these cases it receives the whole, or part, of the common facial vein.

Superficial Nerves. The skin of this region is supplied by the anterior primary rami of the second, third, and fourth cervical nerves through branches of the cervical plexus. The individual nerves appear superficially at the posterior border of the sternomastoid muscle, for the plexus itself lies under cover of that muscle.

The *Lesser Occipital Nerve* (C. 2) appears about the junction of the middle and upper thirds of the posterior border of the sternomastoid muscle, where it hooks round the accessory nerve. It runs upwards and backwards along the posterior border of the muscle to reach and supply the skin of the lateral part of the occipital region and the cranial surface of the auricle.

The *Great Auricular Nerve* (C. 2 and 3) appears at a slightly lower level, and runs upwards across the sternomastoid, side by side with the external jugular vein. It supplies the skin which covers the angle of the jaw, the parotid gland, the lateral aspect (*excluding the tragus*) and most of the medial aspect of the auricle, and the skin over the mastoid region.

The *Anterior Cutaneous Nerve of the Neck* (C. 2 and 3) appears close to the great auricular nerve and runs transversely forwards across the sternomastoid muscle. It divides into ascending and descending branches to supply the skin of the antero-lateral aspect of the neck. Section of this nerve causes a very extensive loss of cutaneous sensibility.

The *Supraclavicular Nerves* (C. 3 and 4) appear at a slightly lower level than the preceding nerve. The *medial supraclavicular nerves* run downwards and medially across the lower part of the sternomastoid; the *intermediate supraclavicular nerves* run downwards across the clavicle; the *lateral supraclavicular nerves* run downwards and laterally across the trapezius, the acromial end of the clavicle and the acromion. *It is important to remember that these nerves go down beyond the limits of the neck and supply the skin over the first intercostal space—the first intercostal nerve gives no adequate cutaneous branches* (p. 3)—*and the skin over the upper part of the shoulder.*

The Deep Cervical Fascia. The deep fascia of the neck forms a general investing layer, and in addition the areolar and fibrous tissue which is situated more deeply in the neck becomes condensed in certain situations, where it is described as forming the prevertebral and pretracheal layers of the deep cervical fascia, the stylomandibular ligament and the carotid sheath.

The *Investing Layer* roofs in the anterior triangle of the neck, encloses sternomastoid, roofs in the posterior triangle of the neck, encloses trapezius, and finally reaches the ligamentum nuchæ.

Its upper limit is very irregular. Anteriorly, it is attached to the lower border of the mandible almost as far back as the angle. Then it ascends over the parotid gland, which it provides with a tough sheath, and reaches the lower border of the zygoma and the anterior and inferior margins of the external auditory meatus. It next follows the insertion of sternomastoid to the mastoid process and the highest nuchal line of the occipital bone, along which it is carried to the external occipital protuberance. These latter attachments can usually be traced on the skull by their linear markings.

At the lower part of the neck the investing fascia splits into two layers, like those enclosing sternomastoid. These two layers are attached to the anterior and posterior margins of the upper border of the sternum and clavicle. In the median plane they enclose a small *suprasternal space*, which contains the sternal heads of the sternomastoid muscles, the jugular arch and a lymph node.

Over the lower part of the posterior triangle of the neck the deeper layer ensheathes the inferior belly of the omohyoid and binds it down to the clavicle.

The *Prevertebral Fascia* covers the prevertebral muscles—longus cervicis and longus capitis—and the scalene muscles, and forms a fascial floor for the posterior triangle of the neck.

In the median plane it is closely related to the front of the vertebral column and lies behind the pharynx and œsophagus. Traced laterally, it passes behind the carotid sheath, and extends from the scalenus anterior to the scalenus medius, levator scapulæ and splenius capitis, *i.e.*, it covers the muscular floor of the posterior triangle. On the surface of the two latter muscles it passes deep to the trapezius and reaches the ligamentum nuchæ. It is connected to the carotid sheath by fibro-areolar tissue which opposes little resistance to the exploring finger.

Near the median plane it can be traced upwards to the basilar part of the occipital bone on the surface of the longus capitis, and downwards into the thorax on the surface of the longus cervicis. In the latter situation it soon blends with the anterior longitudinal ligament. More laterally, its upper and lower limits are very indefinite.

It is important to recognise that *the anterior primary rami of the cervical nerves lie behind the prevertebral fascia*, and the following points all have an important practical bearing:—

(*a*) The loops of the cervical plexus lie behind the fascia.

(*b*) The *phrenic nerve*, as it runs downwards from the plexus on the scalenus anterior, is plastered on to the muscle by the prevertebral fascia.

(*c*) The trunks of the brachial plexus and the subclavian artery, as they emerge between the scalenus anterior and the scalenus medius, thrust the fascia downwards and laterally through the apex of the axilla to form the axillary sheath.

(*d*) The *Thoracodorsal Nerve* and the *Dorsal Scapular Nerve* are plastered on to the muscular floor of the posterior triangle by the prevertebral fascia.

It follows that in operations in the posterior triangle of the neck, the important phrenic nerve, the nerve to serratus anterior and the trunks of the brachial plexus are safe from injury so long as the fascial floor of the triangle is not disturbed.

The *Pretracheal Fascia* is much less extensive than the prevertebral fascia. It lies in front of the trachea and larynx, but behind the infrahyoid muscles. Superiorly, it reaches the thyroid cartilage, but inferiorly, it can be traced into the thorax, where it becomes connected to the outer fibrous coat of the arch of the aorta. Traced laterally the pretracheal layer passes in front of the carotid sheath, and fades away on the deep surface of the sternomastoid.

The relationship of the fascia to the thyroid gland is the only reason for its description. It provides a complete fascial sheath for the gland, which also encloses the parathyroids and the terminal parts of the superior and inferior thyroid arteries, but *neither the recurrent nor the external laryngeal nerve.*

The *Carotid Sheath* is a condensation of fibro-areolar tissue around and between the common and internal carotid arteries, the internal jugular vein and the vagus nerve. These structures must be regarded as being embedded in the tissue and not as being enclosed within a hollow tube. The upper and lower limits of the sheath are very indefinite. Where it covers the arteries the sheath is thick and strong, but it is very much thinner over the internal jugular vein.

The *Stylomandibular Ligament* is a process of the deep cervical fascia which extends between the styloid process and the angle of the jaw. It forms the infero-medial part of the sheath of the parotid gland and intervenes between it and the submandibular gland.

The **Sternomastoid** arises by (1) a rounded tendon from the front of the manubrium sterni, and (2) a musculo-tendinous origin from the medial third of the upper surface of the clavicle. The fibres run upwards and backwards, the clavicular head disappearing under the rapidly widening sternal head, to reach their insertion, which extends from the tip of the mastoid process upwards along its anterior border and then backwards, across the mastoid portion of the temporal bone, to the adjoining part of the superior nuchal line of the occipital bone.

Actions. Both muscles, acting together, draw the head forwards and, in so doing, impose some degree of flexion on the neck. They come into play for this purpose in eating and to elevate or hold the unsupported head when the body is supine. The contraction of one, if acting alone, would tilt the head to the opposite side and draws it down towards the chest. In actual use, the commonest action of the muscle is in rotating the head to the opposite side, particularly in visual movements. The muscle forms a conspicuous landmark in the living subject and its sternal head of origin stands out prominently when the head is turned, especially against resistance.

Nerve Supply. The muscle derives its nerve supply from the accessory nerve (*motor*) and the second cervical nerve (*proprioceptor*).

It should be observed that many of the structures which are described with the contents of the anterior and posterior triangles of the neck are deep to the sternomastoid. The common and internal carotid arteries, the internal jugular vein, the vagus nerve, the scalenus anterior and its related structures, the cervical plexus, etc., are all covered by the sternomastoid in whole or in part.

The **Posterior Triangle** is a gap between muscles, bounded, *in front* by the posterior border of the sternomastoid, *behind*, by the anterior border of the trapezius, and *below*, by the intermediate third of the clavicle. Its apex lies on the superior nuchal line of the occipital bone, and when the anterior and posterior borders fail to meet in that situation the area is occupied by the uppermost part of the semispinalis capitis muscle.

The triangle is roofed in by the investing layer of the deep cervical fascia, and its muscular floor, which is covered by the prevertebral fascia, is formed by the splenius capitis, the levator scapulæ and the scalenus medius. Small portions of the scalenus posterior and the first digitation of the serratus anterior also enter into the formation of the floor in its infero-lateral angle.

Between the fascial roof (investing layer) and the fascial floor (prevertebral fascia) lie numerous deep cervical lymph nodes, the accessory nerve and other vessels and nerves embedded in a layer of fat. The inferior belly of the omohyoid crosses the lower part of the triangle and separates an upper, occipital triangle from a lower, supraclavicular triangle.

The Contents of the Occipital Triangle. The most important structure in the occipital triangle is the *accessory nerve.* It enters the triangle from the deep aspect of sternomastoid at about the junction of the upper and middle thirds, where it is intimately related to the lesser occipital nerve, and runs almost vertically downwards on the levator scapulæ. In this part of its course it is related to the upper and posterior lymph nodes of the deep cervical group. Enlargement of these lymph nodes may displace the nerve from its normal position. Inferiorly, the nerve disappears under cover of the anterior border of the trapezius at the junction of its lower and middle thirds, and its terminal fibres supply that muscle.

The descending branches of the cervical plexus, which appear from beneath sternomastoid at a slightly lower level, run parallel to the accessory nerve. The course and distribution of the cutaneous branches have already been detailed (p. 217), but some of the descending branches pass deep to the trapezius and assist in its innervation (proprioceptive).

The *Transverse Cervical Artery*, which is a branch of the thyrocervical trunk (first part of the subclavian artery), appears first in the supraclavicular triangle. Crossing in front of the trunks of the brachial plexus and behind the inferior belly of the omohyoid, it enters the lower part of the occipital triangle, where it ends by dividing into superficial and deep branches.

The *superficial branch* ramifies on the deep surface of the trapezius muscle, while the *deep branch* accompanies the levator scapulæ to the medial border of the scapula and takes part in the scapular anastomosis (p. 17).

The Contents of the Supraclavicular Triangle. The **Brachial Plexus,** which is formed by C. 5, C. 6, C. 7, C. 8 and T. 1 (anterior primary rami), occupies the antero-inferior angle of the posterior triangle and can be recognised on palpation in this situation in the living subject. Its upper part lies in the occipital triangle, but most of the plexus—so far as it is found in the neck—lies behind the inferior belly of the omohyoid and in the supraclavicular triangle.

The anterior primary rami of the fifth, sixth and seventh cervical nerves lie each in the groove on the upper surface of the transverse process of the corresponding cervical vertebra. They are placed between the anterior and posterior tubercles on the transverse processes and, consequently, as they pass to the surface they run behind the muscles attached to the anterior tubercles, but in front of those attached to the posterior tubercles. When the posterior border of the sternomastoid is drawn forwards the nerves are found emerging between the scalenus anterior and medius. This relationship is a very useful landmark, as it enables these two muscles to be identified with certainty and rapidity (at operation).

Before the nerves reach the posterior triangle of the neck the fifth and sixth cervical have united to form the *upper trunk* of the plexus, and the eighth cervical and first thoracic have united to form the *lower trunk*. Between them lies the seventh cervical, which itself constitutes the *middle trunk* of the plexus. The lower trunk is usually placed behind the third part of the subclavian artery, which emerges from the same intermuscular interval, and the nerves and vessel thrust the prevertebral fascia towards the apex of the axilla, thus acquiring a connective tissue sheath.

As they lie in the supraclavicular triangle each trunk breaks up into an *anterior* and a *posterior division*, and these reunite to form the *cords of the brachial plexus* in the axilla (p. 9).

Four supraclavicular branches of the brachial plexus lie, in some part of their course, in the posterior triangle of the neck.

(*a*) The *Dorsal Scapular Nerve* (C. 5) pierces the substance of the scalenus medius on a level with the thyroid cartilage. Running downwards, it disappears under cover of the levator scapulæ, to which it usually gives a branch, and its terminal branches supply the rhomboid muscles (p. 12). The nerve lies *behind the prevertebral fascia.*

(*b*) The *Long Thoracic Nerve* (*Nerve to Serratus Anterior*) (C. 5, 6 and 7) arises by three roots. The upper two pierce the scalenus medius muscle just above, or deep to, the inferior belly of the omohyoid. After uniting, they run downwards behind the brachial plexus and the subclavian vessels on the surface of the scalenus medius, and enter the axilla through its apex. The lowest root arises from C. 7 and runs downwards on the scalenus medius, but does not pierce it. It joins the rest of the nerve in the axilla. Throughout its course in the neck the thoracodorsal nerve lies *behind the prevertebral fascia.* It is distributed entirely to the serratus anterior muscle.

(*c*) The *Suprascapular Nerve* (C. 5 and 6) arises from the upper trunk of the plexus behind, or below, the inferior belly of the omohyoid. When the plexus is approached from the lateral side this is the first branch to be encountered. It runs laterally and downwards, and passes behind the clavicle, where it meets the suprascapular vessels, which it accompanies to the suprascapular notch. It supplies the supra- and infra-spinatus muscles.

(*d*) The *Nerve to the Subclavius Muscle* (C. 5 and 6) runs downwards in front of the plexus to its destination.

The **Third Part of the Subclavian Artery** begins at the lateral border of the scalenus anterior, from behind which it emerges, and runs downwards and laterally to disappear behind the middle of the clavicle, where it enters the axilla. It is covered by the posterior border of the sternomastoid at its commencement and by the clavicle at its termination, but is comparatively superficial between these two points. Here it is crossed by the external jugular vein and by its tributaries, the transverse cervical and suprascapular veins and by the suprascapular artery. Apart from the prevertebral fascia, no other structures of importance intervene between the vessel and the fascial roof of the posterior triangle and its pulsations can easily be felt, and even seen, in the living subject.

Posterior to the artery lie the lower trunk of the plexus, which often rests on the upper surface of the first rib, and the scalenus medius muscle. *Below*, the artery lies in a groove on the upper surface of the first rib. *Antero-inferior* is the subclavian vein.

As a rule no branches come off from the third part of the artery.

The *Suprascapular Artery* arises from the thyrocervical trunk and runs transversely into the supraclavicular triangle. At the posterior border of the sternomastoid it can be seen crossing in front of the third part of the subclavian artery and the brachial plexus. It passes behind the clavicle and meets the corresponding vein and nerve, which it accompanies to the suprascapular notch. Its terminal branches take part in the scapular anastomosis (p. 17).

The **Subclavian Vein** rarely bulges upwards *above* the clavicle because it lies lower than its companion artery, and, in addition, it is anterior to it. It is supported, below and behind, by a shallow groove on the upper surface of the first rib, and in this situation it is joined from above by the external jugular vein.

The *Suprascapular Vein* runs medially behind, or just above, the clavicle, below and parallel to the transverse cervical vein. Both vessels end in the external jugular vein.

DORSAL ASPECT OF NECK AND TRUNK

The skin and muscles of this region are supplied by the dorsal rami of the spinal nerves. A typical dorsal (posterior primary) ramus breaks up into a medial and a lateral branch. With certain exceptions, the medial branches of the dorsal rami, above and including T. 6, are distributed to both muscles and skin, while the lateral branches supply muscles only. Below and including T. 7, the medial branches supply muscles only, while the lateral branches supply both muscles and skin.

The dorsal ramus of the first cervical nerve does not divide into lateral and medial branches, and, like the ventral ramus of the same nerve, none of its fibres reach the skin. In this connexion, it is interesting to note that the ganglion on the posterior nerve root of C. 1 is always small and may not be visible to the naked eye.

Further, the dorsal rami of C. 7 and C. 8, and L. 4 and 5, are restricted to the supply of muscles.

The *Greater Occipital Nerve* is the large medial branch of the posterior ramus of C. 2. It becomes superficial by piercing the trapezius muscle 1 inch below and lateral to the external occipital protuberance, and is distributed to the skin covering the posterior part of the scalp in company with the terminal branches of the occipital artery.

The medial branch of the dorsal ramus of C. 3 ascends to the scalp, medial to the greater occipital, and is sometimes known as the third occipital nerve.

The trapezius and the latissimus dorsi, which cover the deeper muscles and the rhomboids, have been described on pp. 11 and 12. When they have been reflected, the splenius, the serrati, and the thoracic part of the lumbar fascia, associated with the sacrospinalis, come into view.

The **Splenius** arises from the lower half of the cervical spines through the ligamentum nuchæ and from the upper thoracic spines. It passes upwards and laterally, forming the upper part of the muscular floor of the posterior triangle of the neck, and is inserted into the mastoid process and the adjoining part of the occipital bone, under the sternomastoid muscle.

Action. When both muscles act together they extend the head on the trunk. One muscle, acting alone, rotates the head and neck to the same side, commonly in visual movements (*Cf.* sternomastoid, p. 219).

The *Serratus Posterior Superior* is a thin, flat muscle, which lies under cover of the rhomboids and superficial to the lumbar fascia. It extends from the lower cervical and upper thoracic spines to the upper ribs.

The *Serratus Posterior Inferior* presents a similar appearance. It is placed under cover of the latissimus dorsi, and extends from the lower thoracic and upper lumbar spines to the lower ribs. Its expanded tendinous origin is blended with the thoracolumbar fascia.

The serratus posterior superior elevates, while the inferior depresses, the ribs into which it is inserted.

These two muscles are supplied by the corresponding *intercostal nerves* (*anterior primary rami*). From this it may be inferred that they are derivatives of the ventral portions of the myotomes and that they have migrated dorsally and medially to gain attachment to the vertebral spines. Their actions are not easy to assess.

The **Thoracic Part of the Thoracolumbar Fascia** extends between the vertebral spines and the angles of the ribs, covering the sacrospinalis. Above, it is lost amongst the muscles of the neck; below, it is continuous with the posterior lamella of the lumbar part.

The **Lumbar Part of the Thoracolumbar Fascia** is a strong aponeurotic sheet and has already been described in part in connexion with the posterior abdominal wall. It occupies the interval between the iliac crest and the last rib, and its lateral border gives origin to the middle fibres of the transversus and the upper fibres of the internal oblique muscle. It is more conveniently and appropriately termed the lumbar aponeurosis.

When traced medially, the lumbar aponeurosis splits into three lamellæ. The *posterior lamella* covers the posterior surface of the sacrospinalis, and is attached to the lumbar spines. Superiorly, it is continuous with the thoracic part of the thoracolumbar fascia. The *middle lamella* passes medially, anterior to the sacrospinalis but posterior to the quadratus lumborum, and so reaches the tips of the transverse processes of the lumbar vertebræ. The *anterior lamella* covers the anterior surface of the quadratus lumborum muscle, and is attached to the anterior aspects of the transverse processes of the lumbar vertebræ under cover of the psoas.

The **Sacrospinalis** forms an elongated group of muscles which extend upwards from the dorsum of the sacrum and the posterior parts of the iliac crest. It occupies the groove between the vertebral spines and the ribs, medial to the angles, and can be subdivided into three columns:—

1. The *Iliocostocervicalis*, which consists of lumbar, thoracic and cervical portions, is the most lateral column.
2. The *Longissimus* (thoracis, cervicis and capitis) is intermediate in position, and is much the widest and bulkiest of the three sub-divisions. Its uppermost part (*longissimus capitis*) forms a narrow, strap-like muscle, which ascends under cover of the splenius to be inserted into the lower and back part of the mastoid process.
3. The *Spinalis*, which constitutes the most medial column, is the shortest of the three and is compressed against the sides of the vertebral spines.

The sacrospinalis forms a conspicuous projection on each side of the median furrow which overlies the lower thoracic and lumbar spines (Plate III, p. 16). Its lateral border, also marked by a furrow, covers the transverse processes of the lumbar vertebræ and, in the thoracic region, extends over the ribs as far as their angles. Below, the muscle becomes tendinous and the median furrow merges into a flattened triangular area, the apex of which lies on the third sacral spine at the upper end of the natal cleft. The upper, basal, angles of this triangle are marked by surface dimples which overlie the posterior superior iliac spines. The base of the triangle crosses the second sacral spine (Plate III, p. 16).

It should be noted that the lateral border of the muscle intersects the lower border of the twelfth rib where it is crossed by the lower limit of the pleural sac (p. 101), and in the interval between the muscle and the cartilaginous end of the rib the lower and lateral part of the kidney can be exposed.

The **Semispinalis Capitis** forms an important landmark in the upper part of the back of the neck. It may appear in the apex of the posterior triangle, but it may be completely hidden by the trapezius and splenius muscles. When the trapezius is reflected the *vertical* fibres of the semispinalis capitis are seen above the upper border of the splenius, and when that muscle is reflected the whole of the semispinalis is brought into view.

It arises from the transverse processes of the upper thoracic vertebræ and from the articular processes of the lower cervical vertebræ. The fibres converge to be inserted into the occipital bone between the superior and inferior nuchal lines and close to the median plane.

Both muscles, acting together, extend the head on the trunk. One muscle, acting alone, bends the head to the same side so that the face looks to the opposite side.

In its upper part the semispinalis capitis overlies the medial half of the suboccipital triangle. Its lower part conceals the *semispinalis cervicis*, the uppermost fibres ot which converge to be inserted into the stout spine of the axis vertebra.

The **Suboccipital Triangle** is a small intermuscular regional bounded inferiorly by the inferior oblique, laterally by the superior oblique, medially by the rectus capitis posterior major. The roof of the space is formed by the semispinalis capitis, medially, and by the longissimus capitis, laterally. Between these muscles appear the posterior arch of the atlas and the posterior atlanto-occipital membrane. The *vertebral artery* occupies the lateral angle of the triangle, as it runs medially after emerging from the foramen in the transverse process of the atlas vertebra. It grooves the posterior surface of the lateral mass of the atlas, and then disappears under the lateral border of the posterior atlanto-occipital membrane and pierces the dura mater.

The *Dorsal Ramus of the First Cervical Spinal Nerve* emerges between the vertebral artery and the posterior arch of the atlas, and supplies branches to the superior and inferior oblique, the rectus capitis posterior major and minor, and the semispinalis capitis. The *greater occipital nerve*, which is the main continuation of the medial branch of the dorsal ramus of C. 2, appears at the lower border of the inferior oblique and runs upwards across that muscle before piercing the semispinalis capitis. These two nerves are connected to each other by a communicating branch.

The dorsal rami of the remaining cervical nerves are found between the semispinalis capitis and the semispinalis cervicis. In the same intermuscular interval there occurs an important anastomosis which links up the external carotid with the subclavian artery. The participating vessels are descending branches, which run downwards from the occipital, and the deep cervical artery, which ascends from the costocervical trunk (p. 249).

The *Inferior Oblique* extends from the spine of the axis to the transverse process of the atlas (p. 381), while the *Superior Oblique* extends from the latter point to the occipital bone below the superior nuchal line.

The *Rectus Capitis Posterior Major* passes upwards and laterally from the spine of the axis to the occipital bone. The *Rectus Capitis Posterior Minor* passes upwards from the posterior tubercle of the atlas to the occipital bone immediately below the insertion of the semispinalis capitis.

The remaining muscles of the back, the multifidus spinæ, the rotatores, etc., lie on a plane deep to the sacrospinalis and semispinalis cervicis. The student is warned not to waste time in endeavouring to memorise the attachments of these muscles.

THE FRONT AND SIDE OF THE NECK

The **Anterior Triangle** of the neck is bounded in *front* by the median plane, *behind* by the anterior border of the sternomastoid, and *above* by the lower border of the mandible and a line drawn backwards from its angle to reach the posterior boundary.

The usual subdivision of this area is unnecessary and tends rather to introduce fresh complications than to facilitate the study of the region. It must also be borne in mind that in actual practice the anterior triangle of the neck is always widened by the retraction of the anterior border of the sternomastoid in order to bring certain large vessels and nerves into view.

The **Infrahyoid Group** of muscles comprises the sternohyoid, the omohyoid, the sternothyroid and the thyrohyoid. The former two lie side by side and cover the latter two, which are situated on a deeper plane.

The *Sternohyoid* arises from the posterior surface of the manubrium sterni and the adjoining part of the clavicle, and runs upwards and medially to be inserted into the medial part of the lower border of the body of the hyoid bone. In its lower part it lies deep to the sternomastoid muscle, and covers the lower end of the carotid sheath. Its *action* is to depress the hyoid bone following its elevation in the act of swallowing.

The *Omohyoid* consists of an inferior belly (p. 220), a common tendon and a superior belly. The inferior belly arises from the upper border of the scapula and the suprascapular ligament. Having crossed the lower part of the posterior triangle of the neck, it passes deep to the sternomastoid, where it ends in the common tendon. This structure lies on the surface of the carotid sheath (internal jugular vein), and is bound down to the clavicle by the deep cervical fascia (p. 217). It continues into the superior belly, which runs upwards and medially, superficial to the common carotid artery and along the lateral border of the sternohyoid, to be inserted into the lower border of the body of the hyoid bone in its lateral part. Its *action* is similar to that of the sternohyoid.

The *Sternothyroid* arises from the posterior aspect of the manubrium sterni and runs upwards deep to the sternohyoid and covering the lobe of the thyroid gland. It is inserted into the oblique line on the lamina of the thyroid cartilage. Its action is to depress the larynx after it has been elevated in the act of swallowing.

The *Nerve Supply* of all these muscles is derived from the cervical plexus through the ansa hypoglossi (p. 234).

The *Thyrohyoid* muscle arises from the oblique line of the thyroid cartilage and ascends, covering the lamina of the thyroid cartilage and the thyrohyoid membrane, to be inserted into the lower border of the body of the hyoid bone.

Action. The thyrohyoid depresses the hyoid bone, but, when that structure is fixed by the suprahyoid muscles, it acts as an elevator of the larynx.

Its *Nerve Supply* comes direct from the hypoglossal nerve (C. 1, p. 234).

The **Common Carotid Artery** enters the neck behind the sternoclavicular joint and runs upwards and backwards, behind the anterior border of the sternomastoid muscle, until it reaches the level of the upper border of the thyroid cartilage, where it divides into the external and internal carotid arteries.

Throughout its course it is embedded, together with the internal jugular vein and the vagus nerve, in the carotid sheath (p. 219). The vein lies on the lateral side of the artery and, when full of blood, overlaps it anteriorly; the vagus nerve lies between the two vessels, but is placed on a posterior plane.

Posteriorly, the artery is related to the anterior tubercles of the transverse processes of the lower four cervical vertebræ and the muscles attached to them (scalenus anterior and longus capitis). The enlarged anterior tubercle of the sixth cervical vertebra is termed the *carotid tubercle*, since the artery can be compressed against it. From these structures the common carotid artery is separated by the prevertebral fascia and the trunk of the sympathetic, which lies in the connective tissue between the prevertebral fascia and the carotid sheath.

In the lower part of the neck the common carotid lies in front of the vertebral artery as it ascends to the foramen in the transverse process of the sixth cervical vertebra, and in front of the inferior thyroid artery as it arches medially to reach the thyroid gland. In addition, on the left side, the thoracic duct crosses behind the vessel, below the inferior thyroid artery, but proceeding in the opposite direction (p. 247).

Anteriorly, in addition to the superficial structures, the artery is covered throughout its course by the anterior border of the sterno-mastoid muscle and, when the muscle is not actively contracted, its pulsations can readily be felt. Certain structures intervene between them. In the lower part of the neck these include the superior belly of the omohyoid, the sternohyoid and sternothyroid muscles (p. 227). In the upper part of its course the ramus descendens hypoglossi and the ansa hypoglossi are embedded in the anterior wall of the sheath, and the common facial vein may cross the artery at its termination, or it may lie at a slightly higher level.

Medially the common carotid is related to the thyroid gland and the inferior constrictor muscle of the pharynx. Its *lateral* relationship to the internal jugular vein and the vagus nerve has already been emphasised.

As a rule the common carotid artery gives off no branches excepting the two terminal vessels. At its point of bifurcation, the common carotid artery may show a localised dilatation, or this dilatation may be limited to the commencement of the internal carotid artery. In either event, it is termed the *carotid sinus*. In this situation the middle coat of the artery is thinner than it is elsewhere, but the adventitia, which is relatively thick, receives a very rich innervation from branches of the glossopharyngeal and sympathetic nerves. The structure of the wall of the sinus is well adapted to enable it to act as part of a reflex mechanism for regulating the blood-pressure in the cerebral arteries.

The *Carotid Body* is a small oval structure, less than $\frac{1}{4}$ inch long, placed on the posterior aspect of the bifurcation of the common carotid artery. It receives an abundant nerve supply, derived principally from the glossopharyngeal nerve, and it contains numerous polyhedral cells and sinusoidal vessels, branches of the carotid. Derived from the mesoderm of the third branchial arch, the carotid body retains its intimate relation to the third aortic arch (proximal part of internal carotid artery) and its relation to the carotid sinus probably has more than a topographical significance.

The **Internal Jugular Vein** begins at the jugular foramen, where it is continuous with the sigmoid sinus. It runs downwards and forwards through the neck to end behind the upper border of the sternal end of the clavicle, where it joins the subclavian to form the brachiocephalic vein.

About $\frac{1}{2}$ inch above the clavicle the vein possesses a bicuspid valve, which is often incompetent. That part of the vein which lies below the valve is situated opposite to the interval between the sternal and the clavicular heads of the sternomastoid, and is readily accessible for the purpose of taking tracings of the venous pulse.

Posteriorly, as it descends, the vein crosses the transverse process of the atlas, but it lies lateral to the tips of the lower transverse processes and rests, in succession, on the levator scapulæ, the scalenus medius and the scalenus anterior muscles. From these muscles it is separated by the carotid sheath and the prevertebral fascia, and the latter structure intervenes between it and the loops of the cervical plexus above, and the phrenic nerve below.

In the lower part of the neck, the internal jugular vein comes to lie on the medial side of the scalenus anterior, and it is here placed in front of the thyrocervical trunk, the inferior thyroid artery, the first part of the subclavian artery and, on the left side, the thoracic duct (p. 247).

Medially, the internal jugular vein is related to the vagus nerve and the common carotid artery below, and to the ninth, tenth, eleventh and twelfth cranial nerves and the internal carotid artery above.

The *Superficial* relations are rather more complicated. Throughout the greater part of its course the vein lies under the sternomastoid muscle, but in the uppermost part it lies deep to the parotid gland. Inferiorly, the infrahyoid muscles intervene between the vessel and the sternomastoid.

At about the level of the angle of the jaw the vein is crossed by the posterior belly of the digastric, the stylohyoid muscle, the occipital artery and the accessory nerve. Above this point it lies deep to the parotid gland, from which it is usually completely separated by the styloid process and the stylopharyngeus muscle.

Examination of the skull will show that the lower opening of the carotid canal lies anterior to the jugular foramen. It follows, therefore, that the internal carotid artery, as it enters the skull, lies no longer to the medial side of the vein, but is antero-medial to it, the ninth, tenth, eleventh and twelfth cranial nerves still intervening between them.

Tributaries. (*a*) The *Inferior Petrosal Sinus*, which helps to drain the cavernous sinus (p. 279), passes out of the skull through the anterior part of the jugular foramen and joins the upper end of the internal jugular vein.

(*b*) The (*Common*) *Facial Vein*, which is the largest tributary, receives the anterior branch of the retromandibular (posterior facial) vein in its lower part lying on the submandibular gland. It runs downwards and backwards to join the internal jugular vein just above the level of the upper border of the thyroid cartilage. In its course it crosses superficial to the hypoglossal nerve as that structure crosses the loop of the lingual artery (p. 233), and then crosses the external and internal carotid arteries close to their origin.

The pharyngeal, lingual and superior thyroid veins may, and as a rule at least one of them does, join the common facial vein.

(*c*) The *Pharyngeal Veins* and (*d*) the *Lingual Vein*, when they are not tributaries of the common facial vein, enter the internal jugular opposite the greater cornu of the hyoid bone.

(*e*) The *Superior Thyroid Vein* ascends from the upper pole of the thyroid gland in company with the corresponding artery. It crosses superficial to the common carotid artery, and joins either the common facial or the internal jugular vein.

(*f*) The *Middle Thyroid Vein* runs laterally from the lobe of the thyroid gland, deep to the infrahyoid muscles. It crosses superficial to the common carotid artery, and terminates in the internal jugular vein opposite to the cricoid cartilage.

The **Digastric Muscle** is an important landmark in the upper part of the neck. As its name implies, it consists of two bellies connected by a common tendon.

The *Posterior Belly* arises from the mastoid notch on the mastoid part of the temporal bone. Consequently, it at first lies deep to the mastoid process and the sternomastoid muscle. It runs downwards, forwards and medially, crossing superficial to the internal jugular vein, the accessory, the vagus and hypoglossal nerves, the occipital, the internal and external carotid, and the facial arteries. The *common tendon*, which it joins, lies just above the greater cornu of the hyoid bone and is held down to it by a slip of fascia. It is placed on the surface of the hyoglossus muscle and is overlapped by the submandibular gland.

The *Anterior Belly* runs forwards, medially and slightly upwards from the common tendon to be attached to the lower border of the mandible, near the median plane. It is placed on the surface of the mylohyoid muscle, and is partly overlapped by the submandibular gland.

Nerve Supply. The two bellies receive their nerves from different sources. The posterior belly is supplied by the facial nerve as it emerges from the stylomastoid foramen; the anterior belly is supplied by the nerve to the mylohyoid (p. 268), which is derived ultimately from the trigeminal nerve. The reason for the difference in nerve supply is found in the developmental origin of the two bellies. The anterior belly is a derivative of the first visceral arch, while the posterior belly is derived from the second, and each muscle is innervated by the nerve of the arch to which it belongs.

Action. When the hyoid bone is fixed, the digastric acts as a depressor of the mandible. On the other hand, when the mandible is fixed the muscle assists the mylohyoid to elevate the hyoid bone in the first stages of deglutition.

The *Stylohyoid Muscle* is closely associated with the posterior belly of the digastric. It arises from the posterior aspect of the styloid process and is inserted into the hyoid bone, at the junction of the body with the cornua, by means of two fleshy slips between which the common tendon of the digastric runs.

It is supplied by the facial nerve and acts as an elevator of the hyoid bone.

The **External Carotid Artery** commences under cover of the anterior border of the sternomastoid muscle, on a level with the upper border of the thyroid cartilage. In the lower part of its course the artery forms a gentle curve, convex forwards, and on this account it emerges from under cover of the sternomastoid. Near the angle of the jaw it is crossed by the posterior belly of the digastric muscle and the stylohyoid. Above this level the artery is at first deep to and then enclosed within the parotid gland, and it terminates opposite to the neck of the mandible by dividing into the superficial temporal and the maxillary arteries.

Below the Posterior Belly of the Digastric the external carotid is comparatively superficial, being only partly overlapped by the anterior border of the sternomastoid muscle. In this part of its course the vessel is crossed superficially by the *common facial vein* and *the hypoglossal nerve.*

To its medial side lie the middle and inferior constrictors of the pharynx and the internal and external laryngeal nerves.

On its postero-lateral side the external carotid is related to the internal carotid artery.

Branches. 1. The *Superior Thyroid Artery* arises from the anterior aspect of the external carotid near its origin. It runs downwards and forwards, parallel with, but superficial to, the external laryngeal nerve. It passes deep to the superior belly of the omohyoid and to the sternothyroid, and reaches the upper pole of the lobe of the thyroid gland. Its terminal branches supply the upper third of the lobe and the upper border of the isthmus of the gland. One fairly constant branch runs down the posterior border of the lobe and anastomoses with an ascending branch from the inferior thyroid artery.

Some of the branches of the superior thyroid artery have gained a totally undeserved importance. Apart from the terminal branches the only branches worthy of note are the *superior laryngeal artery*, which accompanies the internal nerve and with it pierces the lateral part of the thyrohyoid membrane, and the *crico-thyroid artery* (p. 303).

2. The *Lingual Artery* arises opposite the greater cornu of the hyoid bone. It at once makes a short upward loop and then disappears under cover of the hyoglossus muscle, to enter the submandibular region (p. 272). The loop, which is very characteristic, is crossed superficially by the hypoglossal nerve and, still more superficially, by the facial vein.

3. The *Facial Artery* arises just above the lingual, and running upwards, deep to the posterior belly of the digastric, comes into close relationship with the submandibular gland (p. 269).

4. The *Occipital Artery* springs from the posterior aspect of the external carotid opposite to the facial artery, and runs upwards and backwards deep to, or just below, the posterior belly of the digastric. At its origin it is crossed by the transverse part of the hypoglossal nerve. In its course it crosses the internal carotid artery, the vagus nerve, the descending part of the hypoglossal nerve and the internal jugular vein. As it crosses the last-named structure it also crosses the accessory nerve, which runs downwards and backwards in front of the internal jugular vein to reach the sternomastoid muscle.

Following the posterior belly of the digastric, the artery comes to lie in contact with the skull medial to the mastoid notch, and in this part of its course the vessel lies deep to the mastoid process and the muscles attached to it. In this situation it gives off descending branches which run downwards, in the interval between the semispinalis capitis and the semispinalis cervicis, to anastomose with the deep cervical artery from the costo-cervical trunk. This anastomosis constitutes a link between the subclavian and the carotid systems.

Emerging from under cover first of the splenius capitis, and then of the sternomastoid, the occipital artery appears at the apex of the posterior triangle, on the surface of the semispinalis capitis muscle. Its terminal branches run in company with the branches of the greater occipital nerve to supply the posterior part of the scalp. The anastomosis between the terminals of the occipital and the superficial temporal arteries is very free (p. 251).

5. The *Ascending Pharyngeal Artery* springs from the deep aspect

of the external carotid close to its origin and runs upwards medial to the internal carotid on the side-wall of the pharynx. Usually small in size, it gives off branches to the neighbouring structures.

6. The *Posterior Auricular Artery* usually springs from the external carotid above the level of the digastric and runs upwards and backwards under cover of the parotid gland. Gradually becoming more superficial, it crosses the base of the mastoid process and ascends behind the auricle (p. 251). It is distributed mainly to the auricle and the back of the scalp.

The **Hypoglossal (Twelfth Cranial) Nerve,** which is the motor nerve of the tongue muscles, emerges from the skull through the anterior condylar canal in the occipital bone and at once comes into close contact with the ninth, tenth and eleventh cranial nerves. Consequently it lies between the internal jugular vein and the internal carotid artery, and it descends in this position, being closely related to the vagus nerve, until it appears at the lower border of the posterior belly of the digastric. It then turns forwards and medially and crosses successively the internal carotid, the occipital and the external carotid arteries and the loop of the lingual artery. As it crosses the last-named vessel, the nerve is itself crossed superficially by the common facial vein. Passing deep to the stylohyoid, the common tendon of the digastric and the submandibular gland, it enters the submandibular region, where it is distributed to the muscles of the tongue (p. 271).

Communications. (*a*) Like the vagus and the glossopharyngeal nerves, the hypoglossal nerve communicates with the superior cervical ganglion of the sympathetic.

(*b*) In the upper part of the neck the hypoglossal nerve is joined by a branch from the cervical plexus (C. 1). This communication ultimately leaves the hypoglossal as its descending branch, and as the nerves to the thyrohyoid and the geniohyoid.

Branches. 1. The *Descending Branch* (C. 1) leaves the nerve as it bends forwards to cross the carotid vessels and runs downwards on the surface of the internal and common carotid arteries, embedded in the anterior wall of the carotid sheath. It is joined from its lateral side by the *descending cervical nerve* (C. 2 and 3), which arises from the cervical plexus, and the loop so formed is termed the *ansa hypoglossi* (C. 1, 2 and 3). Branches arise from the loop to be distributed to the sternohyoid, the sternothyroid, and both bellies of the omohyoid.

2. The *Nerve to the Thyrohyoid* (C. 1) leaves the hypoglossal as it crosses the carotid vessels and runs downwards and medially to the muscle.

3. The terminal branches to the muscles of the tongue are described on p. 275.

The **Vagus (Tenth Cranial) Nerve** leaves the skull through the jugular foramen. At its exit it is closely related to the ninth, eleventh and twelfth cranial nerves, to the internal jugular vein, which is posterior to it, and to the internal carotid artery, which is anterior to it. A little below the skull the internal carotid artery comes to lie on the medial side of the vein, and the vagus nerve retains its position between the two vessels and on a posterior plane. Lower in the neck it maintains the same relative position to the common carotid artery, and before entering the thorax it is placed *anterior* to the first part of the subclavian artery.

The relationship of the ninth, tenth, eleventh and twelfth cranial nerves can be considered conveniently at this stage. All four are in close proximity immediately below the skull, the hypoglossal being on the medial side. The accessory, after giving a large communicating branch to the vagus, diverges in a lateral direction. The glosso-pharyngeal, at a slightly lower level, diverges in a medial direction, crossing the internal carotid in company with the stylopharyngeus muscle. The hypoglossal makes a half-spiral turn round the vagus, and is closely related to that nerve until it bends forwards and medially, across the carotid vessels.

Two ganglia are found on the vagus nerve. The *superior ganglion* (somatic) is situated on the nerve in the jugular foramen. The *inferior ganglion* (visceral) lies on the nerve immediately below the foramen. *It receives the whole of that portion of the accessory nerve* (p. 240) *which arises from the medulla oblongata.*

Branches. 1. The *Auricular Branch* arises from the superior ganglion and traverses a small bony canal which brings it out on the exterior of the skull just behind the external auditory meatus. It is distributed to the skin lining the deep part of the external auditory meatus and to the skin over the base of the mastoid process. Stimulation of its terminal branches may produce reflex retching through the gastric branches of the vagus.

2. The *Pharyngeal Branch* arises from the inferior ganglion, runs downwards and medially in front of the internal carotid artery, and gains the side-wall of the pharynx, where it forms the pharyngeal plexus, with branches from the glossopharyngeal and the sympathetic.

3. The *Superior Laryngeal Nerve* also arises from the inferior ganglion and runs downwards and medially, but it crosses behind the internal carotid artery. It divides into the internal and external laryngeal nerves. (*a*) The *Internal Laryngeal Nerve* is the larger of

the two. Accompanied by the corresponding branch of the superior thyroid artery, it pierces the thyrohyoid membrane at the posterior border of the thyrohyoid muscle. *It is a purely sensory nerve*, and its terminals supply the floor of the piriform fossa (p. 293) and the mucous membrane of the larynx above the vocal folds. (*b*) The *External Laryngeal Nerve* accompanies the superior thyroid artery, but is placed on a deeper plane. It passes deep to the upper pole of the lobe of the thyroid gland, and its terminal branches are distributed to the *cricothyroid* (p. 302) *inferior constrictor muscle.*

4. Two *Cardiac Branches*, a superior and an inferior, arise on each side from the vagus in the neck and run downwards to the thorax. They are the *inhibitory nerves* of the *heart.*

5. The *Recurrent Laryngeal Nerve*, on the right side, leaves the vagus as it crosses the first part of the subclavian artery, and turns upwards and medially behind that artery and the common carotid, to reach the groove between the trachea and the œsophagus. It ascends in this groove deep to the lobe of the thyroid gland and crosses, or is crossed by, the inferior thyroid artery. Reaching the lower border of the inferior constrictor muscle, the nerve passes deep to it in order to gain access to the muscles of the larynx. Its branches supply the muscles which act on the vocal folds, but it also supplies sensory branches to the mucous membrane of the larynx below the vocal folds.

The *left recurrent laryngeal nerve* arises within the thorax (p. 124), and it ascends into the neck in the groove between the trachea and the œsophagus.

The **Internal Carotid Artery** begins opposite the upper border of the thyroid cartilage and runs upwards to the carotid canal in the petrous part of the temporal bone. Its commencement is usually marked by a localised dilatation, termed the *carotid sinus* (pp. 229, 231). Together with the internal jugular vein and the vagus nerve, it is embedded in the upward prolongation of the carotid sheath. In the lower part of its course, where it lies under cover of the anterior border of the sternomastoid muscle, it is comparatively superficial. Above the posterior belly of the digastric the vessel lies on a deeper plane, and is separated from the surface by the parotid gland and the muscles attached to the styloid process, together with other structures.

Posteriorly, the artery rests for most of its course on the anterior surface of the longus capitis, but is separated from the muscle by the carotid sheath, the superior laryngeal nerve, the superior cervical ganglion of the sympathetic, and the prevertebral fascia. Just before it enters the temporal bone the artery lies anteromedial to the internal jugular vein, and the ninth, tenth, eleventh and twelfth cranial nerves (p. 230).

On its *medial* side the artery is related to the constrictors of the pharynx and the ascending pharyngeal artery, but the relationship to the pharynx is not intimate. The external carotid artery lies anteromedial to the internal carotid until the parotid gland is reached.

To its *lateral* side lie the internal jugular vein and the vagus nerve.

The *superficial relations* are very numerous, and it is simpler to consider the lower and the upper parts of the vessel separately.

(*a*) Below the posterior belly of the digastric, the artery is overlapped by the anterior border of the sternomastoid and the more superficial structures. The carotid sheath, in which the vessel is embedded, the hypoglossal nerve, the occipital artery and the common facial vein intervene between it and the muscle.

(*b*) In the upper part of its course the artery ascends deep to the posterior belly of the digastric and the stylohyoid. It then passes under cover of the styloid process and the stylopharyngeus muscle. These two structures are placed between the artery and the parotid gland, in which the external carotid artery, the posterior facial vein and the facial nerve are embedded at this level. As it lies deep to the stylopharyngeus, the vessel is crossed by the glossopharyngeal nerve and the pharyngeal branch of the vagus.

No branches arise from the internal carotid artery in the neck.

The **Autonomic System** is responsible for the innervation of involuntary structures such as glands and unstriped muscle throughout the body. It is subdivided into two functionally antagonistic systems—(*a*) the sympathetic and (*b*) the parasympathetic.

Sympathetic activity is always widespread and is characterised by increased secretion of adrenalin. The cutaneous vessels are constricted and, as the heart rate is accelerated and the blood-pressure raised, there is an increased flow of blood to the brain, the muscles and to the heart itself. At the same time, other visceral activities are diminished. Peristalsis is inhibited and the sphincters closed. The whole body is braced to meet any emergency by the free expenditure of mental and muscular energy.

Parasympathetic activity, on the other hand, tends to produce a local rather than a general manifestation. For example, the pupils become constricted when exposed to a bright light, but this reaction is not accompanied necessarily by any other sign of parasympathetic activity. However, more general effects, such as slowing of the heart rate, increased peristalsis and the opening of sphincters occur, and these tend towards the *conservation* of energy, and to restoration of the body from the excited, "sympathetic", state.

(*a*) The *Sympathetic System* comprises the two ganglionated trunks, their offshoots and subsidiary ganglia. *Each ganglion on the trunk is connected to one or more spinal nerves by a grey ramus communicans. In addition, from T.*1 *to L.*2 *or* 3, *each ganglion is connected to the corresponding spinal nerve by a white ramus communicans.* The *efferent fibres* which are distributed by the sympathetic originate in the lateral column of the grey matter of the spinal cord, and pass out along the anterior nerve roots of the thoracic and upper lumbar spinal nerves (Plate XIII, p. 128). These fibres leave the ventral rami of the nerves concerned in the white rami communicantes, and pass to the corresponding ganglia on the sympathetic trunk. They may end there in connexion with one of the cells of the ganglion, or they may pass through the ganglion into an adjoining ganglion or they may not terminate until they reach the cœliac or some other subsidiary ganglion. These are termed *preganglionic fibres* and they possess medullated sheaths. The fibres which relay the impulses from the ganglion are described as non-medullated, though they may in fact possess a thin myelin sheath; they are termed *postganglionic* fibres. They may travel by the medial branches of the sympathetic or in the various plexuses to the viscera concerned, or *they may travel by the grey rami communicantes back to the spinal nerves* (Plate XIII, p. 128), by which they are distributed to the blood-vessels, sweat-glands, etc., of the body-wall and limbs.

The *afferent fibres* of the sympathetic system travel from the viscera through the sympathetic ganglia without being relayed, traverse the white rami communicantes and reach their cell-stations in the ganglia on the *posterior nerve roots* of the corresponding spinal nerves. They possess medullated sheaths.

(*b*) The *Parasympathetic System* comprises (1) those constituents of certain of the cranial nerves (third, seventh, ninth, tenth and eleventh) which are distributed to glands and unstriped muscle, and (2) the pelvic splanchnics (p. 206), from certain of the sacral nerves.

It is characteristic of the parasympathetic system that its fibres are relayed in peripherally situated ganglia, many of which lie on or in the walls of the viscera innervated. Like the corresponding fibres of the sympathetic system, the preganglionic fibres are medullated, while the postganglionic fibres are non-medullated.

The **Cervical Part of the Sympathetic Trunk** is embedded in the fibro-areolar tissue between the prevertebral fascia and the carotid sheath. It lies behind the common and the internal carotid arteries, and is consequently medial to the vagus, but it occupies a more posterior plane.

Typically, there should be one sympathetic ganglion corresponding to each spinal nerve, but in the cervical region, the upper four, the fifth and sixth, and the seventh and eighth become fused to form the superior, the middle and the inferior cervical ganglia, respectively. Each cervical nerve is connected to the corresponding ganglion by at least one *grey ramus communicans. There are no white rami communicantes in the neck.* The efferent fibres from the spinal cord, which are distributed by the sympathetic system, leave the ventral rami in *white rami communicantes only.* In the case of the cervical sympathetic, the efferent fibres leave the spinal cord by the highest white rami communicantes, *i.e.*, T. 1 to 4, and ascend in the sympathetic trunk. Consequently, if the sympathetic trunk be divided between the inferior cervical and the first thoracic ganglion, all efferent impulses originating in the central nervous system will be cut off completely from the cervical sympathetic. A similar condition would result from division of the spinal cord above the first thoracic segment or of the ventral ramus of the first thoracic nerve, proximal to the point of origin of its white ramus communicans, although, in the latter case, much would depend on the number of efferent sympathetic fibres in T. 2–4.

The **Superior Cervical Ganglion,** which lies behind the internal carotid artery immediately below the skull, is about 1 inch long.

Branches. (*a*) Grey rami communicantes pass to the upper four cervical anterior primary rami.

(*b*) A plexus of nerves streams upwards into the skull on the walls of the internal carotid artery. This is distributed to the hypophysis, and the third, fourth, fifth and sixth cranial nerves, as well as to the internal carotid artery and its branches.

(*c*) Included is the sympathetic root to the ciliary ganglion, which innervates the *dilator pupillæ muscle.*

(*d*) Numerous branches are associated with the external carotid artery and its branches. These not only innervate the muscular walls of the blood-vessels, but also carry the sympathetic roots to the submandibular and the otic ganglia.

(*e*) Descending branches join the pharyngeal plexus.

(*f*) The *superior cervical cardiac branch* of the sympathetic runs downwards to the thorax. On the left side, it joins the superficial part of the cardiac plexus; on the right side, it passes to the deep part of the cardiac plexus.

(*g*) In addition, the superior ganglion communicates with the ninth, tenth, and twelfth cranial nerves, and with the external and recurrent laryngeal nerves.

The **Middle Cervical Ganglion** lies behind the lower part of the carotid sheath, and is related to the summit of the loop of the inferior thyroid artery (p. 247). It is usually very small, may be in two or three portions, or it may be more or less fused with the inferior ganglion.

Branches. (*a*) Grey rami communicantes pass to the fifth and sixth cervical anterior primary rami.

(*b*) Thyroid branches accompany the inferior thyroid artery and subclavian branches follow the subclavian artery.

(*c*) The *middle cervical cardiac branch* runs downwards to the deep cardiac plexus.

The **Inferior Cervical Ganglion** may be fused with the first (and often the second) thoracic ganglion, and lies behind the lower end of the vertebral artery. It gives off grey communicating branches to the seventh and eighth cervical anterior primary rami, and a large vertebral plexus, which runs up, partly as a single nerve trunk, posterior to the vertebral artery. The inferior cervical cardiac branch descends into the thorax to join the deep part of the cardiac plexus.

Some of the fibres connecting the middle with the inferior cervical ganglion descend in front of the subclavian artery and then turn upwards behind it. They constitute the *ansa subclavia.*

The **Accessory Nerve** emerges from the jugular foramen and almost at once gives off a large communication to the inferior ganglion of the vagus. This provides the vagus with most of its motor fibres for the pharynx and larynx, and possibly for the heart, etc., and it represents that portion of the nerve which arises from the medulla oblongata. Thereafter the accessory nerve crosses the internal jugular vein as it lies in front of the transverse process of the atlas vertebra, and is itself crossed by the occipital artery. Continuing on its course downwards and backwards, the nerve emerges from under cover of the posterior belly of the digastric in company with a small branch of the occipital artery, and reaches the deep surface of the sternomastoid, which it supplies. After piercing the deep surface of the muscle the nerve enters the posterior triangle of the neck (p. 220).

The **Cervical Plexus** is formed by the ventral rami of C. 1, 2, 3 and 4 and is a simple looped plexus, connecting branches linking up the first with the second, the second with the third, and the third with the fourth cervical nerves. It lies in front of the origins of the levator scapulæ and scalenus medius, both of which arise from the posterior tubercles of the transverse processes. Anteriorly, it is covered by the prevertebral fascia, which intervenes between the plexus and the carotid sheath (internal jugular vein). More superficially it is covered by the sternomastoid muscle.

Branches. The cutaneous branches (p. 217), and branches to trapezius (p. 221), have already been described.

In addition, muscular branches are given off to the prevertebral muscles, the sternomastoid (C. 2), and the levator scapulæ (C. 3 and 4), but the most important motor branch is the phrenic nerve, which supplies the diaphragm.

Communications. Each of the constituent nerves of the plexus receives at least one grey ramus communicans from the superior cervical ganglion of the sympathetic.

The first cervical nerve communicates with the hypoglossal, and this branch (p. 234) is distributed to the geniohyoid and the thyrohyoid, and forms the ramus descendens hypoglossi.

The *Descending Cervical Nerve* (C. 2 and 3) runs downwards and curves round the lateral side (sometimes the medial side) of the internal jugular vein, and gains the front of the common carotid artery, where it joins the descending branch of the hypoglossal nerve to form the ansa hypoglossi (p. 234).

The **Phrenic Nerve** (C. 3, 4 and 5) arises from the lowest loop of the cervical plexus, and runs downwards on the anterior surface of the scalenus anterior muscle. Owing to the obliquity of the muscle, the nerve crosses from its lateral border above, to its medial border below, and in this part of its course *it is plastered on to the anterior aspect of the muscle by the prevertebral fascia.* More superficially, it is overlapped by the internal jugular vein and the sternomastoid muscle. On leaving the surface of the scalenus anterior, the phrenic nerve runs downwards on the cervical dome of the pleura behind the commencement of the brachiocephalic vein. It crosses in front of, but frequently behind, the internal thoracic artery and enters the thoracic inlet behind the first costal cartilage. On the left side the nerve crosses in front of the first part of the subclavian artery. (See also p. 107.)

In the **Middle Line of the Neck** the left and right anterior triangles meet together, the line stretching from the symphysis menti to the suprasternal notch. In its uppermost part of this junction is the *median submental triangle*, which is bounded by the anterior bellies of the digastrics and by the hyoid bone. The floor of this space is formed by the mylohoid muscles with their median raphe. It contains the *Submental Lymph Nodes*, which drain (1) the superficial tissues below the chin; (2) the central part of the lower lip; (3) the adjoining gum; (4) the anterior part of the floor of the mouth; and (5) *the tip of the tongue.* Efferents pass from these glands to join the submandibular lymph nodes (p. 269).

Below the body of the hyoid bone lies the median thyrohyoid

ligament, behind which the epiglottis is situated. It is attached below to the thyroid cartilage, which forms a prominent median landmark in the neck in the male subject.

The gap between the thyroid and cricoid cartilages is occupied by the cricovocal membrane, with its median thickening, named the cricothyroid ligament.

The narrow anterior part of the cricoid cartilage can be felt easily in the living subject. *It lies on a level with the sixth cervical vertebra.* The cricotracheal membrane connects the cricoid cartilage to the trachea but, as a rule, only the first ring of the trachea can be felt, for the succeeding three rings are covered by the isthmus of the thyroid gland. Below this structure the trachea is related to the inferior thyroid veins, which run downwards into the thorax on its anterior surface.

The **Thyroid Gland** is directly related to the trachea and larynx. It consists of right and left lobes, connected to each other by a narrow *isthmus*, and the whole gland derives a sheath from the pretracheal fascia.

The *Isthmus* stretches across the midline in front of the second, third and fourth rings of the trachea. At each end it is partly overlapped by the sternothyroid and, more superficially, by the sternohyoid muscles, and along its upper border terminal branches of the superior thyroid arteries may anastomose with each other. The *Pyramidal Lobe*, when present, projects upwards from the isthmus a little to the left of the median plane. It is connected to the hyoid bone by a fibrous slip, which is often replaced by a small muscle, termed the *levator glandulæ thyroideæ*.

Each *Lobe* is pear-shaped, with its apex above. Its *antero-lateral* or superficial aspect is covered closely by the sternothyroid muscle, and, more superficially, by the superior belly of the omohyoid, the sternohyoid and, to a lesser extent, by the sternomastoid muscle.

Its *postero-lateral* surface is related to the carotid sheath (common carotid artery). Its *deep surface* is related above to the inferior constrictor and the cricothyroid muscles, which separate it from the thyroid and cricoid cartilages, and below to the œsophagus, the upper six rings of the trachea and the recurrent laryngeal nerves. Between the deep surface and the postero-lateral surface, the gland presents a thick, rounded, posterior border, on which is found an anastomosis between the superior and inferior thyroid arteries.

Blood Supply. The gland receives its arterial supply from (1) the superior thyroid artery (p. 232), which supplies the upper third of the lobe, and the upper half of the isthmus; and (2) the inferior thyroid artery (p. 248), which supplies the lower two-thirds of the lobe and the lower half of the isthmus.

Three veins issue from the gland on each side: (*a*) The superior thyroid vein (p. 233) accompanies the artery of the same name, and ends in the internal jugular or the (common) facial vein. (*b*) The middle thyroid vein has no accompanying artery. It runs laterally across the common carotid artery to join the internal jugular vein about the level of the cricoid cartilage. (*c*) The inferior thyroid veins commence at the lower border of the isthmus and are joined by tributaries from the lower pole of the gland. They run downwards *in front of the trachea*, connected by several transverse branches, and end in the left brachiocephalic vein in the thorax.

The *Lymph Vessels*, for the most part, join the antero-superior and antero-inferior groups of the deep cervical lymph nodes, but a few run downwards in front of the trachea and end in the paratracheal lymph nodes.

The thyroid gland develops in the fourth week as an endodermal outgrowth from the ventral wall or floor of the primitive pharynx, just caudal to the point where the tuberculum impar appears. The rudiment grows caudally and becomes bilobar. It soon loses its hollow character and its connexion with the floor of the mouth (*thyroglossal duct*) becomes lost at a very early stage. At the present time it is generally accepted that the whole of the lateral lobe is derived from the median rudiment; a contribution from the fourth or fifth pouches is still *sub judice*.

The **Parathyroid Glands** comprise superior and inferior pairs. They are important in calcium metabolism and the superior pair are intimately related, on each side, to the posterior border of the lobe of the thyroid gland and to the anastomosing vessel which connects the superior thyroid artery with the inferior (p. 249). The superior parathyroid, which is developed from the pharyngeal entoderm of the *fourth* pharyngeal pouch, lies opposite the lower border of the cricoid cartilage. The inferior parathyroid has a similar origin from the *third* pharyngeal pouch and is closely related at first to the rudiment of the thymus. As the latter grows caudally it is accompanied by the inferior parathyroid, which reaches a more caudal level than the derivative of the fourth pouch. In the adult the inferior parathyroid may lie within or outside the fascial sheath of the thyroid gland or it may be embedded in its substance, at or near the lower pole of the lobe, but it is frequently found in close relationship with the inferior thyroid veins.

The **Trachea** (see also p. 120) commences below the cricoid cartilage, on a level with the lower border of the sixth cervical vertebra. It extends downwards in the median plane to enter the thoracic inlet, and is comparatively superficial in the neck. *Anteriorly*, it is crossed by the isthmus of the thyroid gland (second, third, and fourth rings), and below that structure it is related to the inferior thyroid veins, which run downwards upon it, frequently communicating with one another, to open into the brachiocephalic veins. In young children the left brachiocephalic vein may project above the level of the manubrium sterni and form an anterior relation of the trachea in the root of the neck. In addition, the pretracheal fascia, the investing layer of the deep cervical fascia, the jugular arch (p. 216), and the superficial fascia separate the treachea from the skin.

On each side the trachea is related to the lobes of the thyroid gland, and more posteriorly to the recurrent laryngeal nerves (p. 236). Posteriorly, the trachea rests on the œsophagus.

The **Œsophagus** (see also p. 122) commences opposite the sixth cervical vertebra, where it is continuous above with the laryngeal part of the pharynx. As it descends through the neck it diverges slightly to the left side, so that its left margin is more accessible than its right margin, which is frequently behind the trachea.

Posteriorly, the œsophagus lies on the longus cervicis muscles and the vertebral column. *On each side* it is related to the lobe of the thyroid gland and in addition, on the left side, to the thoracic duct (p. 247). *Anteriorly*, it is in contact with the trachea and the recurrent laryngeal nerves.

The **Deep Cervical Lymph Nodes** lie, for the most part, under cover of the sternomastoid muscles, and form upper and lower groups, each of which may be further subdivided into anterior (or medial) and posterior (or lateral) groups. These subdivisions are by no means sharply separated from one another.

(*a*) The *Antero-superior Group* is closely associated with the carotid sheath above the omohyoid muscle. It receives *afferents* from (1) the parotid lymph nodes (p. 261); (2) the submandibular lymph nodes (p. 269); (3) the retropharyngeal lymph nodes (p. 291); and (4) the dorsum of the tongue.

(*b*) The *Postero-superior Group* lies lateral to the upper part of the internal jugular vein, and many of its members are found in the posterior triangle of the neck (p. 220). It receives *afferents* from (1) the mastoid and occipital lymph glands (p. 252); (2) the interior of the cranium, and (3) the deep muscles of the neck.

The *efferents* from the upper deep cervical lymph nodes pass to the lower groups, but some of them unite with efferents from the lower groups to form the jugular lymph trunk.

(*c*) The *Antero-inferior Group* is associated with the lower end of the carotid sheath, and some of its members lie on the cervical dome of the pleura. It receives *afferents* from (1) the upper groups; (2) the prelaryngeal, pretracheal, and paratracheal lymph nodes, and (3) the thyroid gland.

(*d*) The *Postero-inferior Group* extends laterally into the supraclavicular triangle. It receives *afferents* from (1) the upper groups and (2) the deep muscles of the neck.

The *efferents* of the lower groups unite with some of the efferents of the upper groups to form the *jugular lymph trunk.* This vessel may end in the thoracic duct or right lymphatic duct, or it may join the subclavian lymph trunk, or it may open independently into the brachiocephalic vein.

It must be remembered that those deep cervical lymph nodes which are found in the posterior triangle of the neck are situated in the fat between the fascial roof and the fascial floor of the triangle. They, therefore, lie in the same stratum as the accessory nerve (p. 240).

THE ROOT OF THE NECK

The **Sternoclavicular Joint** is synovial, and approximately of the plane type. But the sternal end of the first costal cartilage usually takes part in the articulation in addition to the medial end of the clavicle and the clavicular notch on the manubrium sterni.

The joint is surrounded by a capsular ligament, which is thickened in front, above and behind. The anterior and posterior thickenings are not of great strength, but the superior (*interclavicular ligament*) is something more than a localised thickening of the capsular ligament. Attached to the upper aspect of the sternal end of the clavicle, it is closely blended with the capsular ligament, and is then carried across the suprasternal notch, bound down to the upper border of the sternum, to a corresponding attachment on the opposite side.

An articular disc of fibrocartilage subdivides the joint cavity into medial and lateral compartments. It is attached above to the clavicle and below to the first costal cartilage. Anteriorly and posteriorly it is attached to the capsular ligament. In addition to acting as a buffer to absorb thrust from the shoulder and arm, the articular disc assists in the limitation of movements at the joint.

The *Costoclavicular Ligament* extends upwards, backwards and laterally from the first costal cartilage to an impression on the lower surface of the sternal end of the clavicle. It is an important extracapsular ligament of the joint, for it helps to limit the movements of the clavicle.

Synovial membranes line the two compartments of the joint.

Movements. It should be observed that movements of the sternal end of the clavicle always accompany movements of the acromial end of the bone *in the opposite direction* (except for rotation around its long axis). Thus, when the shoulders are braced back, the sternal ends of the clavicles are thrust forwards, and when the point of the shoulder is depressed, the sternal end of the clavicle is tilted upwards. The movements are therefore associated with movements at the acromioclavicular joint.

In elevation and depression of the shoulder, the clavicle moves on the articular disc. Elevation of the shoulder is limited by tension of the costoclavicular ligament; depression is limited by the articular disc and the interclavicular ligament.

In forward and backward movements the sternal end of the clavicle and the disc move over the facet on the manubrium, and the anterior and posterior sternoclavicular ligaments are rendered taut alternately.

The **Scalenus Anterior** is a surgically important landmark in the lower part of the neck. It arises by slips from the anterior tubercles of the transverse processes of the third, fourth, fifth, and sixth cervical vertebræ. Its fibres are directed downwards and slightly forwards and laterally to be inserted into the scalene tubercle on the inner border of the first rib. Except at its insertion, which lies behind the clavicle, the whole muscle is under cover of the sternomastoid.

The *Anterior Surface* of the muscle is covered by the prevertebral fascia, and the only structure which intervenes between the muscle and the fascia is the *phrenic nerve*. Arising principally from C. 4, with additional twigs from C. 3 and C. 5, the phrenic nerve runs vertically downwards, but, owing to the slight obliquity of the scalenus anterior, it crosses from the upper end of the lateral border of the muscle to the lower part of the medial border. The prevertebral fascia, which plasters the phrenic nerve against the scalenus anterior, separates both these structures from the carotid sheath.

The subclavian vein crosses in front of the muscle near its insertion.

Along the *Lateral Border* of the muscle *the trunks of the brachial plexus and the subclavian artery emerge* to enter the posterior triangle.

Posteriorly, the muscle is separated from the scalenus medius by the trunks of the plexus and from the cervical pleura by the subclavian artery (second part).

The *Medial Border* of the muscle is related to the following structures. It is separated from the lateral border of the lower part of the longus cervicis by a Λ-shaped interval, the apex of the Λ being situated at the carotid tubercle. The lower part of this gap is crossed by the subclavian artery, which disappears behind the medial border of the scalenus anterior. Before it disappears it gives off from its upper border two large branches: (1) the vertebral; and (2) the thyrocervical trunk.

The *Vertebral Artery* runs upwards to the apex of the space and there enters the foramen in the transverse process of the sixth cervical vertebra. Its accompanying vein descends in front of the artery and, deviating to its lateral side, crosses in front of the first part of the subclavian artery. It ends in the posterior aspect of the innominate vein near its commencement.

The *Inferior Thyroid Artery* arises from the thyrocervical trunk and at first runs upwards along, or in front of, the medial border of the scalenus anterior. When it reaches the level of the sixth cervical transverse process, it turns medially and downwards to reach the posterior border of the lobe of the thyroid gland, to which it is finally distributed. The course of this vessel, therefore, resembles an inverted U, and the summit of the curve varies considerably in level. When, as is often the case, it lies below the sixth cervical transverse process, the inferior thyroid artery crosses in front of the vertebral vessels. As it reaches the thyroid gland the artery usually crosses in front of (but frequently behind) the recurrent laryngeal nerve.

Another structure of considerable importance which crosses the gap between the scalenus anterior and the longus cervicis on the left side is the *thoracic duct.* It ascends from the thorax along the left edge of the œsophagus and in front of the longus cervicis to the level of the seventh cervical transverse process. There, or a little lower—the level is subject to variation—the thoracic duct bends laterally, crossing in front of, or insinuating itself between, the vertebral vessels. It then turns downwards along the medial border of the scalenus anterior, in front of the phrenic nerve and the first part of the subclavian artery, and ends in the angle of union of the left internal jugular and subclavian veins. The course of the duct is therefore very similar to that of the inferior thyroid artery, but it loops in the reverse direction and at a lower level.

All the structures which have just been mentioned, viz., the first part of the subclavian artery, the vertebral vessels, the inferior thyroid artery and the thoracic duct, are *covered over by the lower end of the carotid sheath and its contents, and, still more superficially, by the sternomastoid muscle*, which form the roof over the gap between the scalenus anterior and the longus cervicis.

The scalenus anterior elevates the first rib, and when that bone is fixed it bends the neck to the same side.

It receives its *Nerve Supply* from the anterior rami of C. 4, 5 and 6.

The **Subclavian Artery**—on the right side a branch of the brachio-cephalic, on the left a branch from the arch of the aorta—describes a gentle curve, convex upwards, in its course through the neck. As already mentioned, the artery is crossed by the scalenus anterior, and advantage is taken of this fact to divide the vessel into three parts, the second part lying behind the muscle and forming the summit of the curve. The third part of the artery has already been described (p. 222).

The **First Part** runs upwards and laterally to reach the medial border of the scalenus anterior. *Anteriorly*, as it is traced laterally, the following structures are encountered: (1) the common carotid artery; (2) the ansa subclavia (p. 240); (3) the vagus nerve; (4) the internal jugular vein, partially separated from the artery by the vertebral vein and, on the left side, by the phrenic nerve.

Posteriorly, the artery is in direct relation with the suprapleural membrane, the cupola (dome) of the pleura and the apex of the lung. The ansa subclavia, and, on the right side, the recurrent laryngeal nerve, are the only intervening structures.

Branches. 1. The *Vertebral Artery* (p. 226) arises from the upper border of the subclavian artery and ascends to the foramen in the transverse process of the sixth cervical vertebra, crossing in front of the ventral of the eighth cervical nerve, the seventh cervical transverse process and the ventral of the seventh cervical nerve. The inferior cervical ganglion of the sympathetic lies to its postero-medial side, and a large sympathetic plexus, partly in the form of a single trunk, ascends behind the vessel. As it runs upwards it lies behind the medial portion of the carotid sheath, but certain important structures intervene. On the left side the thoracic duct curves laterally in front of the artery about the level of the seventh cervical transverse process and on both sides, at a slightly higher level, the inferior thyroid artery curves medially and forwards in front of it. The vertebral vein lies directly in front of the artery as it emerges from the foramen in the transverse process of the sixth cervical vertebra, but it deviates to the lateral side as it descends.

The subsequent course of the vessel is described on pp. 283 and 367.

2. The *Thyrocervical Trunk* arises from the upper border of the subclavian artery at the medial border of the scalenus anterior muscle, and at once breaks up into (*a*) the suprascapular (p. 223), (*b*) the transverse cervical (p. 221), and (*c*) the inferior thyroid arteries.

The *Inferior Thyroid Artery* ascends close to the medial border of the scalenus anterior muscle and behind the internal jugular vein.

At or a little below the level of the sixth cervical transverse process it turns medially and downwards, passing behind the vagus nerve and the common carotid artery, and in front of the vertebral vessels and the sympathetic trunk. It thus reaches the lobe of the thyroid gland, where it crosses, or is crossed by, the recurrent laryngeal nerve.

As the inferior thyroid artery turns medially behind the carotid sheath, it gives off its *ascending cervical* branch, which runs upwards, medial to the phrenic nerve, in front of the transverse processes of the cervical vertebræ. In addition the inferior thyroid artery supplies branches to the larynx, pharynx, trachea, œsophagus, and the surrounding muscles.

Most of the terminal branches are given to the lower pole of the lobe of the thyroid gland, but a large branch ascends along the posterior border of the gland to anastomose with a descending branch from the superior thyroid artery.

3. The *Internal Thoracic Artery* arises from the lower aspect of the subclavian, near the medial border of the scalenus anterior. It runs downwards on the pleura, crossing, or being crossed by, the phrenic nerve, and passes behind the first costal cartilage. The rest of its course is described on p. 99.

The **Second Part of the Subclavian Artery** lies behind the scalenus anterior and the superimposed structures. Posteriorly, it is in contact with the cupola of the pleura and the apex of the lung.

From its posterior aspect the *Costocervical trunk* arises and passes backwards above the pleura to the neck of the first rib, where it divides into the *superior intercostal* (p. 127) and *deep cervical arteries*. The latter passes backwards between the neck of the first rib and the transverse process of the seventh cervical vertebra, and then ascends, in the back of the neck, deep to the semispinalis capitis muscle. Its terminal branches anastomose with branches of the occipital artery (p. 233).

The **Subclavian Vein,** which lies at a lower level than its companion artery, *is placed wholly behind the subclavius muscle and the clavicle*. Posteriorly it crosses the phrenic nerve and the scalenus anterior near its insertion, and inferiorly it rests on a wide, shallow groove on the upper surface of the first rib.

As the vein reaches the medial border of the scalenus anterior it joins the internal jugular to form the brachiocephalic vein, and there is, therefore, no part of the vein which corresponds to the first part of the subclavian artery. *Consequently the veins corresponding to the branches of the first part of the artery terminate, for the most part, in the brachiocephalic vein.*

The **Scalenus Medius** arises from the posterior tubercles of the transverse processes of the first or second to the sixth cervical vertebræ. *It therefore lies behind the ventral rami of the lower four cervical nerves* as they run laterally and downwards to form the brachial plexus. It is inserted into the first rib behind the groove for the subclavian artery.

The **Scalenus Posterior** lies behind the medius. It arises from the lower cervical vertebræ and is inserted into the second rib. A small part of the muscle appears in the floor of the posterior triangle of the neck between the levator scapulæ and the scalenus medius.

Both these muscles may elevate the ribs into which they are inserted, and they bend the neck to one side. They are supplied by the ventral rami of the lower four or five cervical nerves.

THE SCALP

The scalp forms the covering of the cranial vault. It consists of five layers: (1) skin; (2) superficial fascia, which is firmly attached to the skin and to the aponeurosis of the occipitofrontalis muscle by numerous fibrous septa; (3) the occipitofrontalis muscle and its epicranial aponeurosis; (4) some loose areolar tissue; and (5) the pericranium.

The **Occipitofrontalis** consists of two frontal and two occipital bellies connected to one another by the epicranial aponeurosis. The frontal bellies arise from the skin in the neighbourhood of the eyebrows, while the occipital bellies arise from the highest nuchal lines of the occipital bone. The former are supplied by the temporal branches and the latter by the posterior auricular branches of the facial nerves.

The *Epicranial Aponeurosis* is connected with the frontal bellies anteriorly and with the occipital bellies posteriorly. On each side it passes superficial to the temporal fascia, with which it is blended.

The loose areolar tissue which intervenes between the epicranial aponeurosis and the pericranium permits of free movement of the scalp, and it allows large collections of blood or pus to accumulate under the scalp without undue stretching of the covering skin. This potential sub-aponeurotic space is closed laterally along the temporal lines, posteriorly along the highest nuchal lines, and anteriorly just above the supra-orbital ridges.

The **Blood Vessels** of the scalp *are very numerous and they anastomose freely with one another*. The arteries are derived from both the internal and the external carotid systems.

Anteriorly, the *supratrochlear* and the *supra-orbital arteries* ascend over the forehead in company with the supratrochlear and the supra-orbital nerves. Both are branches of the ophthalmic artery (internal carotid), and their terminal branches anastomose with one another, with their fellows of the opposite side, and with the superficial temporal artery (external carotid) of the same side.

On each side the *superficial temporal artery* ascends in front of the tragus in company with the auriculotemporal nerve. It divides into anterior and posterior branches, which supply a large area of the scalp extending up to the vertex, where they anastomose with the corresponding branches of the opposite side.

Posteriorly, there are two arteries on each side. The *posterior auricular* (external carotid) ascends immediately behind the auricle and supplies that structure and the adjoining part of the scalp. The *occipital artery* (external carotid), in the terminal part of its course, extends over the occipital region in company with the greater occipital nerve. Its branches anastomose with those of the posterior auricular and with the posterior branch of the superficial temporal artery.

The *Supratrochlear* and *Supra-orbital Veins* unite to form the (anterior) facial vein (p. 259), which communicates with the superior ophthalmic vein.

The *Superficial Temporal Vein* unites with the maxillary vein to form the retromandibular (posterior facial) vein (p. 231), while the *posterior auricular* runs into the external jugular vein (p. 216).

The veins which accompany the occipital artery enter the sub-occipital venous plexus, which lies under cover of the upper part of the semispinalis capitis muscle. Thence the blood is drained by the vertebral veins.

The **Nerves** which supply the scalp are derived from the tri-geminal nerve and from the second and third cervical nerves:—

(*a*) The *Supratrochlear Nerve* (ophthalmic division of V.) (p. 254).

(*b*) The *Supra-orbital Nerve* (ophthalmic division of V.) (p. 253).

(*c*) The *Zygomaticotemporal* (maxillary division of V.) (p. 254).

(*d*) The *Auriculotemporal Nerve* (mandibular division of V.) (p. 255).

(*e*) The *Greater Occipital Nerve* (C. 2, dorsal ramus) supplies a large area of skin over the occipital region and extends forwards to the vertex (p. 223).

(*f*) The *Great Auricular Nerve* (C. 2 and 3, ventral rami) supplies the auricle (p. 217) and the skin over the mastoid process, but does not extend to the scalp.

(*g*) The *Lesser Occipital Nerve* (C. 2, ventral ramus) and the *Third Occipital Nerve* (C. 3, dorsal ramus) may or may not extend into the scalp (pp. 217 and 224).

The *Lymph Vessels* from the anterior half of the scalp drain into the *parotid lymph nodes* on the lateral surface and within the fascial sheath of the parotid gland. These nodes also receive afferents from the adjoining part of the cheek, both eyelids, and the root of the nose.

The lymph vessels from the posterior part of the scalp join the *mastoid lymph nodes*, which lie superficial to the insertion of the sternomastoid, and the *occipital lymph nodes*, which are found at the apex of the posterior triangle of the neck.

The efferents from these three groups join the upper deep cervical lymph nodes (p. 244).

THE FACE

The **Eyelids** can easily be examined superficially in the living subject. They are covered by skin on their superficial aspects and by a mucous membrane, termed the *conjunctiva*, on their deep aspects. The eyelashes spring from the mucocutaneous junction, and immediately behind them the mouths of the *tarsal glands* can be seen. Near the *medial angle of the eye*, where the two eyelids meet, the eyelashes and the tarsal glands stop abruptly, and at this point there is a small rounded elevation on the margin of each eyelid. This is termed the *lacrimal papilla*, and when the eyelid is slightly everted, a small opening, termed the *punctum lacrimale*, will be seen on its summit. Under normal conditions the puncta are kept in close apposition with the conjunctiva, and each leads into a minute *lacrimal canaliculus*, which runs for a short distance *at right angles to the margin of the eyelid*, and then turns medially to open into the *lacrimal sac* (p. 279).

The *lacus lacrimalis* is the triangular area separating the two lids at the medial angle of the eye. It is occupied by the *caruncula lacrimalis*, a reddish elevation which is limited laterally by a small fold of conjunctiva, termed the *plica semilunaris*.

The *conjunctiva* is a mucuous membrane which covers the anterior surface of the eyeball, being reduced in thickness over the cornea, and is reflected at the superior and inferior fornices over the deep surfaces of the eyelids. In its upper and lateral part it is pierced by the ducts of the lacrimal gland (p. 279).

Each eyelid is stiffened by a *tarsus* (*tarsal plate*), which consists of dense fibrous tissue. The superior tarsus is much larger than the inferior, and both are more or less blended with the corresponding *palpebral fascia*, which is a thin fibrous sheet extending into the eyelid from the periosteum at the margin of the orbital opening.

Near the margin of the lid, the tarsus is firmly adherent to the skin, and throughout its extent its deep surface is intimately attached to the conjunctiva. The tarsal glands are embedded in it, and their oily secretion provides a protective film over the lid margins and cilia. The opposed lid and corneal surfaces are covered by a thin film of lacrimal fluid, the drainage of which into the lacrimal sac (p. 279) carries away any small particles of dust. The superficial aspect of each tarsus is clothed by the palpebral fibres of the orbicularis oculi muscle.

The face is developed around the stomodœum or primitive mouth, which is bounded at first by the forebrain and the pericardium. The growth of the *mandibular arches* separates the mouth from the pericardium and forms the lower part of the face. The upper part is formed from (1) the *frontonasal process*, which becomes partly divided into a *median and two lateral nasal processes* after the appearance of the olfactory plate and pit, and (2) the *maxillary process*, which develops from the dorsal part of the cephalic border of the mandibular arch. The median nasal process extends beyond the lateral nasal processes and expands into the two *globular processes*. The maxillary process fuses with the lateral nasal process, along the line of the nasolacrimal duct, and with the globular processes. Thereafter the mouth is bounded by the mandibular arches, on the one hand, and the maxillary and globular processes, on the other. The philtrum of the upper lip is formed from the fused globular processes, in which the premaxilla is subsequently formed, while its lateral part is derived on each side from the maxillary process. The ophthalmic nerve is distributed to the frontonasal process and its derivatives; the maxillary nerve to the maxillary process, and the mandibular nerve to the mandibular arch. The skin of the philtrum is supplied by labial branches from the infra-orbital nerve and this is explained by the fact that, subsequent to fusion of the maxillary and globular processes, the latter are invaded by mesenchymal cells of the maxillary process. In *hare-lip* the cleft is almost always lateral to the median plane and is due to failure of the maxillary arch to fuse with the globular process. (See also p. 298.)

THE SENSORY NERVES OF THE FACE

With the exception of the skin over the parotid region and adjoining the angle of the jaw—supplied by the great auricular nerve (C. 2 and 3)—*the whole of the skin of the face is supplied by the trigeminal nerve*. Terminal branches from each of its three divisions reach the face, and they are at fault in cases of facial neuralgia.

The **Ophthalmic Nerve** supplies the skin over the top of the head, the forehead, the upper eyelid and the whole of the conjunctiva, and the anterior two-thirds of the side of the nose, down to and including the tip. No fewer than five of its branches reach the skin.

(*a*) The *Lacrimal Nerve* (p. 275) supplies the lateral part of the upper eyelid.

(*b*) The *Supra-orbital Nerve* leaves the orbit through the *supra-orbital* notch, or foramen, as the case may be, about two fingers' breadth from the median plane. It divides into lateral and medial branches, which supply the central part of the upper eyelid and ascend under cover of the orbicularis oculi and the frontal belly of the occipitofrontalis. They supply the conjunctiva and the skin of the forehead and the scalp *as far back as the vertex*.

(*c*) The *Supratrochlear Nerve* emerges from the orbit one finger's breadth from the median plane. It supplies the medial part of the upper eyelid and a small area of the forehead above the root of the nose.

(*d*) The *Infratrochlear Nerve* emerges from the orbit above the medial palpebral ligament and supplies a small area of skin of the upper eyelid and the adjoining part of the nose.

(*e*) The *External Nasal Nerve*, which has a complicated intracranial course (p. 276), emerges on the face at the lower border of the nasal bone and supplies the skin of the nose down to the tip.

The **Maxillary Nerve** is distributed, roughly, to the skin over the upper jaw. It includes the posterior part of the side of the nose, the upper lip, the anterior and upper part of the cheek, the lower eyelid, and the skin on the lateral side of the orbital opening. This it does by means of one large and two small branches.

(*a*) The *Infra-orbital Nerve* is the direct continuation of the maxillary nerve. It emerges from the infra-orbital foramen, which lies half an inch below the lower margin of the orbital aperture and vertically below the supra-orbital notch, or foramen. Under cover of the levator labii superioris it divides into (1) palpebral branches, for the lower eyelid; (2) nasal branches, for the posterior part of the side of the nose; (3) labial branches, for the upper lip; and (4) buccal branches, for the cheek.

(*b*) The *Zygomaticofacial Nerve* (p. 281) emerges from a small foramen on the lateral surface of the zygomatic bone and supplies the skin in its immediate neighbourhood.

(*c*) The *Zygomaticotemporal Nerve* pierces the temporal fascia close to the zygomatic bone on a level with the lateral palpebral ligament and supplies a small area of skin in that situation.

The **Mandibular Nerve** supplies, roughly, the skin over the lower jaw, but it extends on to the auricle and upwards on to the side of the head. Three branches of this nerve reach the skin.

(*a*) The *Mental Nerve* emerges from the mental foramen of the mandible (p. 398) and supplies branches to the lower lip, the chin, and the skin over the immediately adjoining part of the body of the bone.

(*b*) The *Buccal Nerve* reaches the surface in front of the masseter muscle and gives off branches to the cheek.

(*c*) The *Auriculotemporal Nerve* passes from under cover of the parotid gland in company with the superficial temporal artery. It crosses the pre-auricular point, and ascends over the side of the head. It gives branches to the skin of the tragus and the skin of the scalp above the auricle, and it also supplies the modified skin which lines the external auditory meatus and covers the outer surface of the tympanic membrane. The terminal branches on the scalp may reach almost to the vertex.

The Muscles of the Face. Under this heading are included all the muscles which act, directly or indirectly, on the skin of the face. Most of them have a bony origin, but as the deep fascia is absent from the face, except in the region of the masseter muscle, they all lie in the superficial fascia.

All the facial muscles, including the buccinator and the platysma, receive their nerve supply from the facial nerve.

The muscles of this group arrange themselves (1) around the orbital openings; (2) around the nose; and (3) around the mouth.

1. The *Orbicularis Oculi* forms a sphincter muscle for the palpebral fissure. It consists of a palpebral portion, confined to the two eyelids, an orbital portion, which extends upwards on to the forehead and downwards on to the face, and a lacrimal portion.

(*a*) The *Palpebral Portion* arises from the medial palpebral ligament, a short fibrous cord which stretches horizontally from the medial commissure of the eyelids to the adjoining part of the maxilla, and its fibres curve laterally in both eyelids. They mingle at their insertion to form the lateral palpebral raphe.

Contraction of this muscle can be carried out without contraction of the orbital portion, and it results in simple closure of the palpebral fissure.

(*b*) The *Orbital Portion* arises from the medial end of the medial palpebral ligament and from the adjoining bone. Its fibres form a series of concentric rings immediately outside the palpebral portion.

Contraction of this muscle may or may not be associated with contraction of the palpebral portion. In the former case the "eye is shut tightly." In the latter case the skin around the orbital apertures is thrown into wrinkles.

(*c*) The *Lacrimal Portion* lies deep to the medial part of the palpebral portion of the muscle. It arises from the lacrimal fascia, which bridges over the groove lodging the lacrimal sac, and from the adjoining parts of the lacrimal bone. Passing laterally it divides into upper and lower portions, which mingle with the fibres of the palpebral portion, some fibres being inserted into the upper and others into the lower tarsus.

Contraction of the muscle draws the eyelids medially and directs the lacrimal puncta (p. 253) into the lacus lacrimalis. At the same time traction is exerted on the lacrimal fascia with resulting dilatation of the lacrimal sac.

The *Corrugator*, partly intermingled with the orbicularis oculi, arises from the medial end of the superciliary arch and runs upwards and laterally. It is contracted in frowning.

2. The muscles which are grouped around the nose act on the skin of the nose and on the movable alar cartilages. Thus the alæ may be dilated, elevated or depressed. Elevation of the alæ is accompanied by wrinkling of the skin of the nose—this being the popular mode of expressing disgust, particularly when an offensive odour is detected. This action is produced by the levator labii superioris alæque nasi, a vertically running fleshy slip, which is partly inserted into the ala of the nose and partly into the upper lip. The wrinkling of the skin over the nose is always accompanied therefore by some elevation of the upper lip.

3. The muscles which are grouped around the mouth are called into play in eating and in speech and also in facial expression,

The *Risorius* may be continuous with the posterior fibres of the platysma, or it may arise independently from the fascia covering the masseter muscle. Its fibres converge on the angle of the mouth, where they are inserted into the skin.

By drawing the angle of the mouth in a lateral direction the risorius plays a large part in the production of a smile.

The *Zygomaticus Major* arises from the zygomatic bone and runs downwards and medially to the angle of the mouth.

The *Levator Labii Superioris* arises from the lower border of the orbital opening and is inserted into the skin of the upper lip.

The *Levator Labii Superioris Alæque Nasi*, which has been already mentioned, lies along the medial border of the levator labii superioris.

The *Zygomaticus Minor* is a small slip which arises from the zygomatic bone and is closely related to the lateral margin of the levator labii superioris.

The *Levator Anguli Oris* lies deep to the levator labii superioris. It arises from the upper jaw below the infra-orbital foramen, and is inserted partly into the skin of the angle of the mouth, and partly blends with the orbicularis oris.

The *Depressor Anguli Oris* is placed superficially. It is triangular in shape, the base corresponding to the origin from the body of the mandible, and the apex corresponding to the insertion in the neighbourhood of the angle of the mouth.

The *Depressor Labii Inferioris* has a linear origin from the front of the body of the mandible, and its fibres are inserted into the skin of the lower lip. The two muscles meet each other in the median plane.

The **Buccinator** forms the fleshy stratum of the cheek. It is more deeply situated, and its fibres run horizontally forwards to the angle of the mouth. It arises from the outer alveolar margins of both the upper and lower jaws in the region of the molar teeth. These comprise the upper and lower fibres of the muscle, but intermediate fibres arise from the pterygomandibular ligament (p. 288). At the angle of the mouth the muscle blends with the orbicularis oris in a definite manner. The uppermost and lowermost fibres pass directly into the upper and lower lips, respectively, but the middle fibres decussate, the upper half running into the lower lip and the lower half into the upper lip.

Contraction of the buccinator compresses the cheek against the gum and so prevents partially masticated food from lodging in that situation—an unpleasant concomitant of *facial paralysis*.

The buccinator is innervated by the facial nerve.

The *Orbicularis Oris* is a true sphincter muscle. Its fibres encircle the oral aperture and extend upwards to the nose and downwards to the groove between the lower lip and the chin. Many of its fibres are derived directly from the buccinator, while others are provided by the depressors and elevators of the angles of the mouth.

The **Facial Nerve** (p. 373) emerges from the stylomastoid foramen and at once gives off (1) a branch to supply the posterior belly of the digastric and the stylohyoid, and (2) the posterior auricular nerve. The latter ascends behind the ear and supplies the posterior and superior auricular muscles and the occipital belly of the occipitofrontalis. Having given off these branches, the facial nerve enters the parotid gland and runs forwards in its substance, crossing the posterior facial vein and the external carotid artery. In the gland, the nerve breaks up into its terminal branches.

(*a*) The *temporal branch* appears at the upper border of the gland and runs upwards and forwards to supply the facial muscles above the zygoma and the frontalis. (*b*) The upper *zygomatic branch* is usually small. It runs forwards from the upper part of the anterior border of the parotid gland to the zygomatic bone and supplies the adjoining facial muscles. The lower *zygomatic branch* appears at the anterior border of the parotid gland above the duct and runs forwards in company with the transverse facial vessels to supply the muscles of the nose and upper lip. (*c*) The *buccal branch* appears at the anterior border of the parotid gland and runs forwards below the duct to supply the *buccinator* and the orbicularis oris. It communicates freely with the buccal nerve from the mandibular division of the trigeminal (p. 264). (*d*) The *mandibular branch* also appears at the anterior border of the parotid gland and runs forwards towards the lower lip and chin, supplying the risorius and the neighbouring muscles. (*e*) The *cervical branch* appears at the lower border of the parotid gland and curves downwards and forwards below the angle of the jaw. It supplies the platysma, and its terminal fibres are distributed to the depressors of the lower lip.

It will be seen that of the five named branches of the facial nerve, one emerges from the upper border, three from the anterior border, and one from the lower border of the parotid gland. In a dissected specimen they give the appearance of radiating out from a point on the neck of the mandible.

One other point about these branches should be mentioned. Free communications are established between them and the neighbouring branches of the trigeminal nerve.

The Facial Nerve supplies all the facial muscles. It contains no cutaneous branches. In the embryo it is the nerve of the second visceral arch.

The **Facial Artery** (pp. 233 and 269) leaves the submandibular region and enters the face by curling round the lower border of the mandible immediately in front of the masseter muscle. Its course in the face is characterised by its tortuosity, but the general line of the vessel runs from the point at which it enters the region to a point just behind the angle of the mouth, and from there it ascends along the side of the nose to the medial side of the eye.

In the lower part of the face the artery rests on the mandible and is covered only by the skin, a little fat and the risorius muscle. It is therefore conveniently situated for the anæsthetist when he wishes to examine the pulse.

Leaving the mandible, the artery ascends on the surface of the buccinator and is crossed by the zygomaticus major, but in the interval between the latter muscle and the risorius it is covered only by skin and superficial fascia. In this situation its pulsations can readily be felt through the mucous membrane when the lower part of the nasolabial furrow is grasped between the finger and thumb.

In the upper part of the face the vessel is usually placed more deeply. At first under cover of, though often superficial to, the levator labii superioris, it ends in the substance of the levator labii superioris alæque nasi by anastomosing with the nasal branch of the ophthalmic artery.

Branches. Superior and *Inferior Labial* arteries arise from the facial artery and run medially in the upper and lower lips. They run in the submucous tissue about $\frac{1}{4}$ inch from the mucocutaneous junction, and their pulsations can easily be felt. Each anastomoses with its fellow of the opposite side.

The (**Anterior**) **Facial Vein** is formed near the medial angle of the eye by the union of the supra-orbital and supratrochlear veins. As these veins correspond to branches of the ophthalmic artery, it is not surprising to find that at its commencement *the facial vein communicates with the superior ophthalmic vein.* It takes an almost straight course downwards and backwards to the lower part of the anterior border of the masseter muscle, and so is placed behind the facial artery. It receives tributaries which correspond to the branches of the artery, and it also receives a *deep facial vein*, by which it establishes a connexion with the pterygoid venous plexus.

At the lower border of the mandible it crosses superficial to the submandibular gland and is joined by the anterior ramus of the retromandibular (posterior facial) vein.

The facial vein communicates with the cavernous sinus, through the superior ophthalmic vein and through the deep facial with the pterygoid plexus (p. 264).

The **Superficial Temporal Artery** arises from the external carotid artery opposite the neck of the mandible and under cover of the parotid gland. It emerges at the upper border of the gland, in company with the corresponding vein and the auriculotemporal nerve, and ascends across the root of the zygoma (pre-auricular point), where its pulsations can readily be felt. It runs upwards on the temporal fascia and divides into anterior and posterior branches to supply the scalp. The former anastomoses with its fellow and with the supra-orbital and supratrochlear branches of the ophthalmic artery (internal carotid). The latter anastomoses with its fellow and with the occipital and posterior auricular arteries.

Branches. In addition to numerous small branches which supply the structures in their immediate vicinity (parotid gland, auricle and facial muscles), the superficial temporal artery gives off a *transverse facial* branch, which runs forwards on the masseter and, emerging at the anterior border of the parotid gland, is continued onwards above and parallel to the parotid duct. It anastomoses with branches of the facial artery.

The **Parotid Gland** occupies a deep hollow between the sternomastoid and the ramus of the lower jaw, but its superficial facial part extends beyond the limits of this area and overlaps the masseter.

It is surrounded by a connective tissue sheath, which is derived from the investing layer of the deep cervical fascia.

The *superficial* or lateral aspect of the gland is related to the skin, subcutaneous connective tissue, the branches of the great auricular nerve and the parotid lymph nodes.

Examine a subject in which the parotid has been completely removed, and explore the "bed" of the gland. The *posterior wall* of the hollow, and therefore the *postero-medial relations* of the gland, are formed by the mastoid process and the anterior border of the sternomastoid, the posterior belly of the digastric and the styloid process, with the stylohyoid attached. The styloid process can be felt readily in the floor of the hollow, and the portion of the gland which rests upon it is often termed the *pterygoid lobe.* The *upper boundary* is formed by the cartilaginous part of the external auditory meatus, a relationship which is sometimes of considerable practical importance. The anterior edge of the upper surface of the gland passes upwards behind the mandibular condyle and in front of the external auditory meatus. It is sometimes termed the *glenoid lobe* and it is closely related to the auriculo-temporal nerve.

The anterior part of the deep surface of the gland, or *antero-medial surface*, is moulded round the posterior border of the ramus of the mandible. It is in contact with the masseter, the tempero-mandibular ligament, the medial surface of the ramus and the medial pterygoid.

The *Parotid Duct* emerges from the facial process of the gland and runs forwards and slightly downwards across the masseter to its anterior border. There it turns medially through the suctorial pad of fat, pierces the buccinator muscle obliquely, and opens through the mucous membrane of the cheek opposite the second molar tooth of the upper jaw. The openings through which the duct passes in the mucous membrane and the buccinator muscle are not placed opposite each other, so that a valve-like arrangement is provided which may prevent inflation of the duct in violent blowing.

At the point where it crosses the anterior border of the masseter, the duct can be easily felt through the skin in the living subject, provided that the masseter is thrown into contraction by clenching the teeth.

Frequently a portion of the superficial part is detached from the rest of the gland and lies immediately above the duct. It is termed the *accessory parotid.* It occasionally happens in "mumps," which is an acute infection of the parotid gland, that the accessory parotid is the only part of the gland to become involved.

Several structures penetrate the substance of the parotid gland. These include the external carotid artery, the retromandibular vein, and the facial nerve.

The external carotid at first lies between the postero-medial surface of the gland and the origin of the stylohyoid muscle. It then pierces the substance of the gland and emerges on the antero-medial surface, where, on a level with the neck of the mandible, it ends by dividing into the superficial temporal and the maxillary arteries. The retromandibular vein accompanies the artery, lying superficial to it.

The facial nerve, on emerging from the stylomastoid foramen, at once pierces the postero-medial aspect of the gland and then runs horizontally forwards in its substance, superficial to the external carotid artery and the retromandibular vein. Within the gland it divides into its terminal branches (p. 257).

The parotid gland is developed from a groove which appears on the inside of the cheek near the angle of the mouth. The groove becomes converted into a tube, and its blind end grows dorsally, its cells proliferating to form the gland.

The *Parotid Lymph Nodes* lie partly superficial to and partly within the salivary gland. They drain the auricle (lateral aspect), the side of the scalp, the external auditory meatus, the tympanic cavity, the parotid gland, the upper part of the cheek, part of both eyelids and the root of the nose.

THE TEMPORAL AND INFRATEMPORAL REGIONS

The muscles of mastication include the Masseter, the Temporal, the Lateral and Medial Pterygoid, the Mylohyoid, and the Anterior Belly of the Digastric. They are all supplied by the mandibular branch of the trigeminal nerve.

The **Masseter** covers nearly the whole of the lateral surface of the ramus of the mandible. It has superficial and deep portions attached to the lower border and deep surface of the zygomatic arch. The deep fibres are practically vertical, while the others are directed obliquely downwards and backwards. The muscle is inserted into the whole of the lateral surface of the ramus, including the coronoid process but excluding the neck of the mandible, which is hidden by the parotid gland.

Its *Nerve Supply* is derived from the masseteric branch of the mandibular nerve, which reaches the deep surface of the muscle by passing through the mandibular notch.

Action. The masseter is a powerful elevator of the jaw in biting and chewing.

The **Temporal Fascia** is a strong aponeurotic layer which covers the upper four-fifths of the temporal muscle. It is attached, above, to the superior temporal line on the side of the skull. Below, the fascia splits into two layers, which are attached to the lateral and medial margins of the upper border of the zygoma, and a small amount of fat and some small blood vessels occupy the interval. That the fascia is denser below than it is above can be demonstrated readily by clenching the teeth; the contraction of the underlying temporal muscle can easily be felt along the temporal line, but less easily immediately above the zygoma, where it is also becoming tendinous.

The **Temporalis** arises from the whole of the temporal fossa (frontal, parietal, squamous temporal and greater wing of sphenoid) down to the infratemporal crest of the greater wing of the sphenoid, and its fibres converge on the gap between the zygoma and the side of the skull. They pass at first deep to the arch and then to the masseter, to be inserted into the margins and deep surface of the coronoid process. The anterior fibres descend beyond the coronoid process to reach the anterior border of the ramus.

A full view of the muscle can be obtained only when the temporal fascia is removed and the zygoma is divided and turned downwards, together with the masseter muscle.

The *Nerve Supply* is derived from the deep temporal branches of the mandibular nerve.

Action. The temporalis is a powerful elevator of the mandible. The fibres which arise from the posterior part of the temporal fossa run horizontally forwards before they turn downwards to reach the coronoid process. These fibres act as retractors of the mandible.

The pterygoid muscles lie deeper, and they are almost completely hidden by the temporalis and the ramus of the mandible. Only a small part of the lateral pterygoid can be seen through the mandibular notch unless the detached coronoid process and temporal muscle are turned upwards and a large piece of the ramus taken away.

The **Lateral Pterygoid** arises by (1) an upper part from the infratemporal surface of the greater wing of the sphenoid; and (2) a lower part from the lateral surface of the lateral pterygoid plate. There is scarcely any interval between the two parts and the fibres run backwards and laterally, converging to be inserted into a small depression on the front of the neck of the mandible and the anterior border of the articular disc of the temperomandibular joint.

Its *Nerve Supply* is from the mandibular nerve.

Action. In considering the action of this muscle (which, of course, cannot be palpated in life), it must be remembered that, in the movement of opening the mouth, the mandibular condyle does not merely rotate in its articular fossa, but passes forwards on to the articular eminence, and this movement cannot be effected without a downward movement of the condyle as well. The lower fibres of the lower head of the lateral pterygoid have to ascend to reach their insertion, and they are responsible for the latter movement. The lateral pterygoids, therefore, take part in depressing the mandible and so opening the mouth. When the lateral and medial pterygoids of both sides contract the mandible is protruded. Lastly, when the two pterygoid muscles of one side act together, the condyle of that side is drawn forwards and at the same time rotated, so that the mandible as a whole is protruded to the opposite side. This constitutes the lateral chewing movement.

Both the maxillary artery and the mandibular nerve, with its terminal branches, are closely related to the lateral pterygoid muscle. The artery crosses the lower head obliquely; it may be either superficial or deep to it. The nerve, as it emerges from the foramen ovale, lies deep to the upper part of the muscle, a relationship which can easily be confirmed by reference to a skull. Its terminal branches emerge along the upper border of the upper head, between the two heads, and at the lower border of the lower head.

The **Medial Pterygoid** is placed, for the most part, on a somewhat deeper plane. It possesses (1) a superficial head, which arises from the tuberosity of the maxilla and the bone adjoining, and runs downwards and backwards on the surface of the lower part of the lower head of the lateral pterygoid muscle; and (2) a deep part, which arises from the medial surface of the lateral pterygoid plate. The fibres run downwards, backwards and laterally, and the deep head emerges at the lower border of the lateral pterygoid. The muscle is inserted into a roughened area on the deep surface of the angle of the mandible.

Its *Nerve Supply* is derived from the main trunk of the mandibular nerve.

Action. The medial pterygoid assists the temporal and masseter muscles to elevate the mandible. Working in association with the lateral pterygoid of the same side, it rotates the mandible so that it is protruded to the opposite side. All four pterygoids working together protrude the mandible.

The **Maxillary Artery** arises from the external carotid opposite to the neck of the mandible under cover of the parotid gland. Running forwards deep to the neck of the bone and superficial to the sphenomandibular ligament, it reaches the lower border of the lateral pterygoid muscle. In the next part of its course the vessel runs forwards, with an upward inclination, either between the lateral pterygoid and the temporal muscle, or deep to the lateral pterygoid. In the former event it disappears by passing between the two heads of the lateral pterygoid to gain the pterygopalatine fossa. In the latter event it crosses the lingual and the inferior dental nerves before it reaches the fossa.

Branches. (*a*) The *Inferior Dental Artery* runs downwards behind the nerve of the same name, between the sphenomandibular ligament and the mandible. It gives off a *mylohyoid branch*, and then enters the mandibular foramen to supply the teeth of the lower jaw. Its terminal branch appears on the face in company with the mental nerve.

(*b*) The **Middle Meningeal Artery** arises from the upper border of the maxillary and runs upwards and medially deep to the lateral pterygoid. As it ascends to reach the *foramen spinosum* it lies postero-lateral to the mandibular nerve and is embraced by the two roots of the auriculotemporal nerve. The intracranial course of this vessel and its surgically important relationship to the motor cortex are described on p. 368.

(*c*) The *Accessory Meningeal Artery* has a similar course, and may be a branch of the foregoing vessel. It enters the skull through the foramen ovale in company with the mandibular nerve.

(*d*) Muscular branches supply all the neighbouring muscles.

(*e*) Numerous small branches arise from the terminal part of the vessel in the pterygopalatine fossa, and are associated with the infra-orbital nerve and the branches of the sphenopalatine ganglion.

The **Pterygoid Venous Plexus** forms a rich vascular network around the lateral pterygoid muscle. Into this plexus flow veins which correspond to the branches of the maxillary artery, and from its posterior end the maxillary vein passes backwards to unite with the superficial temporal vein and so form the retromandibular vein.

The plexus communicates (1) with the *inferior ophthalmic veins* through the inferior orbital fissure; (2) with the *cavernous sinus* through the foramen ovale; and (3) with the *facial* through the deep facial vein (p. 259).

The **Mandibular Division of the Trigeminal Nerve** leaves the skull through the *foramen ovale* in the greater wing of the sphenoid. It differs from the other two divisions in being a *mixed* nerve, for it carries with it the whole of the *motor root* of the trigeminal nerve. As it leaves the skull it is covered by the lateral pterygoid and lies on the surface of the tensor veli palatini (palati), which separates the nerve from the pharyngotympanic tube and the nasal pharynx. The middle meningeal artery lies behind and to the lateral side. Almost at once the nerve breaks up into a small anterior and a large posterior division, so that its extracranial course is very short. It lies at a depth of 4 cm. from the surface of the face. The mandibular nerve is the principal nerve to the mandibular arch in the embryo.

The *Nerve to the Medial Pterygoid* arises from the main trunk and at its origin is close to the *otic ganglion* (p. 266).

The *Anterior Division* gives off the nerve to the lateral pterygoid, the masseteric and the deep temporal branches. The latter appear at the upper border of the lateral pterygoid and run upwards on the bone on the deep surface of the temporal muscle.

The *Buccal Nerve* passes downwards between the two heads of the lateral pterygoid and is the only branch which follows this route. It then very commonly pierces the anterior part of the temporal muscle, and, traversing the suctorial pad of fat, sends branches outwards *to the skin of the face*, and inwards *to the mucous membrane of the cheek.*

The *Posterior Division* gives origin to three large branches:—

1. The **Lingual Nerve** runs downwards deep to the lateral and on the surface of the medial pterygoid muscle. It appears at the lower border of the lateral pterygoid in front of the inferior dental nerve. Running downwards and forwards, it leaves the lower border of the medial pterygoid and comes to lie on the styloglossus under the mucous membrane on the medial side of the gum opposite the third lower molar tooth. In this situation it is closely related to the mandible, and it lies above the posterior end of the mylohyoid line. It then passes on to the lateral surface of the hyoglossus (p. 269), and is ultimately distributed to the mucous membrane of the *anterior part of the tongue* and the floor of the mouth.

2. The **Inferior Alveolar (Dental) Nerve** also runs downwards deep to the lateral pterygoid, but superficial to the sphenomandibular ligament. Near the mandibular foramen it gives off a *mylohyoid branch*, and then enters the mandibular canal to supply the *lower teeth* and to emerge through the mental foramen as the mental nerve (p. 254).

The *Mylohyoid Branch* runs downwards and forwards between the ramus and the medial pterygoid and, reaching the posterior edge of the mylohyoid, passes superficial to that muscle. It ends by supplying the *mylohyoid* and the anterior belly of the *digastric* muscle.

3. The **Auriculotemporal Nerve** has usually two roots of origin, which run backwards, one on each side of the middle meningeal artery, and unite to form a single trunk. The nerve passes between the neck of the mandible and the sphenomandibular ligament, above the maxillary artery. It then turns upwards behind the condyle and appears at the upper border of the parotid gland in company with the superficial temporal vessels. Its *auricular branch* supplies (1) the skin of the tragus and (2) the modified skin which lines the external auditory meatus and covers the outer surface of the tympanic membrane. The *temporal branch* supplies the skin of the scalp behind the areas supplied by the zygomaticotemporal and the supra-orbital nerves, but it does not extend upwards so high as the vertex.

The *Otic Ganglion* is a small *parasympathetic* ganglion which lies immediately below the skull, between the mandibular nerve and the tensor veli palatini. It receives preganglionic fibres from the glossopharyngeal through the lesser superficial petrosal nerve. These fibres are relayed in the ganglion and leave it as postganglionic fibres in branches which communicate with the auriculotemporal nerve. They are thus conveyed to the parotid gland and provide it with secretomotor fibres.

Postganglionic *sympathetic* fibres from the plexus on the middle meningeal artery pass *uninterruptedly* through the ganglion into the auriculotemporal nerve to supply the blood vessels of the parotid gland. The nerves of supply to the tensor veli palatini and the tensor tympani arise from the mandibular nerve or its medial pterygoid branch and traverse the ganglion on their way.

The **Chorda Tympani** is a small nerve which leaves the facial nerve in the temporal bone (p. 373), traverses the tympanic cavity on the inner surface of the tympanic membrane, and runs through a small canal in the petrotympanic fissure. It then runs downwards and forwards, deep to the middle meningeal artery, and joins the lingual nerve, by which its fibres are ultimately carried to the submandibular ganglion and the mucous membrane of the anterior part of the tongue. It conveys the special sense of taste for this part of the tongue, and when the fibres are traced centrally they are found to join the facial nerve in the temporal bone (p. 373). They leave the nerve at its ganglion and run in its sensory root and ultimately end by arborising round cells in the upper end of the nucleus solitarius. The taste fibres from the posterior part of the tongue travel in the glossopharyngeal nerve and reach the lower part of the same nucleus (p. 318).

The **Temporomandibular Joint** is a synovial joint, the cavity of which is divided into upper and lower parts by an *articular disc.*

The *Capsular ligament* is thin and lax except on its lateral aspect, where it is considerably strengthened by the lateral (*temporomandibular*) *ligament.* The fibres of this run downwards and backwards from the posterior part of the zygoma to the posterior border of the neck of the mandible. The lateral ligament is covered by the upper part of the parotid gland, and is related to the superficial temporal vessels and the auriculotemporal nerve.

The articular disc is attached circumferentially to the capsular ligament, except in front, where it receives part of the insertion of the lateral pterygoid muscle.

The joint is separated from the tympanic plate behind by the small glenoid lobe of the parotid gland.

Save when the disc is incomplete, non-articular surfaces in the two joint cavities are lined by separate synovial membranes. Owing to the greater size of the articular fossa of the temporal bone, the upper synovial cavity is the more extensive of the two.

Movements. When the mouth is opened widely the articular disc moves forwards on to the articular eminence, but at the same time the condyle rotates forwards on the lower surface of the cartilage, and when the mouth is closed the reverse movements take place. In protrusion of the jaw the condyle and the cartilage maintain the same position relative to each other, but the cartilage and the condyle together move forwards and downwards on the articular fossa. Lateral chewing movements are a combination of the above movements, modified by the fact that corresponding muscles of the two sides work alternately and not in unison.

The *Sphenomandibular Ligament* is usually described as an accessory ligament of the temporomandibular joint, and is often referred to as the "internal lateral ligament." It is in fact a vestigial structure, representing the remains of the upper part of Meckel's cartilage. It must be clearly understood that the ligament is on a deeper plane than the joint and that it is quite distinct from the medial part of the capsule. Above, it is attached to the spine of the sphenoid, and it forms a thin, flattened band as it descends to the margins of the mandibular foramen. It is crossed by the auriculotemporal nerve and the maxillary artery above, and the inferior dental vessels and nerve run downwards on its surface below. Just above the lingula it is pierced by the mylohyoid vessels and nerve.

THE SUBMANDIBULAR REGION

The submandibular gland occupies almost the whole submandibular region, and it is not until it has been displaced that a good view of the muscles, etc., can be obtained.

The **Mylohyoid** arises from the whole length of the mylohyoid line of the mandible, which extends from the region of the last molar tooth to the lower border of the genial tubercle in the median plane. The fibres run medially and forwards and slightly downwards. The posterior fibres are inserted into the body of the hyoid bone, but the anterior fibres reach the median plane between the symphysis menti and the hyoid bone, and there form a median raphe.

The *Nerve Supply* is derived from the mandibular nerve through the mylohyoid branch of the inferior dental nerve.

Action. The two mylohyoids form a muscular floor for the mouth, and when they contract they elevate the hyoid bone and with it the root of the tongue. If, however, the hyoid bone is fixed by the depressor muscles, the mylohyoids act on the mandible, and by depressing it they open the mouth.

The mylohyoid muscle is the key to the submandibular region, and its relations should be considered carefully. The muscle possesses a free posterior border, stretching from the posterior end of the mylohyoid line to the lateral extremity of the body of the hyoid bone. This border is covered to a large extent by the submandibular gland, and it is crossed, near its upper end, by the mylohyoid vessels and nerve, and near its lower end by the common tendon of the digastric. The hyoglossus muscle, with the hypoglossal nerve on its surface, disappears under this border at its lower end, while the styloglossus runs forwards deep to its upper end.

The superficial, or inferior, surface of the mylohyoid muscle forms the floor of the submental triangle and is covered partly by the anterior belly of the digastric. Behind this it is closely related to the submandibular gland.

The deep, or superior, surface of the muscle is related to the geniohyoid, the genioglossus and the sublingual gland in front and to the hyoglossus, and the numerous structures which lie on it, behind.

The **Submandibular Gland** is a large salivary gland, which lies partly under the body of the mandible and partly under cover of the investing layer of the deep cervical fascia. The deeper portion of its posterior end passes forwards under the posterior border of the mylohyoid muscle and is known as the *deep part* of the gland. It will be considered later (p. 271).

The *Superficial Part* of the gland is in contact, *laterally*, with the submandibular fossa on the inner surface of the body of the mandible. *Infero-laterally* it is covered by the investing layer of the deep cervical fascia and crossed by the anterior facial vein. Its *deep surface* rests on the anterior belly of the digastric, the mylohyoid muscle, the common tendon of the digastric and the stylohyoid.

The *Submandibular Lymph Nodes* lie mainly between the salivary gland and the deep fascia. They receive *afferents* from (1) the submandibular salivary gland; (2) the sublingual gland; (3) the submental lymph nodes; (4) *most of the anterior part of the tongue, excluding the tip* (p. 287); (5) the upper lip and maxillary gum, the nose and anterior part of the cheek, and those portions of the lower lip and mandibular gum which do not drain into the submental lymph nodes (p. 241). Their *efferents* pass to the upper deep cervical lymph nodes.

The submandibular gland develops as a groove in the alveolo-lingual sulcus in the floor of the mouth. The groove becomes converted into the duct, which proliferates at its blind end to form the gland.

The **Facial Artery** arises from the external carotid a little above the greater cornu of the hyoid bone, and runs upwards, deep to the posterior belly of the digastric and the stylohyoid muscle. It then comes into relation with the posterior part of the submandibular gland and ascends in a groove on its medial surface. In this way the artery rises to a level above the lower border of the jaw and may come into relation with the styloglossus as that muscle crosses the lateral aspect of the tonsil (p. 293). It curves forwards and downwards, grooving the lateral aspect of the gland, to reach the lower border of the mandible at the anterior margin of the masseter muscle. There it turns upwards into the face (p. 258).

When the submandibular gland is removed the artery can be replaced—provided it has not been divided—and it will then be seen to form an upward loop very similar to the loop of the lingual artery.

Before it reaches the submandibular gland, the facial artery gives off tonsillar and palatine branches, and subsequently it supplies branches to the gland and the adjoining muscles.

The **Hyoglossus** arises from the upper border of the body and greater cornu of the hyoid bone, and it runs upwards, deep to the mylohyoid, to reach the side of the tongue, where it intermingles with the horizontal fibres of the styloglossus.

It receives its nerve supply, *like all the other muscles of the tongue, from the hypoglossal nerve.*

Action. The two hyoglossi depress the tongue against the floor of the mouth.

The relations of the hyoglossus are important. It possesses a free anterior and a free posterior border. Along the latter the glossopharyngeal nerve, the stylohyoid ligament and the lingual artery disappear as they pass forwards, and the middle constrictor emerges. Along the anterior border the rapidly deepening genioglossus disappears from view, and the lingual artery emerges.

The lateral, or superficial, aspect of the hyoglossus muscle is related to the lingual nerve above, and to the hypoglossal nerve below, while the deep part of the submandibular gland, from which the submandibular duct emerges, occupies an intermediate position. Above the commencement of the duct, the submandibular ganglion is suspended from the lingual nerve.

The deep, or medial, surface of the muscle is related to the genioglossus in front, and to the middle constrictor of the pharynx behind. The lingual artery intervenes between them, as it runs forwards above the greater cornu of the hyoid bone.

The **Styloglossus** arises from the tip of the styloid process and runs forwards and downwards at first on the surface of the stylopharyngeus, and then on the lateral aspect of the superior constrictor of the pharynx, which separates it from the tonsil. At the lower border of the superior constrictor the styloglossus reaches the side of the tongue and intermingles with the vertical fibres of the hyoglossus.

Action. The two styloglossi, working together, retract the tongue.

The **Lingual Nerve** has already been described in the upper part of its course. Opposite the last molar tooth it comes into relation with the inner surface of the mandible above the posterior end of the mylohyoid line. It then runs downwards and forwards on the styloglossus and the upper part of the hyoglossus muscles. In this part of its course it lies immediately above the deep part of the submandibular gland and is connected to the *submandibular ganglion.* At the anterior border of the hyoglossus the nerve crosses superficial to the submandibular duct, and both structures disappear under cover of the sublingual gland, lying on the genioglossus muscle. Finally it enters the substance of the tongue.

Branches. 1. The *Lingual Nerve* distributes its terminal branches to the mucous membrane of the anterior part of the tongue and to the mucous membrane of the corresponding part of the floor of the mouth and of the gums. As it traverses the submandibular region the nerve contains ordinary sensory fibres and special taste fibres, but, as has been already described, the latter leave the lingual in the infratemporal region and travel *via* the chorda tympani to the facial nerve and its sensory root (p. 373).

2. Communicating branches connect the nerve (*a*) to the hypoglossal nerve, and (*b*) to the submandibular ganglion.

The *Submandibular Ganglion* is a small *parasympathetic* ganglion which lies on the hyoglossus muscle at the upper border of the deep part of the submandibular gland. It is connected to the lingual nerve, which lies above it, by two communicating branches. The first of these conveys *preganglionic* fibres from the chorda tympani (facial nerve) and these, after being relayed in the ganglion, are distributed as *postganglionic secretomotor fibres* to the submandibular and sublingual glands. Some of the sensory fibres from the anterior part of the tongue travel in the second branch to the ganglion, through which they pass *without relay*, and return in the first branch to the lingual nerve. Postganglionic sympathetic fibres from the plexus on the facial artery traverse the ganglion and then supply the blood vessels of the two salivary glands.

The **Deep Part of the Submandibular Gland** lies on the upper part of the hyoglossus muscle near its posterior border, and is placed under cover of the mylohyoid muscle. Above, it is related to the lingual nerve and the submandibular ganglion. Below, it is related to the hypoglossal nerve.

The *Submandibular Duct* emerges from the anterior extremity of the deep part of the gland and runs forward on the hyoglossus, deep to the mylohyoid muscle. At the anterior border of the hyoglossus the duct is crossed by the lingual nerve, and disappears under cover of the sublingual gland. It opens through the mucous membrane of the floor of the mouth on the summit of a small papilla situated close to the frenulum of the tongue.

The **Hypoglossal Nerve** (p. 234) passes forwards on the surface of the hyoglossus just above the greater cornu of the hyoid bone, in company with a *vena comitans*. Its terminal branches turn upwards along the anterior border of the muscle to reach the genioglossus and the intrinsic muscles of the tongue. In this part of its course the nerve supplies the styloglossus, the hyoglossus, the geniohyoid (C. 1, p. 234), the genioglossus and the intrinsic muscles of the tongue, and it communicates with the lingual nerve.

The **Geniohyoid** is a short strap-like muscle which arises from the lower part of the genial tubercles, and is inserted into the body of the hyoid bone under cover of the mylohyoid. Its medial border is closely related to the corresponding muscle of the opposite side, and its deep surface is applied to the lower fibres of the genioglossus.

Its *Nerve Supply* is directly from the hypoglossal nerve, but is ultimately derived from C. 1.

Action. The geniohyoid assists the mylohyoid (1) to elevate the hyoid bone, and (2) to depress the mandible (p. 268).

The **Genioglossus** arises from the upper of the genial tubercles and extends backwards, widening out in a fan-shaped manner. The upper fibres pass to the tip of the tongue, and the others to the dorsum. A few of the lowest fibres reach the body of the hyoid bone.

Action. The lower fibres protrude the tongue from the mouth, the intermediate fibres depress the tongue, while the upper fibres retract the tip.

The **Sublingual Gland** is the smallest of the three salivary glands. Its anterior end is relatively wide, but, as it is traced backwards the gland diminishes in size, its lower border accommodating itself to the obliquity of the mylohyoid line. It is placed under the mucous membrane of the floor of the mouth, with its long axis directed forwards and medially below the *plica sublingualis*, so that its anterior end nearly reaches the median plane. In front, and to its lateral side, the gland is related to the sublingual fossa on the inner surface of the mandible. To its medial side the gland rests on the genioglossus muscle and is related to the lingual nerve and the submandibular duct, whilst inferiorly it is supported by the mylohyoid.

The *Ducts* of the sublingual gland are numerous (8–20). They may open into the submandibular duct or directly into the floor of the mouth along the plica sublingualis.

The **Lingual Artery,** after making its characteristic loop (p. 233), passes under hyoglossus and runs forwards above the greater cornu of the hyoid bone. It lies at first on the middle constrictor of the pharynx, and subsequently on the genioglossus. Here it gives off two or more *dorsal lingual* arteries, which ascend into the substance of the tongue. At the anterior border of the hyoglossus the artery turns upwards, supplies the sublingual gland, and ends as the *profunda* artery, which runs forwards in the lower part of the tongue to its tip.

The *Veins* of the tongue form *venæ comitantes*, which accompany the lingual artery, and a *vena comitans*, which runs with the hypoglossal nerve. They are joined by tributaries which correspond to the branches of the artery, and they terminate by joining either the facial or the internal jugular vein.

The **Glossopharyngeal Nerve** winds round the stylopharyngeus muscle, and divides into a pharyngeal and a lingual branch. The latter enters the tongue below the styloglossus at the posterior border of the hyoglossus, and *supplies the mucous membrane of the* *posterior part of the tongue* both with ordinary sensibility and with the special sense of taste, *extending forwards to include the area of the vallate papillæ.* In addition, this nerve supplies the mucous membrane over the tonsil, the soft palate and the front of the epiglottis.

The difference in the nerve supply of the two parts of the tongue can be demonstrated easily in the living subject. So long as a spatula, introduced into the mouth, is in contact with the anterior two-thirds of the tongue, no unpleasant sensation is aroused. As soon, however, as it is carried backwards so as to come into contact with the glossopharyngeal area the sensation is very disagreeable and the pharyngeal reflex is induced. For a similar reason the mucous membrane of the cheek, the gums, and of the hard palate (supplied by the trigeminal nerve) differs in its response to stimulation from the mucous membrane over the tonsil and the soft palate (glosso-pharyngeal nerve).

THE ORBIT AND MIDDLE CRANIAL FOSSA

Before revising the structures contained in the orbit, examine the walls of the bony orbit and the openings which traverse them (p. 392).

The **Muscles of the Orbit** include the four *recti* (superior, inferior, medial and lateral), two *obliques* (superior and inferior), and the *levator palpebræ superioris.* The latter acts on the upper eyelid, as indicated by its name, while all the others act on the eyeball, rotating it so as to make the eye look upwards, downwards, laterally or medially, or any combination of these.

In the posterior part of the orbit the four recti arise from a *common annular tendon*, which surrounds the optic foramen and crosses the medial end of the superior orbital fissure. The superior rectus arises from the upper part of the ring, the medial rectus from its medial part, and the inferior rectus from its lower part, while the superior oblique arises just above the medial rectus. The lateral rectus arises by two heads, the lower adjoining the inferior rectus and the upper springing from the part of the ring which crosses the superior orbital fissure.

As these muscles pass forwards through the orbit they become wider and diverge from one another, so as to form a sort of muscular cone around the optic nerve and the posterior half of the eyeball. Owing to the manner of origin of the lateral rectus, those structures which enter the orbit through the lower end of the superior orbital fissure pass between its two heads and find themselves within the muscular cone, whereas the structures entering through the upper part of the same fissure lie outside it.

The insertions of the recti are uncomplicated. Each tendon pierces the fascial sheath of the eyeball (p. 278) opposite its coronal equator, and is inserted into the sclera a little in front of that line. The actions of the lateral and medial recti are as uncomplicated as their insertions. The former rotates the eyeball so as to make the pupil look laterally; the latter produces rotation in the opposite direction. The actions of the superior and inferior recti are not so simple. In these cases the line of pull of the muscle is medial to the vertical axis of the eyeball, and as a result contraction of the superior rectus does not produce a pure upward rotation, but a combination of upward and medial rotation. Similarly, the inferior rectus produces a combination of downward and medial rotation.

The *Superior Oblique* runs forwards above the medial rectus in the angle between the roof and the medial wall, and ends in a tendon, which passes through a fibrocartilaginous sling attached to the antero-medial part of the orbital roof. Having passed through the sling, the tendon runs backwards and laterally to be inserted into the sclera immediately *behind* the coronal equator of the eyeball. The *action* of this muscle is to rotate the eyeball so as to make the pupil look downwards, but in addition it produces a certain amount of lateral rotation, since the line of pull of the tendon passes medial to the vertical axis.

It is now clear that a pure downward rotation of the eyeball can be produced only when the inferior rectus and the superior oblique work in association with each other.

The *Inferior Oblique* arises from the antero-medial part of the floor of the orbit, and passes backwards and laterally below the eyeball. It is inserted into the sclera immediately *behind* the equator, and its line of pull passes behind and to the medial side of the vertical axis. As a result the inferior oblique rotates the eyeball so as to make the pupil look upwards and laterally. Consequently, *when it is desired to look straight upwards, the inferior oblique and the superior rectus must work together.*

The *Levator Palpebræ Superioris* arises near the apex of the orbit in front of the superior rectus, and passes forwards on the upper surface of that muscle. Its broad, thin tendon is inserted (1) partly into the skin of the upper eyelid, (2) partly into the front of the tarsus of the upper eyelid, and (3) partly, by means of a fine sheet of unstriped muscle fibres, into the upper border of the tarsus. In addition, the muscle gains an indirect attachment to the superior fornix of the conjunctiva through the medium of the fascial sheath.

The *Nerve Supply* of these muscles is derived from the third, fourth and sixth cranial nerves. Of these, the abducens, or sixth, is restricted to the supply of the lateral rectus, and the trochlear, or fourth, to the superior oblique. The other three recti, the inferior oblique and the levator palpebræ superioris are all supplied by the oculomotor or third nerve.

The **Lacrimal Nerve** arises from the ophthalmic division of the trigeminal in the cavernous sinus, and enters the orbit through the upper part of the superior orbital fissure. It runs forwards along the upper border of the lateral rectus, passes deep to the lacrimal gland, to which it gives some branches (p. 278), and ends in the lateral part of the upper eyelid. It is a very small nerve.

The **Frontal Nerve** arises from the ophthalmic division of the trigeminal in the cavernous sinus, and enters the orbit in company with the lacrimal nerve. It runs forwards on the upper surface of the levator palpebræ superioris, soon dividing into a small supra-trochlear branch and a large supra-orbital branch, which have already been described (p. 253).

The **Trochlear (Fourth Cranial) Nerve,** enters the orbit in company with the two foregoing nerves. It runs forwards and medially to supply the superior oblique, the upper border of which it pierces close to the origin of the muscle.

These three nerves enter the orbit above the upper head of the lateral rectus. Consequently they remain outside the muscular cone referred to on p. 274.

The **Abducent (Sixth Cranial) Nerve,** enters the orbit from the cavernous sinus through the lower part of the superior orbital fissure, *i.e.*, between the two heads of the lateral rectus. It therefore lies within the muscular capsule, and it runs forwards on the ocular surface of the lateral rectus muscle and sinks into its substance.

The **Nasociliary Nerve** arises from the ophthalmic division of the trigeminal in the cavernous sinus, and enters the orbit through the lower part of the superior orbital fissure and in close relationship with the third and sixth nerves and the ophthalmic veins. It runs forwards and medially, inside the muscular capsule, and crosses above the optic nerve, parallel to and usually behind the ophthalmic artery. Gaining the medial wall of the orbit, the nerve follows the interval between the superior oblique and the medial rectus, and finally ends by dividing into the infratrochlear nerve and the anterior ethmoidal.

Branches. 1. A *Ramus Communicans to the Ciliary Ganglion* arises from the nasociliary nerve as it enters the orbit and joins the ciliary ganglion (p. 277).

2. The *Long Ciliary Nerves*, two in number, run forwards medial to the optic nerve and pierce the sclera. They probably contain *sympathetic fibres* which join the ophthalmic nerve from the internal carotid plexus in the cavernous sinus. Running forwards in the perichoroidal space, they reach the iris and *supply the dilator pupillæ muscle.*

3. The *Infratrochlear Nerve* continues the course of the nasociliary nerve and, passing below the trochlea of the superior oblique, reaches the medial part of the upper eyelid and the adjoining part of the nose.

4. The *Anterior Ethmoidal Nerve* leaves the orbit through the anterior ethmoidal foramen, and appears on the cribriform plate of the ethmoid in the floor of the anterior cranial fossa. It then turns downwards through the nasal slit and reaches the nasal cavity, where it supplies a small area of mucous membrane. Finally, passing between the lower border of the nasal bone and the upper lateral cartilage, it appears on the face, where it gives off external nasal branches to the skin of the nose (p. 284).

The **Ophthalmic Artery** arises from the internal carotid immediately after that vessel leaves the cavernous sinus, and it proceeds forwards through the optic foramen, lying below the optic nerve. In the orbit the artery makes a spiral turn round the lateral side of the nerve and, crossing above it, runs forwards parallel to the nasociliary nerve. Near the medial angle of the eye the ophthalmic artery ends by dividing into supra-orbital and supratrochlear branches.

Branches. 1. The *Arteria Centralis Retinæ* arises from the ophthalmic artery while it still lies below the optic nerve. It actually enters the nerve (p. 377) and runs in its substance to the optic disc, where it divides into branches to supply the retina. These branches can be seen and identified in the living eye by means of the ophthalmoscope. *They are end arteries.*

2. The *Ciliary Arteries* form a posterior and an anterior group. The former pierce the sclera around the optic nerve and ramify in the choroid coat. Two of them, however, known as the *long posterior ciliary arteries*, run forwards to the ciliary zone, where they form an anastomotic circle with the anterior ciliary arteries. The latter arise from muscular branches in the anterior part of the orbit and pierce the sclera near the corneoscleral junction. The arterial ring so formed supplies branches to the ciliary body and the iris. It can be seen through the conjunctiva in cases of inflammation of the ciliary body.

3. The supratrochlear and (4) the supra-orbital arteries leave the orbit in association with the supratrochlear and the supra-orbital nerves respectively. They ramify in the superficial tissues of the forehead, where they anastomose with branches of the superficial temporal artery (external carotid).

In addition, the ophthalmic artery supplies muscular and palpebral branches and a branch to the lacrimal gland.

The **Ophthalmic Veins** are two in number. The *superior* accompanies the artery and, at its origin, communicates freely with the commencement of the facial vein. The *inferior* lies below the optic nerve and communicates with the pterygoid plexus through the inferior orbital fissure. Usually both veins leave the orbit through the lower part of the superior orbital fissure, where they are closely related to the oculomotor, the abducent and the nasociliary nerves. They terminate by joining the anterior end of the cavernous sinus.

The **Oculomotor (Third Cranial) Nerve** enters the orbit from the cavernous sinus through the lower part of the superior orbital fissure. It at once divides into an *upper division*, which supplies the levator palpebræ superioris and the superior rectus, and a *lower division*, which supplies the medial and inferior recti and the inferior oblique. It is from the nerve to the last-named that the short motor root of the ciliary ganglion arises.

The **Optic Nerve** enters the orbit through the optic foramen and runs forwards and laterally to pierce the sclera at a point *medial* to the *posterior pole* of the eyeball. Its relationship to the nasociliary nerve, the ophthalmic artery and the ophthalmic veins has already been indicated. Together with these structures it is embedded in the orbital fat.

Traced backwards, the optic nerve enters the anterior cranial fossa and joins the corresponding anterolateral angle of the optic chiasma (p. 337). Within the orbit the nerve is surrounded by a triple sheath consisting of dura, arachnoid and pia mater, which carry with them a prolongation of the subarachnoid space. The nerve fibres are derived from the cells of the ganglionic layer of the retina and, as they pass to the optic disc, they form the stratum opticum or innermost layer of the retina. Developmentally (p. 378) the retina and the optic nerve are outlying parts of the brain and the nerve fibres, like those of the white matter of the cerebrum (p. 345), have *no neurolemmal sheaths*. They do not become myelinated until a few weeks after birth.

The *Ciliary Ganglion* is a parasympathetic ganglion which lies in the posterior part of the orbit, on the lateral side of the optic nerve.

It is very minute and is not easy to recognise in the orbital fat. It receives a communicating branch from the nasociliary nerve, a *motor root* from the oculomotor (nerve to the inferior oblique), and a *sympathetic root* from the cavernous plexus.

From its anterior border the *short ciliary nerves* arise. They pierce the sclera and eventually supply vasomotor branches to the blood vessels of the eyeball (sympathetic) and the *sphincter pupillæ and ciliary muscles* (*oculomotor—parasympathetic*). *Only the parasympathetic fibres are relayed in the ganglion.*

The **Bulbar Sheath (Fascia Bulbi)** forms an investment for the posterior five-sixths of the eyeball. *Anteriorly*, it blends with the sclera near the corneoscleral junction. *Posteriorly*, it blends with the sheath of the optic nerve. A small amount of loose areolar tissue and numerous lymph-spaces intervene between the sheath and the eyeball. At each side the fascial sheath is connected to the bony wall (zygomatic and lacrimal bones), and these connexions constitute the *check ligaments*, which some consider prevent excessive action of the lateral and medial recti. *Inferiorly*, the anterior part of the facial sheath is thickened to form the *suspensory ligament*, the extremities of which are attached to the bony walls of the orbit in the vicinity of the check ligaments.

The tendons of the ocular muscles must pierce the sheath before they can reach their insertions. As they do so, the sheath is carried backwards on the tendons, and, in the cases of the medial and lateral recti, is attached to the orbital wall, constituting "*check*" *ligaments.*

Owing to the attachments of the check and suspensory ligaments to the bony walls of the orbit, and to the connexion of the fascial sheath to the eyeball at the corneoscleral junction, the movements of the eyeball do not exceed what is strictly necessary. (N.B. It is more probable that these attachments help to ensure that the globe is *rotated* and not *displaced* by its muscles.)

The **Lacrimal Gland** lies in the anterior and upper part of the orbit. It is placed above the eyeball and to the medial side of the zygomatic process of the frontal bone. Its *palpebral process* is partially separated from the rest of the gland and projects into the upper eyelid above the conjunctiva.

Numerous small ducts open from the inferior surface of the gland into the upper and lateral part of the conjunctival sac.

The gland receives its secretomotor nerve supply from the sphenopalatine ganglion *via* the maxillary and zygomatic nerves and thence by a communicating branch to the lacrimal nerve.

The *puncta lacrimalia* and the *lacrimal canaliculi* have already been described (p. 252). The latter open into the *lacrimal sac*, which occupies the deep lacrimal groove in the anterior part of the medial wall of the orbit and is covered on its lateral aspect by the lacrimal fascia (p. 252). The *nasolacrimal duct* emerges from the lower end of the lacrimal sac and descends in a bony canal to open into the inferior meatus of the nose, under cover of the anterior part of the inferior nasal concha. *It is only half-an-inch in length.*

The **Cavernous Sinus** lies in the floor of the middle cranial fossa on the side of the body of the sphenoid. Like the other intracranial venous sinuses, its walls consist of a single layer of endothelium, supported by dura mater. The oculomotor and trochlear nerves, as well as the ophthalmic and maxillary divisions of the trigeminal, are interposed between the endothelial wall and the dura mater. These structures are described as lying in the lateral wall of the sinus. The internal carotid artery and the abducent nerve lie more definitely within the sinus.

The anterior end of the sinus lies immediately behind the superior orbital fissure and is joined by the ophthalmic veins. Posteriorly, the sinus ends opposite the dorsum sellæ of the sphenoid, where it gives origin to the superior and inferior petrosal sinuses, which carry off the blood to the transverse sinus and to the internal jugular vein, respectively. Medially, the sinus is related to the hypophysis cerebri, and both in front of, and behind, the stalk of the hypophysis the two cavernous sinuses communicate with each other through the intercavernous sinuses. Laterally and superiorly the sinus is related to the uncus (p. 345). *Inferiorly, it communicates with the pterygoid venous plexus, the connecting veins passing through the foramen ovale* and, when present, a small foramen near its anteromedial corner.

The **Oculomotor Nerve** runs forwards from the midbrain (p. 330) through the cisterna interpeduncularis, and pierces the arachnoid and the dura mater at the posterior end of the cavernous sinus. It then runs forwards in the upper part of the lateral wall of the sinus to the superior orbital fissure, and enters the orbit between the two heads of the lateral rectus muscle.

The **Trochlear Nerve** has a precisely similar course, lying slightly below and to the lateral side of the oculomotor. At the superior orbital fissure it enters the orbit above the muscles.

The **Internal Carotid Artery** enters the skull through the carotid canal in the petrous part of the temporal bone. The canal runs at first upwards and then forwards, and its upper end lies in the posterior wall of the foramen lacerum. When the internal carotid artery leaves its canal it traverses the upper portion of the foramen lacerum and then enters the lower and posterior part of the cavernous sinus. It runs forwards within the sinus, occupying the carotid groove on the lateral aspect of the body of the sphenoid. Opposite to the anterior clinoid process it bends sharply upwards and backwards, and pierces the dura mater in the roof of the cavernous sinus on the medial side of the process. Its subsequent history is described on p. 365.

The **Abducent Nerve** lies below and medial to the trochlear as it crosses the cisterna interpeduncularis. In this part of its course, it runs upwards and slightly forwards. It then bends forwards sharply as it pierces the lower part of the posterior wall of the sinus near the apex of the petrous part of the temporal bone. It lies at first to the lateral side of the internal carotid artery and to the medial side of the ophthalmic nerve, but as it approaches the superior orbital fissure the nerve lies below the artery. There it enters the orbit through the fissure and within the annular tendons.

The **Trigeminal Ganglion** is on the large sensory root of the trigeminal nerve and corresponds to the dorsal root ganglion of a spinal nerve. It lies on the apex of the petrous portion of the temporal bone in a small recess of the dura mater, which is termed the *cavum trigeminale*. This recess is placed under the dura mater of the floor of the middle cranial fossa, and extends upwards for a variable distance on the lateral wall of the cavernous sinus. Its cavity communicates with the posterior cranial fossa, through an opening which is placed below the attached margin of the tentorium cerebelli, and which is largely occupied by the roots of the trigeminal nerve. On its postero-medial aspect the ganglion is joined by the sensory root, and from its antero-lateral border the three divisions of the nerve arise. The much smaller *motor root* of the trigeminal lies below the ganglion and takes no part in its formation, but subsequently *joins the mandibular division* at the foramen ovale.

(A) The **Ophthalmic Nerve** runs forwards in the lower part of the lateral wall of the cavernous sinus (p. 279). On reaching the superior orbital fissure it divides into lacrimal, frontal and nasociliary branches, all of which pass through the fissure into the orbit, where they have already been examined (pp. 275, 276).

(B) The **Maxillary Nerve,** like the ophthalmic, is a purely sensory nerve. It runs forwards to the foramen rotundum, through which it passes to gain the pterygopalatine fossa. Having crossed the upper part of the fossa, the nerve next passes through the inferior orbital fissure and occupies the infra-orbital groove, and subsequently the infra-orbital canal, in the floor of the orbit.

As it lies in the pterygopalatine fossa, the maxillary nerve is connected by two short roots to the *pterygopalatine* (sphenopalatine) *ganglion*, which lies below it, surrounded by the terminal branches of the maxillary vessels. *This ganglion, like the ciliary, the otic and the submandibular ganglia, belongs to the parasympathetic system.* From it arise secretomotor fibres to the lacrimal gland (p. 278). In addition, the ganglion communicates with the carotid sympathetic plexus and with the facial nerve, through the nerve of the pterygoid canal, which probably conveys the secretomotor fibres. Sensory branches from the mucous membrane (1) of the nasal cavity, (2) the hard palate and (3) the soft palate *traverse the ganglion—but have no cell-station in it*—on their way to the maxillary nerve.

Before entering the orbit the maxillary nerve gives off two branches:—

1. The *Posterior Superior Alveolar Nerve* enters the posterior aspect of the maxilla, and ultimately supplies the three upper molar teeth and the adjoining area of the gum.

2. The *Zygomatic Nerve* enters the orbit through the inferior orbital fissure, and ascends on the lateral wall, where it passes into a canal in the zygomatic bone. There it divides into (*a*) *zygomaticotemporal*, and (*b*) *zygomaticofacial branches*, which are distributed to the skin of the face (p. 254).

As it lies in the infra-orbital groove, the nerve gives off the *middle superior dental nerve*, which runs downwards in a small bony canal in the lateral wall of the maxillary sinus, and supplies the two upper premolars and adjoining area of the gum.

As it lies in the infra-orbital canal, the nerve gives off the *anterior superior alveolar nerve*, which runs downwards in a minute bony canal to supply the upper canine and incisors. Thereafter the terminal branch, which is known as the *infra-orbital nerve*, supplies a *large area of skin on the face* and the mucous membrane of the upper lip and cheek (p. 256).

Summary of Distribution. 1. Through sphenopalatine ganglion:—

(*a*) Secretomotor to lacrimal gland (preganglionic fibres come from facial and *not* from trigeminal).
(*b*) Sensory to mucous membrane of nasal cavity.
(*c*) Sensory to mucous membrane of soft and hard palate and tonsil.
(*d*) Sensory to mucous membrane of pharyngeal roof.

These sensory branches traverse the ganglion but have no cell-station in it.

2. Directly:—
   (*a*) Teeth of maxilla.
   (*b*) Mucous membrane of upper gum, upper lip, and upper part of cheek.
   (*c*) Skin of lower eyelid, posterior part of nose, upper lip, cheek, zygomatic region, and lower and anterior part of temporal region.

(C) The **Mandibular Nerve** (p. 264) has a short intracranial course, and as it enters the foramen ovale it is joined by the small motor root of the trigeminal. It is, therefore, a mixed nerve.

Summary of Distribution. (*a*) Through otic ganglion:—
Secretomotor to parotid gland (*preganglionic fibres come from glossopharyngeal nerve*, p. 266).

(*b*) Through submandibular ganglion (*preganglionic fibres come from chorda tympani and* not *from trigeminal*):—
1. Secretomotor to submandibular gland.
2. Secretomotor to sublingual gland.

(*c*) Directly:—
1. Mucous membrane of anterior part of tongue, floor of mouth, lower gum, lower lip and lower part of cheek.
2. Teeth of mandible.
3. Skin over mandible (except over parotid gland and area below and in front of it), lining external auditory meatus and tympanic membrane, of tragus and side of head (behind supraorbital nerve and in front of occipital nerves).
4. Muscles of mastication.
5. Tensor tympani muscle.
6. Tensor veli palatini muscle.

THE PREVERTEBRAL REGION

The **Longus Capitis** has a precisely similar origin to the scalenus anterior (p. 246), but its fibres ascend, overlapping the longus cervicis and the rectus capitis anterior, to be inserted into the lower aspect of the basilar part of the occipital bone.

Its *Nerve Supply* is derived from the anterior primary rami of the upper four cervical nerves.

The trunk of the sympathetic and the internal carotid artery lie on the anterior surface of this muscle.

The **Longus Cervicis** consists of three parts all connected to one another: (*a*) The *Lower Oblique Portion* arises from the sides of the bodies of the upper two or three thoracic vertebræ, and runs upwards and laterally to be inserted into the anterior tubercles of the transverse processes of the fifth and sixth cervical vertebræ. (*b*) The *Upper Oblique Portion* arises from the anterior tubercles of the third, fourth and fifth cervical vertebræ, and runs upwards and medially to the anterior tubercle of the atlas. (*c*) The *Vertical Portion* lies medial to the oblique portions, and its lateral border is partially blended with them. It arises from the bodies of the upper thoracic and lower cervical vertebræ, and is inserted into the bodies of the upper cervical vertebræ.

It receives its *Nerve Supply* from the ventral rami of C. 3, 4, 5, 6, 7 and 8.

Action. Acting together, or separately, these muscles assist in producing flexion and rotation of the neck and (upper portion) rotation of the head.

The upper half of the muscle is overlapped by the longus capitis; the lower half is related anteriorly to the œsophagus and, on the left side, to the thoracic duct.

The **Rectus Capitis Anterior** is a smaller muscle, which extends from the front of the lateral mass of the atlas to the basilar part of the occipital bone. It lies under cover of the longus capitis.

The **Rectus Capitis Lateralis** does not belong to this group, but can be conveniently considered at this point. It extends from the upper surface of the transverse process of the atlas to the jugular process of the occipital bone.

The internal jugular vein lies on its anterior surface immediately after leaving the jugular foramen, and the anterior primary ramus of C. 1 appears at its medial border.

The **Cervical Spinal Nerves,** as they emerge from the intervertebral foramina, at once divide into ventral and dorsal rami. The latter pass backwards round the articular processes to reach the muscles of the back of the neck.

Each ventral ramus runs laterally behind the vertebral artery and in front of the posterior intertransverse muscle, emerging from behind the longus capitis above, and the scalenus anterior below (*i.e., from behind the muscles attached to the anterior tubercles of the transverse processes*).

The **Vertebral Artery** enters the foramen in the transverse process of the sixth cervical vertebra (p. 247) and ascends, passing successively through the foramina of the transverse processes of the upper six cervical vertebræ. As the transverse process of the atlas is much larger than that of the axis, the vertebral artery has to run laterally as well as upwards in its course from the second to the first cervical vertebra. Having pierced the transverse process of the atlas, it winds medially round the posterior aspect of the lateral mass and pierces the dura mater (p. 285). In this part of its course the artery can be seen only when the anterior intertransverse muscles have been removed. If a specimen is obtained in which this dissection has been carried out, the ventral rami of the cervical nerves will be seen as they run laterally behind the vessel.

The **Vertebral Joints in the Cervical Region.** The bodies of the lower five cervical vertebræ articulate, each with its neighbour, by means of a cartilaginous joint.

The cartilaginous joint involves the greater parts of the opposed surfaces of the vertebral bodies, which are connected to one another by intervertebral discs. This joint is supported by the anterior and posterior longitudinal ligaments (p. 128).

The vertebral arches of the lower five cervical vertebræ are connected, each to its neighbour, by (1) the articular processes; (2) the ligamenta flava; and (3) the ligamentum nuchæ.

1. The opposed articular processes form synovial joints of a plane type.

2. The *Ligamenta Flava*, which are composed of yellow elastic tissue, extend from the upper border of a lamina to the anterior surface and lower border of the lamina above. By virtue of their elasticity they may assist the extensor muscles of the neck.

3. The *Ligamentum Nuchæ* is continuous below with the supraspinous ligaments. It is triangular in shape, the apex being attached to the spine of the seventh cervical vertebra and the base to the external occipital crest. Its anterior border is attached to the cervical spines, while its posterior border is free and blends with the investing layer of the deep cervical fascia. It gives origin to the splenius, the rhomboid and trapezius muscles.

The joints of the atlas and axis with each other and with the skull do not conform exactly to the same type.

Atlanto-axial Joints. 1. The lateral masses of the atlas articulate with the superior articular facets of the axis by means of two simple synovial joints.

2. The anterior surface of the odontoid process of the axis articulates with the posterior aspect of the anterior arch of the atlas by means of a synovial joint, which is also simple in type. This joint, however, is greatly strengthened by the presence of an accessory ligament which spans the interval between the lateral masses, passing behind the odontoid process. This is termed the *transverse ligament of the atlas*. A small bursa intervenes between the ligament and the odontoid process.

The *Atlanto-occipital Joints* are simple synovial joints. They are formed by the occipital condyles on the one hand, and the upper surfaces of the lateral masses on the other. They support the weight of the head.

These joints are strengthened by the *anterior and posterior atlanto-occipital membranes.* The anterior membrane stretches between the upper border of the anterior arch of the atlas and the lower surface of the basilar part of the occipital bone, in front of the foramen magnum. It blends on each side with the capsule of the atlanto-occipital joint, and its central part, which reaches the anterior tubercle of the atlas, is definitely thickened.

The posterior atlanto-occipital membrane extends between the posterior arch of the atlas and the posterior border of the foramen magnum. It is deficient at each lateral extremity, and in this situation the vertebral artery passes under cover of the free lateral edge of the membrane to pierce the dura mater.

Although the axis does not normally articulate with the occipital bone, several ligaments pass between the two bones, and serve indirectly to support the atlanto-occipital and the atlanto-axial joints.

1. The *Membrana Tectoria* represents the upward continuation of the posterior longitudinal ligament. It is attached to the posterior surface of the body of the axis and runs upwards, behind the transverse ligament and the odontoid process, to be attached to the basilar part of the occipital bone just within the foramen magnum.

2. The *Cruciate Ligament* consists of the transverse ligament of the atlas together with a longitudinal band, which runs upwards to join it from the posterior surface of the body of the axis, and extends upwards to the anterior margin of the foramen magnum.

3. The *Apical Ligament* connects the apex of the odontoid process to the anterior margin of the foramen magnum, and is placed in front of the upper limb of the cruciate ligament.

4. The *Alar Ligaments*, two in number, extend between the flattened shoulders of the odontoid process and the medial sides of the occipital condyles. They possess considerable strength, and they limit both flexion and rotation of the head.

It must be remembered that when the head is rotated from side to side the atlas moves with the occipital bone, so that the joints involved in this movement are those between the atlas and the axis. Nodding movements of the head, on the other hand, involve the atlanto-occipital joints only.

THE MOUTH AND PHARYNX

The buccal cavity is subdivided into the *mouth proper*, which lies within the arch of the teeth, and the *vestibule*, which lies between the lips and cheeks on the one hand, and the gums and teeth on the other. When the teeth are clenched, the two communicate by means of a small interval situated behind the last molar tooth.

Posteriorly, the mouth opens into the pharynx through the isthmus of the fauces (*oropharyngeal isthmus*). The *roof* is formed by the hard palate in front, and the soft palate behind. When the mouth is closed the roof is in contact with the tongue, which occupies the floor. The mucous membrane of the palate receives its sensory nerve supply from the maxillary nerve. The anterior part of the hard palate is supplied by the nasopalatine (long sphenopalatine) nerve (p. 294), and the remainder by the greater palatine nerve, which ascends through the greater palatine foramen and canal (p. 393) to traverse the pterygopalatine ganglion and reach the maxillary nerve (p. 281).

The *Cheek*, which constitutes the outer wall of the vestibule, is lined with mucous membrane. Outside the mucous membrane lies the buccinator muscle (p. 257), which forms the fleshy stratum of the cheek. The superficial aspect of the muscle is covered by a dense layer of fascia, termed the *buccopharyngeal fascia*, which is continuous behind with the fascia on the outer surface of the superior constrictor.

The *Floor of the Mouth* is formed anteriorly by the reflection of the mucous membrane from the mandible to the under surface of the tongue. The *frenulum of the tongue* forms a ridge in the median plane, and is rendered prominent when, with the mouth open, the tip of the tongue is pressed against the hard palate. On each side of its lower end there is a small papilla, on the summit of which the duct of the submandibular gland opens. A ridge of mucous membrane runs laterally and backwards from the papilla. It is termed the *plica sublingualis* and it overlies the sublingual gland (p. 272).

The **Tongue** is a solid mass of muscle, covered by mucous membrane where it projects into the floor of the mouth and the anterior wall of the oral pharynx. At the junction of its anterior part with its posterior third or so is a V-shaped groove, the *sulcus terminalis*, the apex of which is directed backwards and coincides with a small blind pit, termed the *foramen cæcum*.

These two parts of the tongue are developed from different parts of the primitive pharynx, and differ from each other (1) in the structure of the covering epithelium, (2) in function, and (3) in sensory nerve-supply.

The presence of papillæ, which the student can readily examine in his own tongue with the aid of a concave mirror, is the characteristic feature of the mucous membrane of the anterior two-thirds of the tongue. These papillæ are of three types. (*a*) The *vallate papillæ* are ten or twelve in number, and lie immediately in front of the sulcus terminalis. They form a V, the apex of which is placed in front of the foramen cæcum. Each consists of a cylindrical projection surrounded by a deep circular trench, the parapet of which is slightly raised above the general level of the dorsum of the tongue. (*b*) The *fungiform papillæ* are most numerous near the tip and margins of the tongue. Smaller than the vallate papillæ, they can be recognised in the living subject by their bright red colour. Each consists of a narrow pedicle with an enlarged, rounded head. (*c*) The *filiform papillæ* cover the anterior part of the tongue, and give it a characteristic, velvety appearance. They are the smallest and most numerous of the lingual papillæ.

The mucous membrane of the posterior part of the tongue shows no similar elevations. It is characterised by the presence of lymphoid tissue (*lingual tonsil*) and of serous and mucous glands in the submucosa.

The muscular substance of the tongue is formed by the muscles already examined in the submandibular region (p. 269), and by a number of intrinsic muscles, *all of which are supplied by the hypoglossal nerve.*

The distribution of the lingual nerve to the anterior part, and of the glossopharyngeal nerve to the posterior part of the tongue has already been emphasised (p. 273).

The *lymphatics* from the *tip of the tongue* pass to the submental lymph nodes (p. 241). Those from the anterior part of the tongue, excluding the tip, pass to the submandibular lymph nodes (p. 269), but many of them run directly to the upper group of the deep cervical lymph nodes (p. 244). Those from the posterior part of the tongue also pass to the upper group of the deep cervical lymph nodes.

The tongue, considered from the developmental point of view, is a composite organ. Roughly its anterior two-thirds are formed, partly by the tuberculum impar—a small median elevation in the floor of the mouth—and partly by bilateral lingual swellings which appear on the entodermal surface of the mandibular arches. This part of the tongue is accordingly supplied by the mandibular nerve. The posterior "third" of the tongue is formed from the ventral ends of the fused second and third arches (anterior part of hypobranchial eminence), which grow forwards with a V-shaped anterior border to join the anterior two-thirds. The foramen cæcum, which marks the site of the original median thyroid outgrowth, is placed at the apex of the V. This part of the tongue is supplied by the glosso-pharyngeal nerve, because the mesenchymal constituents of the third arch grow over and bury the mesenchyme of the second arch.

The muscles of the tongue are derived from the occipital myotomes and they migrate into the tongue, bringing their nerve of supply—the hypoglossal—with them.

The **Isthmus of the Fauces (Oropharyngeal Isthmus)** connects the mouth and pharynx. It is bounded above by the soft palate and uvula, and below by the dorsum of the tongue. On each side it is bounded by the *palatoglossal arch*, which starts in front of the base of the uvula and arches laterally and downwards to reach the side of the tongue. It contains the small palatoglossus muscle.

The Teeth. The child is provided with deciduous ("milk") teeth, which begin to erupt *between the sixth and ninth months*, and which should all be present in a healthy child *by the end of the second year or soon after*. The teeth of the lower jaw usually appear before those of the upper jaw, and the central incisors are followed at intervals of a few weeks by the lateral incisors, the first molars, the canines and the second molars, in that order.

The first permanent tooth to erupt is the first molar. It usually appears during the *sixth year*, and its presence enables the child to continue to masticate while the deciduous molars are becoming extruded to make room for the premolar teeth. The permanent central incisor erupts during the seventh year, and is followed by the lateral incisor. During the ninth and tenth years the first and second pre-molars appear, and they are followed in the eleventh year by the canine. After the eruption of the second molar tooth, during the twelfth or thirteenth years, the process ceases for a time; the third molar ("wisdom") tooth, which is very variable in its time of appearance, does not erupt until between the seventeenth and thirtieth years. Occasionally the third molar fails to erupt and remains buried in its bony crypt, and even this may be absent.

The incisors, canines and premolars have single roots, with the exception of the first upper premolar, the root of which is bifid. The upper molars have three roots, of which two are lateral and one is medial. The lower molars, on the other hand, have only two roots, one being anterior and the other posterior.

The enamel of the teeth is ectodermal in origin and is derived from the enamel germs which bud off from the dental lamina. The dentine cement and pulp are all derived from the mesenchyme.

The *Pterygomandibular Ligament* is a fibrous band which extends between the pterygoid hamulus and the posterior end of the mylohyoid line of the mandible. The buccinator muscle arises from its anterior border, and the superior constrictor from its posterior border, so that these two muscles, the one in the cheek and the other in the pharyngeal wall, are on the same plane.

The **Pharynx** is placed behind the nose, mouth and larynx. It extends from the base of the skull downwards to the level of the sixth cervical vertebra, where it becomes continuous with the œsophagus. The muscular wall of the pharynx is entirely deficient anteriorly, where the choanae (posterior nasal apertures), the isthmus of the fauces, and the inlet of the larynx are situated.

The *Superior Constrictor Muscle* arises from the lower third or less of the posterior border of the medial pterygoid plate, the pterygoid hamulus, the pterygomandibular ligament, the posterior end of the mylohyoid line, and from the side of the tongue. Reference to a skull will show that this constitutes a linear and nearly vertical origin. The upper fibres run medially and upwards to reach the pharyngeal tubercle on the lower surface of the basilar part of the occipital bone, and the succeeding fibres constitute, with those of the opposite side, a median raphe on the dorsal wall. The more inferior fibres have a downward inclination, and are overlapped by the upper border of the middle constrictor. A group of horizontal fibres, often termed the palatopharyngeal sphincter, arises from the palatal aponeurosis and passes round the pharynx on the deep surface of the superior constrictor at the level of the raised soft palate. By their contraction they approximate the posterior wall of the pharynx to the free edge of the raised soft palate and cut off communication between the oral and nasal parts of the pharynx.

The superior constrictor muscle is on the same plane as the buccinator, and the buccopharyngeal fascia is continued from the one to the other.

The *Middle Constrictor Muscle* arises from the upper border of the greater cornu of the hyoid bone, from the lesser cornu, and from the stylohyoid ligament. From this narrow origin the fibres radiate medially and are inserted into a medium raphe on the dorsal wall of the pharynx. The upper fibres overlap the superior constrictor, and the lower fibres are, in turn, overlapped by the inferior constrictor muscle.

The *Inferior Constrictor Muscle* arises from the lamina of the thyroid cartilage behind the oblique line, and from the side of the cricoid cartilage. The fibres diverge, and the upper fibres overlap the middle constrictor, while the lower run horizontally medially. All are inserted into a median raphe on the dorsal wall of the pharynx. The lowermost fibres are believed to exercise a sphincteric action to prevent the entry of air into the œsophagus during inspiration.

When the attachments of the three constrictor muscles are examined, it will be apparent that there are three places where the lateral muscular wall of the pharynx is deficient. One of these gaps is placed between the upper border of the superior constrictor and the base of the skull. Another lies between the lower border of the superior constrictor and the upper border of the middle constrictor. The third is placed between the lower border of the middle and the upper border of the inferior constrictor.

1. The gap above the superior constrictor is bounded in front by the upper part of the posterior border of the medial pterygoid plate, below by the oblique upper border of the superior constrictor muscle, and above by the base of the skull. It forms a large part of the lateral wall of the nasal pharynx, and is occupied by the tensor and the levator veli palatini muscles and the pharyngotympanic tube.

The *Tensor Veli Palatini* arises from the spine of the sphenoid, the lateral side of the pharyngotympanic tube, and the scaphoid fossa. The fibres descend outside the superior constrictor and converge on the pterygoid hamulus. There the triangular muscle ends in a small tendon, which, as it twists round the bone, passes through a small gap in the upper and posterior part of the origin of the buccinator and so enters the soft palate. It is inserted into the palatal aponeurosis.

Its *Nerve Supply* is derived from the mandibular nerve (p. 264).

The *Levator Veli Palatini* lies on a deeper plane than the tensor. It arises from the inferior aspect of the petrous part of the temporal bone and descends medial to the pharyngotympanic tube. Unlike the tensor, the levator passes within the upper border of the superior constrictor, and so has no obstacle to its entry into the soft palate, where it is inserted into the palatal aponeurosis.

Its *Nerve Supply* is derived from the pharyngeal plexus.

The *Auditory Tube* (p. 372) runs forwards and medially in the interval between the two muscles.

2. In the gap which is left between the lower border of the superior constrictor and the upper border of the middle constrictor muscle, the stylopharyngeus muscle, the glossopharyngeal nerve and the stylohyoid ligament are found.

The *Stylopharyngeus* arises from the medial side of the styloid process near its base and descends across the internal carotid artery to reach the superior constrictor muscle. It passes within the upper border of the middle constrictor and runs downwards deep to that muscle, the greater cornu of the hyoid bone and the inferior constrictor, to be inserted into the upper and posterior borders of the thyroid cartilage.

Its *nerve supply* is derived from the glossopharyngeal nerve, and it assists in elevating the larynx and pharynx during the act of swallowing.

The *Glossopharyngeal Nerve* (p. 272) comes into relation with the deep surface of the stylopharyngeus as they both cross superficial to the internal carotid artery. It supplies the stylopharyngeus and gives off branches to join the pharyngeal plexus. It also supplies minute twigs to the carotid sinus (p. 229) and the carotid body. Its terminal branch curls round the posterior border of the stylopharyngeus, and enters the tongue below the styloglossus muscle, to be distributed to the *mucous membrane of the posterior part of the tongue* (*both general sensibility and the special sense of taste*) *and to the mucous membrane of the tonsillar region and soft palate*.

3. The gap between the middle and inferior constrictors is of small size. It is traversed by the internal laryngeal nerve and its accompanying vessels as they pierce the thyrohyoid membrane (p. 302).

The *Pharyngeal Plexus* of nerves is placed on the outer surface of the middle constrictor muscle. It is formed by pharyngeal branches of the glossopharyngeal and vagus nerves with one another, and with branches from the superior cervical ganglion of the sympathetic. From the plexus branches are given off to supply the constrictor muscles and the muscles of the soft palate, with the exception of the tensor veli palatini. In addition, numerous sensory branches supply the mucous membrane of the pharynx.

The *lymph vessels* of the pharynx terminate in the retropharyngeal lymph nodes, which occupy the areolar interval between the pharyngeal wall and the prevertebral fascia. Their efferents join the upper and anterior group of the deep cervical lymph nodes.

The Interior of the Pharynx. Its **Nasal Part** is limited above by the base of the skull. When the soft palate is raised, it is shut off from the oral part of the pharynx, but at other times the two chambers communicate freely, an arrangement rendered necessary by its respiratory function.

The *Roof* and *Posterior Wall* form a continuous surface which slopes downwards and backwards. It is supported by the inferior surfaces of the body of the sphenoid and the basilar part of the occipital bone above, and by the anterior arch of the atlas, below. In the young child a collection of lymphoid tissue, which is termed the *pharyngeal tonsil*, is found in the anterior part of the roof. It may become hypertrophied and spread backwards and downwards, so as to occlude the cavity of the nasal part of the pharynx. This condition, which clinically is termed "*adenoids*," may render nasal breathing impossible.

The *Anterior Wall* is occupied by the posterior nasal apertures separated from each other by the posterior edge of the nasal septum. Each opening measures 1 inch long by $\frac{1}{2}$ inch wide.

The *Lateral Wall* presents the *opening of the auditory tube*, which is directed forwards, medially, and slightly downwards. The *posterior lip of the opening forms a thickened elevation*, which is known as the tubal elevation. It is produced by the free anterior edge of the cartilage in the wall of the tube. The *pharyngeal recess*, which lies behind the elevation, varies considerably in depth.

The **Oral Part of the Pharynx** lies below the level of the raised soft palate and above the upper border of the epiglottis. Its *posterior wall* adjoins the body of the axis, but the two are separated by the prevertebral fascia and the longus cervicis and longus capitis muscles, in addition to the constrictors and the buccopharyngeal fascia. Scattered nodules of lymphoid tissue are found in the submucous tissue.

The *Anterior Wall* is occupied by the isthmus of the fauces and the posterior aspect of the tongue.

The *Lateral Wall* is important owing to the presence of the tonsil and the palatopharyngeal arch.

The *palatopharyngeal arch* begins on the posterior aspect of the base of the uvula and disappears below on the side wall of the oral pharynx. It contains the palatopharyngeus muscle (p. 297).

The triangular interval between the palatoglossal and the palatopharyngeal arches is occupied in its lower part by the **Tonsil.** Up to the age of puberty the tonsil forms a prominent projection on the lateral wall of the oral pharynx. It consists of a mass of lymphoid tissue, covered by mucous membrane, which shows numerous little *pits* or crypts. The upper pole of the tonsillar mass is covered by a hood-like fold of mucous membrane and the narrow interval between them is termed the *intratonsillar cleft*, because the deep surface of the fold contains a layer of lymphoid tissue continuous laterally with the lymphoid tissue of the tonsil, of which it is in fact an outlying part. In the operation of tonsillectomy the tonsillar mass and the hood-like fold are removed in one piece. In the normal condition the tonsil does not possess a limiting capsule, but when it is diseased the surrounding fibroareolar tissue, which intervenes between it and the superior constrictor muscle, becomes condensed on its outer surface. Outside the superior constrictor the styloglossus crosses the lower part of the tonsil and, when the upward loop of the facial artery is pronounced, the vessel reaches the styloglossus and so comes into indirect relation with the tonsil. In that event the vessel may be injured during the removal of the tonsil, but the accident is very rare.

The tonsil receives its blood supply from the *tonsillar artery*, a branch of the facial artery, which enters its lateral aspect near its lower pole. A number of small vessels, which anastomose freely with one another in the neighbourhood of the tonsil, are often described as helping the tonsillar artery, but it seems very doubtful whether they actually reach the tonsil in most cases.

A relatively large vein issues from the soft palate and runs downwards and forwards in the bed of the tonsil, lying on the fibro-areolar tissue which clothes the inner surface of the superior constrictor muscle. It pierces the pharyngeal wall in company with the tonsillar artery, after receiving the tonsillar veins near its point of exit. (Injury to this vein is the usual cause of severe hæmorrhage from the tonsillar bed following tonsillectomy).

The *lymph vessels* of the tonsil pass to the upper anterior group of the deep cervical lymph nodes, one of which occupies the angle between the internal jugular vein and the common facial vein, lying a little below and a little behind the angle of the jaw. It is this node which is first involved when the tonsil is affected.

The crypts of the tonsil develop as a number of endodermal out-growths in the wall of the second pharyngeal pouch. The lymphoid tissue which surrounds them is mesodermal in origin.

The **Laryngeal Part of the Pharynx** is the longest of the three subdivisions. Its *anterior wall* is occupied, above, by the inlet of the larynx (p. 300). In its lower part it is formed by the mucous membrane covering the posterior aspect of the arytenoid and cricoid cartilages and their associated muscles. The *posterior wall* is in contact with the anterior wall below the laryngeal inlet, except during the passage of food. It is supported by the bodies of the third, fourth, fifth and sixth cervical vertebræ.

The *Lateral Wall* is supported by the posterior part of the lamina of the thyroid cartilage, and it presents a small recess termed the *piriform fossa*, which is bounded on its medial side by the ary-epiglottic fold. Terminal branches of the internal laryngeal nerve supply its mucous membrane, and consequently the lodgment of a crumb or any small particle of food in the piriform fossa gives rise to an uncontrollable fit of coughing.

THE NOSE

The **Nasal Cavity** is divided into right and left halves by the nasal septum, a structure which is rarely strictly median.

The **Nasal Septum** is an osteocartilaginous partition, covered on each side by closely adherent mucous membrane. Its upper half is formed by the perpendicular plate of the ethmoid and its posterior part by the vomer. The very oblique anterior border of the vomer articulates with the perpendicular plate and below this with the septal cartilage. The latter structure constitutes the lower and anterior part of the septum.

It should be observed that deflection of the nasal septum does not affect the median position of its borders, but is usually restricted to the central area and is produced by overgrowth of one or more of the constituent parts.

The mucous membrane of the septum is supplied by branches of the olfactory and trigeminal nerves. The *olfactory nerves* are restricted to the upper part, while the trigeminal branches are distributed over the whole of its extent. The latter are an *internal nasal branch from the anterior ethmoidal* (ophthalmic nerve) and the *nasopalatine* (*long sphenopalatine*) *nerve*, which arises from the pterygopalatine ganglion (maxillary nerve). This nerve runs downwards and forwards on the septum, and, as its name indicates, its terminal branches pass through the incisive foramina and supply the mucous membrane of the anterior part of the hard palate.

Each cavity extends from the piriform aperture to the choana, and from the hard palate to the base of the skull. The transverse width is greatly diminished by the presence of the projecting conchæ on the lateral wall, and it is greatest below.

The *Floor*, which has a slight downward inclination, is formed by the palatine process of the maxilla and the horizontal plate of the palatine bone, and the *medial wall* is formed by the nasal septum.

The *Roof* slopes downwards, both in front and behind. Its central portion is horizontal and is formed by the cribriform plate of the ethmoid. The posterior sloping part is formed by the body of the sphenoid, while the anterior sloping part is formed, in turn, by the frontal, the nasal bone, and the nasal cartilages.

The *Lateral Wall* may be subdivided into a small anterior, and a large posterior part. The anterior part is almost featureless. Immediately above the anterior nasal aperture it is lined by modified skin and hollowed out to form the *vestibular portion* of the lateral wall, and it is in this area that the short, curved hairs or *vibrissæ* are found. Above the vestibular portion the lateral wall is very slightly hollowed out, and this area forms the *atrium of the middle meatus.*

The posterior part of the lateral wall is characterised by the presence of the conchæ and the meatuses of the nose.

The *Superior and Middle Nasal Conchæ* are simply projections from the medial surface of the labyrinth of the ethmoid. The former is situated on the upper and back part of the lateral wall of the nasal cavity, and it does not overhang sufficiently to hide the superior meatus of the nose, of which it constitutes the upper boundary.

The *Middle Nasal Concha* is placed below the superior meatus, and, by its overhang, it completely conceals the middle meatus. It possesses a free anterior and a free inferior border.

The *Inferior Nasal Concha* is a separate bone, which articulates with the maxilla and the perpendicular plate of the palatine bone, and so forms part of the medial wall of the maxillary sinus. It overhangs the inferior meatus, and its lower border almost reaches the floor of the nasal cavity.

The *Inferior Meatus* of the nose lies between the overhanging inferior nasal concha and the floor. In the anterior part of its lateral wall the *nasolacrimal duct* opens.

The *Middle Meatus* lies between the middle nasal concha and the adjoining part of the labyrinth of the ethmoid, and it cannot be examined unless the middle concha has been detached or has been fractured and turned upwards. A rounded elevation, termed the *ethmoidal bulla*, is situated on its lateral wall. It is formed by the underlying middle ethmoidal sinuses, which open into the middle meatus at the upper border of the elevation. A deep sulcus, termed the *hiatus semilunaris*, lies immediately below the bulla. Its anterior end leads into the *infundibulum*, a short passage by means of which the *frontal sinus* opens into the middle meatus. The anterior ethmoidal sinuses may open directly into the fore-part of the groove or they may open into the infundibulum. The *maxillary sinus* opens into the posterior part of the hiatus semilunaris, and its orifice is concealed by the flange-like medial border of the groove. Not infrequently the sinus opens into the middle meatus by an additional orifice placed behind the hiatus semilunaris.

The *Superior Meatus* is very short in comparison with the middle and inferior meatuses. It receives the openings of the posterior ethmoidal sinuses.

The *Spheno-ethmoidal Recess* lies above the superior nasal concha, and its posterior wall, which is formed by the anterior aspect of the body of the sphenoid, presents the opening of the *sphenoidal sinus*.

The *Mucous Membrane*, which covers the whole of the lateral wall except the vestibular portion, is especially thick and vascular over the respiratory part of the cavity (the middle and inferior conchæ), where the submucous tissue is more plentiful and contains a plexus of veins. These characters enable the air to obtain warmth and moisture in its passage through the nose, and they account for the manner in which one or both halves of the cavity become completely blocked up in the early stages of a common cold.

The *Nerves* which are found on the lateral wall of the nose are derived from two sources:—

1. Numerous *Olfactory Nerves* arise from the special olfactory cells scattered throughout the mucous membrane in the upper part of the cavity and ascend through the cribriform plate to reach the olfactory bulb. *They are non-medullated.*

2. The nerves of ordinary sensibility are branches of the trigeminal. (*a*) The *Anterior Ethmoidal* (ophthalmic nerve) gives off a branch to the septum and runs downwards on the inner surface of the nasal bone over the atrium of the middle meatus. It supplies the mucous membrane in this region and the integumentary lining of the vestibular part, and emerges between the nasal bone and the upper nasal cartilage to supply the skin (p. 276). Its terminal part is termed the *external nasal nerve.*

(*b*) The *Posterior superior nasal branches* (short sphenopalatine nerves) and (*c*) the *Nasal branches of the greater palatine nerve* are both derived, indirectly, from the maxillary nerve. The former, after passing through the pterygopalatine ganglion, are distributed to the mucous membrane of the superior meatus. The latter are distributed by the mucous membrane of the middle and inferior meatuses.

The *Blood Supply* of the nasal mucous membrane is derived, principally, from the terminal part of the maxillary artery, which lies in the pterygopalatine fossa. Its largest branch, the *sphenopalatine artery*, enters the nasal cavity through the sphenopalatine foramen and, after giving off branches to supply the lateral wall, runs downwards and forwards on the septum, in company with the corresponding nerve.

Before leaving this region, observe that all the cranial air-sinuses open into the nasal cavity or the nasal pharynx. (1) The tympanic antrum, the mastoid air-cells and the tympanic cavity open into the nasal pharynx through the pharyngotympanic tube. (2) The sphenoidal sinus opens into the spheno-ethmoidal recess. (3) The posterior ethmoidal sinuses open into the superior meatus of the nose. (4) The maxillary sinus, the anterior and middle ethmoidal sinuses and the frontal sinus open into the middle meatus.

As a result, all these air-sinuses are lined by mucous membrane—firmly adherent to the periosteum, and therefore termed mucoperiosteum—which is directly continuous with the mucous membrane of the nasal cavity. Further, since the nasolacrimal duct opens into the inferior meatus, the nasal mucous membrane is also continuous with the conjunctiva.

The **Soft Palate** is a fleshy flap, covered by mucous membrane on both its upper and lower surfaces. Its anterior border is attached to the hard palate, but its posterior border is free and presents, in the median plane, a downward projection which is termed the uvula. On each side the soft palate is attached to the lateral wall of the pharynx.

During respiration the soft palate is relaxed and offers no obstruction to the passage of air. During the second stage of deglutition, on the other hand, the soft palate is rendered tense, it is raised and its posterior border comes firmly into contact with the posterior pharyngeal wall. In this way the passage of food or drink into the nasal pharynx is effectively prevented but, when the muscles of the soft palate are paralysed, the regurgitation of fluids through the nose is a distressing and characteristic symptom.

The fleshy substance of the soft palate contains the insertions of the tensor and levator veli palatini (p. 290), the origins of the palatoglossus and the palatopharyngeus muscles (which form the palatine arches), and the uvular muscle.

The **Palatoglossus** muscle arises from the under surface of the palatine aponeurosis, descends in front of the tonsil in the palatoglossal arch and is inserted into the side of the tongue at the junction of its anterior and posterior parts.

The **Palatopharyngeus** muscle arises from the posterior border of the bony palate and from the palatine aponeurosis, and descends behind the tonsil in the palatopharyngeal arch. As it descends, it is in intimate relation with the inner surfaces of the constrictor muscles and lies postero-medial to, and edge to edge with, the stylopharyngeus. It is inserted, partly, into the posterior border of the thyroid lamina and partly into the posterior wall or median raphe of the pharynx.

The *Nerve Supply* of all these muscles, with the exception of the tensor veli palatini, which is supplied by the mandibular nerve (p. 265), is derived from the pharyngeal plexus (p. 291).

The *actions* of the tensor and levator are indicated by their names. The palatoglossi help to elevate the dorsum of the tongue and to close the oropharyngeal isthmus in the first stage of deglutition. The palatopharyngei help to elevate the larynx and to shorten the pharynx during the second stage of deglutition. The uvular muscle—a small muscle which runs backwards into the uvula from the posterior nasal spine—shortens and raises the uvula.

Numerous mucous glands are present in the soft palate, and they constitute a large part of its substance.

The *Mucous Membrane* of the soft palate derives its nerve supply from branches descending from the pterygopalatine ganglion (maxillary nerve). These are termed the lesser palatine nerves.

The *Blood Supply* of the soft palate is derived from branches of the facial, ascending pharyngeal and maxillary arteries.

The nasal septum is derived from the oral aspect of the median nasal process (p. 253). The palate is formed from right and left palatine processes, which grow from the oral aspects of the maxillary processes and fuse with each other and with the oral border of the nasal septum. Development of the palate may be arrested at any stage. In the grossest form, the palatine processes fail to fuse with each other and with the nasal septum, and the maxillary processes remain separate from the globular processes. As a result, a double hare-lip is present, and the two gaps converge behind on a complete cleft in the palate, through which the lower border of the nasal septum can be seen in the living subject.

THE LARYNX

The **Larynx,** which is placed in front of the lowest subdivision of the pharynx, extends from about the middle of the third to the lower border of the sixth cervical vertebra. It forms the important part of the respiratory passage which is concerned in the production of the voice, and is kept patent by means of a cartilaginous skeleton consisting of several units. These articulate with one another at small joints, which allow of a certain amount of movement.

The **Thyroid Cartilage** consists of two laminæ widely separated behind, but united to each other in front, where they form a projection termed the *laryngeal prominence.* In the male the two laminæ meet at an angle of about 90°, but in the female the angle is nearly 120°. As a result the laryngeal prominence is much more salient in the male. This difference in angulation is reflected in the length of the vocal fold and is therefore associated with the difference in the pitch of the voice in the two sexes. The anterior borders of the laminæ are united only in their lower halves, the upper halves being separated by a V-shaped notch, termed the *thyroid notch,* which can easily be felt through the skin immediately above the laryngeal prominence and a little below the body of the hyoid bone. The posterior border of the lamina is drawn upwards into a superior cornu, and downwards into an inferior cornu. The latter articulates at its extremity with the side of the cricoid cartilage. The former is attached to the tip of the greater cornu of the hyoid bone by the lateral thyrohyoid ligament, which is simply the lateral thickened border of the thyrohyoid membrane.

An oblique line marks the posterior part of the lateral aspect of the lamina. It gives insertion to the sternothyroid, and origin to the thyrohyoid muscle. The large area in front of the oblique line is covered by the latter muscle, while the narrower posterior area gives origin to part of the inferior constrictor muscle of the pharynx.

The **Cricoid Cartilage** forms a complete ring, which encircles the larynx below the thyroid cartilage. Its narrow anterior part or *arch*, which can be felt through the skin, lies on a level with the sixth cervical vertebra. The posterior part of the ring, which is termed the *lamina*, is very much deeper, and projects upwards so as to occupy the lower part of the gap between the two laminæ of the thyroid.

The two **Arytenoid Cartilages** articulate with the upper border of the lamina of the cricoid cartilage by means of their expanded basal surfaces. They therefore help to occupy the gap between the two laminæ of the thyroid cartilage. The lateral angle of the base of the arytenoid forms a well-marked projection and is termed the *muscular process*. The anterior angle gives attachment to the vocal ligament, *which constitutes the vibrating medium of the vocal fold*, and it is consequently termed the *vocal process*.

The crico-arytenoid and cricothyroid articulations are simple synovial joints. The arytenoid cartilage is able to glide from side to side on the cricoid, and it is also able to rotate round a vertical axis. With reference to the latter movement, observe that forward movement of the muscular process rotates the arytenoid medially so that the two vocal processes, and therefore the vocal folds, are adducted, while the reverse movement provides the opposite effect.

The **Cricothyroid** muscle is the only intrinsic muscle which lies on the exterior of the larynx. It arises from the side of the cricoid and is inserted into the inferior cornu of the thyroid cartilage. The line of pull of the muscle lies in front of the transverse axis of the cricothyroid joint, and, consequently, when the muscle contracts, the thyroid cartilage is tilted downwards and forwards, while the lamina of the cricoid, carrying the arytenoids with it, is tilted downwards and backwards. The two inferior cornua being more or less fixed by the joint capsules the two cartilages are rotated in opposite directions around a transverse axis. This means that the *anterior attachment of the vocal fold is drawn downwards and forwards, while the posterior attachment is drawn downwards and backwards.* As a result the *vocal folds are rendered tense.*

The **Epiglottis** is a large leaf-shaped cartilage which lies in the anterior wall of the upper part of the larynx. Its pointed lower end is firmly attached to the deep surface of the upper part of the thyroid angle, and its anterior surface is attached to the posterior aspect of the body of the hyoid bone by the *hyo-epiglottic ligament*. The expanded upper end of the epiglottis projects upwards beyond the hyoid bone and, being free, is covered by mucous membrane both anteriorly and posteriorly. The anterior surface is connected to the dorsum of the tongue by a median *glosso-epiglottic fold*, and the corresponding depressions on each side of the median plane constitute the *valleculæ*. Right and left *pharyngo-epiglottic folds* connect the lateral margins of the epiglottis to the side wall of the pharynx below the tonsil. The posterior surface of the epiglottis lies in the anterior wall of the vestibule of the larynx.

The cavity of the larynx is divided into three compartments by the vestibular and the vocal folds. The upper part, or *vestibule*, lies above the former and is the largest subdivision. The middle part lies between the vestibular and the vocal folds, whilst the lower subdivision lies below the vocal folds and is directly continuous with the trachea.

It should be noted that the cricoid and thyroid cartilages, and the lower part of the arytenoid consist of hyaline cartilage, whereas the rest of the arytenoid (including the vocal process), the epiglottis, the corniculate and the cuneiform cartilages consist of yellow elastic fibro-cartilage. *It is only the hyaline cartilages which become calcified and later ossified* as age progresses.

The **Inlet of the Larynx** looks almost directly *backwards*, *i.e.*, it is set at right angles to the long axis of the tube, in much the same way as the opening of a ventilating shaft on the deck of a steamship. It is bounded *above* by the free margin of the epiglottis, *on each side* by the ary-epiglottic fold of mucous membrane, which stretches from the side of the epiglottis to the apex of the arytenoid cartilage, and *below* by the short interarytenoid fold of mucous membrane.

Two small elevations are found in the lower extremity of the ary-epiglottic fold. The higher is produced by a small isolated nodule, which is embedded in the fold and is known as the *cuneiform cartilage*. The lower is produced by the *corniculate cartilage*, which is placed on the apex of the arytenoid cartilage. These elevations are easily visible on laryngoscopic examination.

Owing to the plane of the inlet, the anterior wall of the vestibule of the larynx is much longer than the posterior wall. It is formed throughout by the mucous membrane covering the posterior aspect of the epiglottis, and its central part is marked by a rounded elevation termed the *tubercle of the epiglottis*. This forms a noticeable feature on examination with the laryngoscope, and is frequently all that is seen until the observer learns how to manipulate his mirror.

On each side the vestibule is bounded by the ary-epiglottic fold, which contains between its two layers of mucous membrane the *ary-epiglottic muscle. Posteriorly*, the vestibule is bounded by the arytenoid cartilages and the interarytenoid fold, containing the *transverse arytenoid* muscle.

These two muscles are of great importance, for by their action the inlet of the larynx is closed during deglutition. The *ary-epiglottic muscle* arises from the posterior aspect of one arytenoid cartilage, runs upwards and laterally behind the other, and then enters the ary-epiglottic fold of that side to reach the margin of the epiglottis. When the two muscles contract they approximate the apices of the arytenoids to the lowest aspect of the tubercle of the epiglottis, so that the laryngeal inlet is very markedly diminished. At the same time the contraction of the transverse arytenoid muscle approximates the two arytenoid cartilages, still further diminishing the opening.

At its lower end the vestibule becomes narrowed by the presence of the vestibular folds, which project into the cavity of the larynx and are separated by the *rima vestibuli.* The vestibular fold is a fold of mucous membrane running backwards and laterally from the thyroid angle. It contains a weak fibrous band, termed the *vestibular ligament*, which stretches from the thyroid angle to the side of the arytenoid cartilage.

The **Middle Subdivision of the Larynx** opens into the vestibule through the rima vestibuli. Below, it is bounded by the vocal folds and opens into the lowest subdivision through the *rima glottidis.*

On each side a small pouch, termed the *sinus of the larynx*, intervenes between the vestibular and vocal folds. From it a small diverticulum passes upwards between the vestibular fold and the lamina of the thyroid cartilage. It is termed the *saccule* of the larynx.

The **Vocal Fold** extends from the vocal process of the arytenoid to the thyroid angle. It is a sharp, straight-edged fold, and *is characterised by the pallor of its covering mucous membrane.* This feature is due to (1) the firm adhesion of the mucous membrane to the supporting vocal ligament, (2) the absence of the loose submucous tissue found elsewhere in the laryngeal wall (except over the epiglottis) and (3) the consequent absence of blood vessels.

The *Vocal Ligament* is the upper border of the conus elasticus (cricovocal membrane) (p. 302). Posteriorly it is attached to the vocal process of the arytenoid; anteriorly it is attached to the deep surface of the thyroid angle (cricothyroid ligament). Its lateral aspect is in contact with a sheet of muscle (thyro-arytenoid), which stretches from the arytenoid cartilage behind to the thyroid in front.

The deepest fibres of this muscle are attached to the vocal ligament and constitute the *vocalis muscle*.

The *thyro-arytenoid muscle*, by approximating its two attachments, causes relaxation of the vocal fold, while the fibres of the *vocalis* which are attached to the ligament may act like the finger on a violin string and so alter the pitch of the voice

The vocal folds and the rima glottidis are readily visible to the expert on laryngoscopic examination. The *rima glottidis* consists of an intermembranous part in front, lying between the vocal folds, and an intercartilaginous part behind, lying between the two arytenoid cartilages. When the folds are widely abducted, as in forced inspiration, the rima glottidis presents a diamond-shaped outline, but when they are adducted it becomes slit-like.

The movements of the vocal folds are comparatively simple, and are produced by the intrinsic muscles of the larynx. The folds may be tightened (cricothyroid muscle) or they may be relaxed (thyro-arytenoid muscle). They may be adducted or abducted. The crico-arytenoideus lateralis, which arises from the upper border of the arch of the cricoid cartilage, swings the muscular process of the arytenoid forwards, rotating the cartilage medially around a vertical axis so that the vocal fold is adducted. The crico-arytenoideus posterior, which arises from the lamina of the cricoid cartilage, swings the muscular process backwards, rotating the arytenoid cartilage laterally so that the vocal fold is abducted.

All the muscles of the larynx, with one exception, receive their nerve supply from the recurrent laryngeal nerve. The solitary exception is the cricothyroid muscle, which, as already described (p. 236), is innervated by the external laryngeal nerve.

It is a curious and important fact that, when the recurrent laryngeal nerve is injured without being completely divided, it is usually the abductor muscles which are paralysed.

The *Thyrohyoid Membrane* fills up the gap between the hyoid bone and the thyroid cartilage. It is attached below to the upper border and the superior cornu of the thyroid, and above to the posterior aspect of the body of the hyoid bone and the greater cornu. In the median plane a small bursa is interposed between the membrane and the body of the hyoid bone. The lateral border of the membrane is thickened and is termed the lateral thyrohyoid ligament.

The thyrohyoid membrane is covered, to a large extent, by the muscle of the same name, and is thus separated from the sternohyoid and the omohyoid muscles. It is pierced in its lateral part by the internal laryngeal nerve and its accompanying vessels (p. 291).

The *Conus Elasticus* (Cricovocal Membrane) of the larynx fills in the gap between the thyroid and cricoid cartilages, but its attachments are not so simple as those of the thyrohyoid membrane. Below, it is attached to the upper border of the cricoid cartilage, as far back as the capsule of the cricoarytenoid joint. Above, and in front, it is attached to the lower border of the thyroid cartilage and to its deep surface close to the thyroid angle. Posteriorly, it is attached to the lower border and tip of the vocal process of the arytenoid. Between these two points of attachment the membrane passes upwards, medial to the lower border of the thyroid lamina, and in a free border, which constitutes the vocal ligament.

The cricothyroid arteries, which are derived from the superior thyroid, meet and anastomose in front of the upper part of the cricovocal membrane.

Section VI

THE CENTRAL NERVOUS SYSTEM

THE central nervous system comprises the brain and spinal cord. It represents the mechanism whereby the individual is able to react to the environment, and whereby the various systems in the body can be regulated, co-ordinated and controlled for the benefit of the individual.

The brain consists of the parts of the central nervous system within the cranium, viz.: (1) the cerebrum, (2) the brainstem, which includes the midbrain, the pons and the medulla oblongata, and (3) the cerebellum. Together, (2) and (3) comprise the hindbrain. Almost all the central nervous system is developed from the ectoderm which forms the neural groove and, later, the neural tube. The cerebrum is derived from the primitive forebrain, which becomes subdivided into a caudal part, termed the *diencephalon*, consisting, roughly, of the limiting walls of the third ventricle, and a cephalic part, termed the *telencephalon*, comprising the rest of the cerebral hemispheres. The lamina terminalis represents the cephalic end of the primitive neural tube, and the lateral ventricles represent the cavities of the diverticula which form the cerebral hemispheres.

The mesencephalon develops from the primitive midbrain, and the cavity of its vesicle becomes reduced to form the aqueduct. The primitive hindbrain, or rhombencephalon, has a complicated history, and ultimately it forms the pons, the medulla oblongata and the cerebellum, and the cavity of its vesicle becomes the fourth ventricle.

The remainder of the neural tube forms the spinal cord, and its lumen is reduced to a minute central canal. It retains its relatively simple structure.

In both the brainstem and the spinal cord, the lateral wall of the tube, as it thickens, shows the presence of a longitudinal *sulcus limitans*, which separates a *basal lamina* from an *alar lamina*. The basal lamina gives origin to groups of motor cells; the cells derived from the alar lamina are sensory. In the spinal cord the basal lamina lies ventral to the alar lamina, but in the hindbrain, owing to the splaying out of the lateral walls of the tube in the early stages of development, the basal lamina lies medial to the alar lamina. As a result, motor cells of the spinal cord occupy the anterior and lateral columns of grey matter, while sensory cells are found in the posterior column, whereas in the hindbrain, the sensory nuclei are placed lateral to the corresponding motor nuclei. Groups of nerve cells which are originally near one another tend to become separated in the course of development and growth, but where one group receives its incoming stimuli from a neighbouring group, it tends to retain its close topographical relationship, even though it may have to migrate in order to do so. The factors which bring this about are unknown, but they are covered by the term *neurobiotaxis*. As a group of cells migrates under this influence, its own axons must lengthen and they subsequently trace out the path along which the group has travelled. The course taken by the fibres of the facial nerve on leaving their nucleus of origin is the best example of this process (pp. 320 and 332).

THE SPINAL CORD

The spinal cord begins at the foramen magnum, where it is continuous with the medulla oblongata, and terminates at or near the lower border of the *first lumbar vertebra*. It is surrounded by its membranes (p. 360) within the vertebral canal. At lower cervical and upper thoracic and again at lower thoracic levels, the spinal cord shows local enlargements. These *cervical* and *lumbar enlargements* correspond to the segments of the cord concerned in innervation of the limb, and are due to the consequent accumulations of nerve cells and fibres at these levels.

As the spinal cord is shorter than the canal in which it lies, the roots of the lower spinal nerves become progressively longer. Consequently, below the first lumbar vertebra the canal is occupied by a leash of lumbar and sacral nerve roots, termed the *cauda equina*. The lower end of the spinal cord tapers off into a conical extremity, the *conus medullaris* from the apex of which a thread, the *filum terminale*, descends among these nerve roots. It is continuous above with the pia mater and its upper end contains a little grey matter and the continuation of the central canal of the spinal cord. Below, it pierces the arachnoid and the dura mater and emerges at the sacral hiatus to blend with the periosteum on the dorsum of the coccyx.

A distinct fissure indents the spinal cord anteriorly. It is termed the *anterior median fissure*.

In the spinal cord the grey matter is arranged centrally and the white matter peripherally. The grey matter forms a fluted column, which on transverse section shows an H-shaped figure, the ventral extremities being short and blunt and the dorsal extremities longer and narrower. These are termed respectively *the ventral* (*anterior*) *and dorsal* (*posterior*) *columns*, and their shape varies in the different regions of the cord. The traverse limb of the H is the *grey commissure* and surrounds the *central canal of the spinal cord*. The ventral column is expanded in the cervical and lumbar enlargements where it contains many more nerve cells than it does in the thoracic and upper cervical segments. These cells, which are typically large and multipolar, constitute the *somatic efferent column* and their axons are distributed to skeletal muscle. In the thoracic region there is a small, pointed *lateral column*, which projects laterally opposite the central canal. Its cells constitute the *general visceral efferent column* and give origin to the preganglionic sympathetic fibres which run into the white rami communicantes (p. 18). The dorsal column, which is narrow and elongated in the cervical and thoracic segments but shorter and broader in the lumbar and sacral segments, contains nerve cells of the second neurones on many of the afferent pathways. Its tip is covered by a cap of grey matter of distinctive appearance, termed the *substantia gelatinosa. Traced upwards this part of the posterior column becomes continuous with the nucleus of the spinal tract of the trigeminal nerve.*

From the large cells of the ventral column the fibres of the anterior nerve roots, *which are purely motor in function*, stream out of the antero-lateral aspect of the spinal cord. Near the tip of the dorsal column the fibres of the dorsal nerve roots, *which are purely afferent*, enter the spinal cord. In this way the white matter can be divided into three white columns. The *ventral white column* lies between the anterior median fissure and the emerging anterior nerve root fibres; the *lateral white column* lies between the anterior and the posterior nerve root fibres; and the *dorsal white column* lies between the posterior nerve root fibres and the *posteromedian septum*, a thin neuroglial partition which stretches forwards from the pia mater in the median plane.

In the immediate neighbourhood of the grey columns, the white columns contain a number of scattered nerve cells and unmyelinated fibres. Owing to the reticular appearance seen under low powers of the microscope it is known as the *formatio reticularis*. (V. p. 354.)

The nerve fibres which constitute the white matter may be divided into two main groups, viz. (*a*) *ascending* and (*b*) *descending*. The former are arranged in fasciculi, or tracts, which become larger as they are traced upwards owing to the addition of new fibres at each higher level. The latter form fasciculi, or tracts, which become smaller as they are traced downwards, since they are constantly giving off fibres as they descend.

In addition to the above groups, there exist shorter fibres. Of these, some are intrasegmental and establish a pathway for local reflexes (Plate XXII); others are intersegmental and also serve to connect the grey matter at different levels. Individual fibres vary in

C.

B.

A.

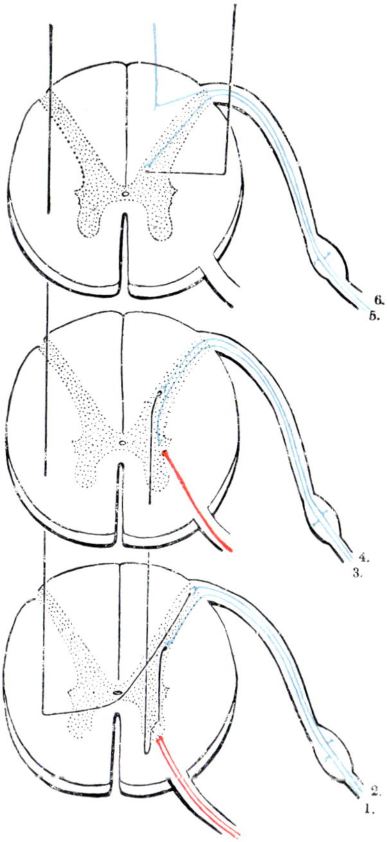

Sections through the Thoracic Part of the Spinal Cord at three different levels.

A. 1. Pathway for an intrasegmental reflex. 2. Pathway for pain.

B. 3. Pathway for a sympathetic reflex. 4. Pathway for an intersegmental reflex.

C. 5. Afferent proprioceptive pathway to cerebellum, *viâ* the posterior spinocerebellar tract. 6. Pathway for tactile and proprioceptive sensibility.

The first neuron is shown in blue, the second in black, and the third in red.

length according as they connect adjoining or widely separated segments of the spinal cord. They are found in and around the *formatio reticularis*, and, in accordance with their position, they are termed the anterior, lateral and posterior *intersegmental tracts*.

Both in front of and behind the central grey matter, anterior and posterior commissural fibres cross the median plane. Some of these fibres are true commissural fibres, *i.e.*, they connect the two halves of the spinal cord with each other—though not necessarily at the same level—but others, after crossing the median plane, may join one or other of the ascending tracts.

ASCENDING TRACTS

The ascending fibres convey afferent impulses, which may or may not be appreciated in consciousness. They may be subdivided into two principal groups: (*a*) *exteroceptive*, *i.e.*, receiving the initial stimulus from something outside the individual, *e.g.*, tactile, painful and thermal sensations; (*b*) *proprioceptive*, *i.e.*, receiving the initial stimulus from an internal source, *e.g.*, muscles, joints, etc.; (c) *interoceptive*, carrying impulses from viscera.

Fibres of exteroceptive sensibility travel by two, possibly three, distinct pathways in the spinal cord. Clinical evidence shows that impulses concerned with pain and temperature ascend in the lateral spinothalamic tract, and that some tactile and pressure impulses ascend in the posterior white columns in company with a large number of propriceptive fibres. Certain types of tactile and pressure sensibility are served by a third path, viz., the *dorsal spinothalamic tract*, although the evidence in favour of this view is not entirely convincing.

1. The fibres conveying impulses concerned with *pain and temperature* are closely related. Their parent cells are placed in the spinal ganglia, the central processes of which form the *postero-lateral tract*, a small bundle situated superficial to the substantia gelatinosa and consisting mainly of finely myelinated fibres. In this tract the incoming fibres ascend for a short distance, giving off ascending and descending collaterals before they enter the substantia gelatinosa, in which they terminate. The second neuron fibres arise in the cells of the substantia gelatinosa and *at once cross the median plane* to turn up in the lateral white column in the *lateral spinothalamic tract*. This fasciculus lies antero-lateral to the lateral cerebrospinal (crossed pyramidal) tract, and is separated from the surface by the anterior spinocerebellar tract (Fig. 3, p. 308). It ascends, constantly receiving additional fibres, to the medulla oblongata, where it joins

the anterior spinothalamic tract (see above), and the two together form the *spinal lemniscus*.

2. Some fibres concerned with *touch* and *pressure* behave in a

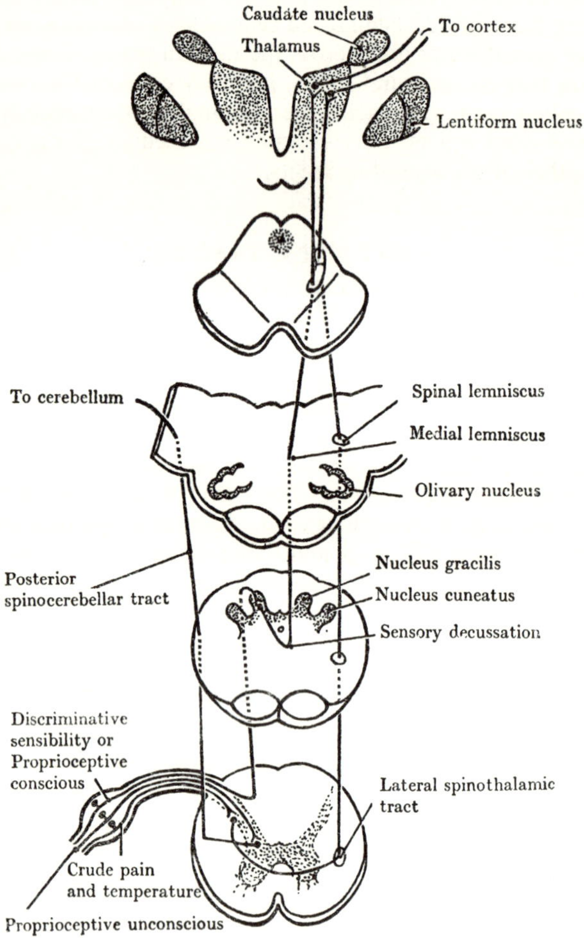

FIG. 3. Schematic Representation of the Paths of some of the Ascending Tracts.

similar manner, but their second neurons ascend in the posterior white column for a few segments before crossing the median plane and turning upwards in the *anterior spinothalamic tract* (Fig. 4, p. 310), which lies in the anterior white column (see above).

The *spinal lemniscus*, formed in the medulla oblongata by the union of the anterior and lateral spinothalamic tracts, conveys all the impulses concerned with pain and temperature from the opposite side of the body. In the medulla oblongata it lies in the formatio reticularis, dorsal to the olivary nucleus and deep to the anterior spinocerebellar tract. At this level the lower limb fibres lie in the lateral or superficial part of the lemniscus, and the upper limb fibres in its medial part. In the pons the spinal lemniscus occupies a corresponding position, and it here becomes associated with the *medial lemniscus* (Fig. 9, p. 321), with which it ascends through the tegmentum of the midbrain and the subthalamic region to end by arborising around cells in the thalamus (p. 386). These cells give rise to new fibres, which ascend through the posterior limb of the internal capsule to reach the cerebral cortex of the postcentral gyrus. Additional connexions are also established by the second and terminal neurons, by means of collaterals.

The corresponding fibres from the trigeminal nerve constitute a separate fasciculus, termed the *trigeminal lemniscus* (p. 331). It establishes similar connexions with the thalamus.

3. The *proprioceptive fibres*, which mediate sensations of movements, active or passive, or of posture, together with the exteroceptive fibres which convey most, if not all, varieties of *tactile sensibility*, have their parent cells situated in the spinal ganglia. The centrally directed fibres of these ganglion cells enter the spinal cord and turn upwards in the posterior white column. They constitute the *fasciculus gracilis* and the *fasciculus cuneatus*, which are therefore functionally identical. The former is placed more medially, since fibres entering at successively higher levels do so from the lateral side of the column. The fasciculus cuneatus occupies the lateral half of the dorsal white column, and naturally consists of fibres from the upper thoracic and the cervical nerves. In the lower part of the medulla oblongata these fibres end by arborising round cells in the gracile and cuneate nuclei (p. 316), two masses of neurons situated side by side in the dorsal region of the closed part of the medulla oblongata. The second neuron fibres, which are termed the *internal arcuate fibres*, sweep ventrally round the central grey matter and cross the median plane (Fig. 7, p. 317), *decussating with the corresponding fibres of the opposite side in the sensory decussation.* They then ascend as the *medial lemniscus*, through the medulla oblongata, the pons, and the midbrain, to the thalamus, where they end. A third neuron arises in the thalamus and extends through the posterior limb of the internal capsule to the postcentral gyrus. The impressions conveyed are therefore appreciated by consciousness. Some of the axons from the gracile and cuneate nuclei enter

into the formation of the inferior cerebellar peduncle either of the same or of the opposite side. They, therefore, reach the cerebellum and the impulses which they convey do not obtrude themselves upon consciousness.

4. Many of the fibres which originate in the spinal ganglia are destined to reach the cerebellum. They form the afferent part of the pathway for spinocerebellar reflexes. These fibres, on entering the spinal cord, terminate in the cells of the *nucleus thoracicus*, and the second neuron fibres ascend in the lateral white column of the

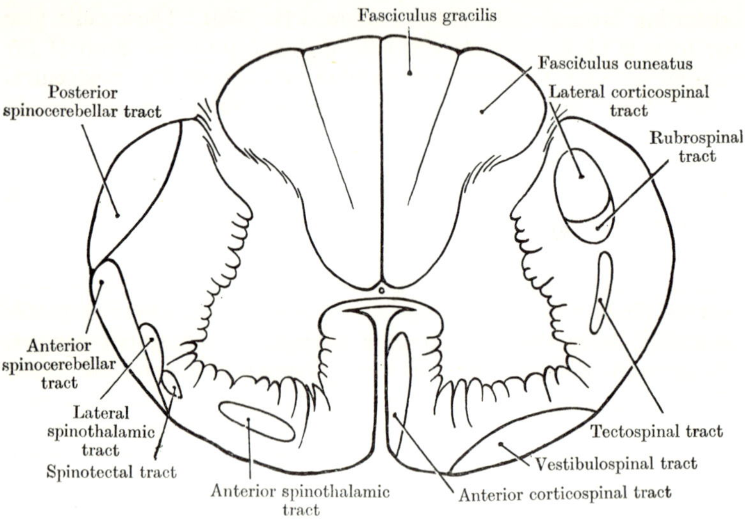

FIG. 4. Diagram of a Transverse Section through the upper part of the Spinal Cord. The Descending Tracts are shown on the right side of the figure, and the Ascending Tracts on the left side.

same side. Here they are arranged in two principal groups, named the posterior and anterior spinocerebellar tracts (Fig. 6, p. 315).

The *nucleus thoracicus* extends throughout the thoracic segments of the spinal cord and lies on the medial aspect of the base of the posterior column of the grey matter. As it does not extend into the cervical segments of the cord, the corresponding incoming fibres from the brachial plexus must follow a different route to reach the cerebellum. They are believed to ascend in the posterior column to the accessory cuneate nucleus, where they are relayed as the dorsal external arcuate fibres (p. 324).

(*a*) The *dorsal spinocerebellar tract* lies near the surface of the spinal cord in the dorsal part of the lateral white column (Fig. 6).

The fibres ascend to the medulla oblongata, where they join the inferior cerebellar peduncle (Plate XXIII, p. 324). They thus reach the cerebellum uncrossed, and they end in the superior vermis and the anterior part of the inferior vermis, where some cross to the opposite side. They are therefore connexions of the palæocerebellum (p. 322).

(*b*) The *ventral spinocerebellar tract* lies close to the margin of the spinal cord, ventral to (*a*). It ascends through the medulla oblongata and the pons, and at the upper end of the latter it turns downwards in the superior cerebellar peduncle of the same side, by which it is conducted to the cerebellum, where its fibres end in the cortex of the superior vermis, for the most part. They are also connexions of the palæocerebellum.

5. Some of the dorsal nerve root fibres establish connexions with the tectum through the medium of the *spinotectal tract* (Fig. 4).

The entering fibres end in cells of the dorsal grey column and the second neuron fibres cross the median plane and ascend with the spinothalamic fibres, leaving these at midbrain levels to curve dorsally into the superior colliculus.

DESCENDING TRACTS

Descending through the spinal cord are tracts which are concerned with the production of movements, both voluntary and visceral, and tracts which form the efferent paths for cerebellar, visual, equilibratory and other reflexes.

1. Voluntary motor impulses travel from the cortex in the **Corticospinal (Pyramidal) Tracts.** The fibres arise in cells in the cortex of the pre-central gyrus and traverse the corona radiata (p. 352), being intersected by fibres of the corpus callosum (p. 346). Becoming more and more closely aggregated together, they enter the genu and posterior limb of the internal capsule (p. 352), and at its lower end they pass as a compact bundle into the crus cerebri, of which they occupy, roughly, the middle third. In the ventral portion of the pons the compact corticospinal tract is broken up into a large number of smaller bundles by the nuclei pontis and transverse fibres of the pons. In the upper part of the medulla oblongata the compact tract is re-established, and it forms a surface projection on the anterior aspect, termed the *pyramid*, which lies immediately lateral to the anterior median fissure. In the lower part of the medulla oblongata the majority of the fibres decussate with the corresponding fibres of the opposite side in the *decussation of the pyramids*, and, having crossed, they take up their final position in the middle of the lateral white column of the spinal cord (Fig. 4). The *lateral corticospinal tract* becomes progressively smaller as it is

traced downwards, for it is constantly giving off fibres, which synapse with the large motor cells in the anterior horn. The fibres of these cells form the anterior nerve roots of the spinal nerves.

Those fibres which do not take part in the pyramidal decussation in the medulla oblongata constitute the *anterior corticospinal tract*, which descends in the anterior white column close to the anterior median fissure. Before they terminate these fibres also cross the median plane, and they end, like the fibres of the crossed tract, by arborising round the large, ventral grey column motor cells (Fig. 5). Few of these fibres descend far in the spinal cord and their number is most variable; in some individuals they may be absent, all corticospinal fibres being then in the lateral tract. In addition, *uncrossed lateral corticospinal fibres* have been described.

It must be remembered that as the corticospinal tract descends through the brainstem, it gives off *corticonuclear* fibres to the motor nuclei of the cranial nerves both of the same and of the opposite side, most of which are therefore bilaterally represented in the cortex.

2. The *vestibulospinal tract*, which is an efferent path for equilibratory reflexes, has its origin in the lateral vestibular nucleus (Fig. 12), and descends near the surface of the spinal cord in the ventral white column (Fig. 4, p. 310). Some of its fibres terminate, *uncrossed*, round the cells of the ventral grey column and are actively motor; others descend on the opposite side and are inhibitory to the corresponding cells of that side. (See also p. 353.)

3. The *rubrospinal tract* has its origin in the red nucleus in the midbrain. It at once decussates with its fellow of the opposite side (Fig. 11, p. 329), and descends through the dorsal part of the pons and the dorsolateral part of the medulla oblongata, to reach the lateral white column of the spinal cord, where it lies in close relationship with the lateral corticospinal tract (Fig. 4, p. 310). Its fibres end in association with the motor cells of the anterior horn of the same side. The tract is an efferent path relayed from the cerebellum and the corpus striatum and it has been suggested that it is concerned functionally with depression of muscle tonus. It is a constituent of the extrapyramidal system (p. 353), but there is a growing body of evidence that the fibres of this tract are relatively few or do not descend far in the cord—at least, not far without relay.

4. The *tectospinal tract*, which, together with the ascending spinotectal tract, provides a pathway for visual reflexes, begins in the superior corpus quadrigeminum of the midbrain and at once decussates with its fellow of the opposite side in front of the aqueduct of the midbrain. It runs downwards in the lateral white column

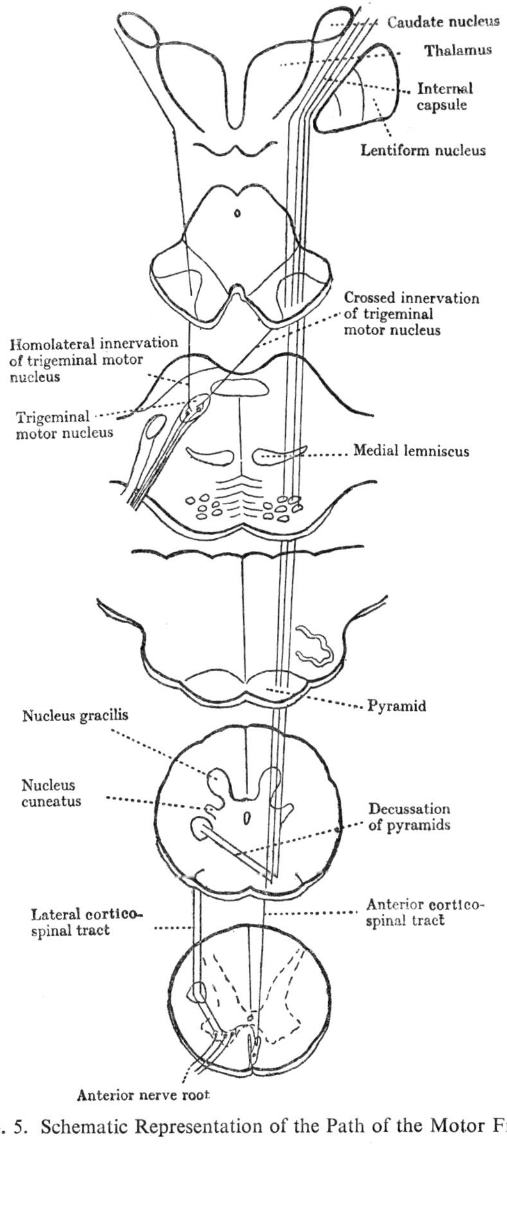

FIG. 5. Schematic Representation of the Path of the Motor Fibres.

of the spinal cord, and its fibres probably end in the same manner as those of the other descending tracts (Fig. 4, p. 310).

THE BRAIN

The brain includes the brainstem, the cerebellum and the cerebrum. The *brainstem*, which comprises the medulla oblongata, the pons and the midbrain, superficially resembles the spinal cord in its structure but contains a number of additional constituents which are not represented in the cord. Though in the central positioning of its nuclear masses it resembles the spinal cord rather than cerebrum or cerebellum (where the grey matter is superficial), it must be remembered that the brainstem is directly continuous with the diencephalon. It is thus very much a part of the primitive vertebrate brain, and therefore much modified as compared with the cord.

The **Medulla Oblongata** lies between the pons and spinal cord, and is related ventrally to the basi-occiput. The anterior median line is indicated by a linear furrow, on each side of which, in the upper part of the medulla, there is an elongated projection termed the *pyramid*, produced by the corticospinal (motor) tract. Lateral to the pyramid is an oval elevation, which is known as the *olive*, and from the groove between this and the pyramid the hypoglossal nerves emerge. The *inferior cerebellar peduncle* projects on the dorsolateral aspect of the medulla, and from the groove by which it is separated from the olive the roots of the ninth and tenth nerves emerge. The roots of the cranial portion of the eleventh nerve leave the surface of the medulla oblongata at a lower level, but are in series with the roots of the ninth and tenth nerves. In its upper half the *posterior aspect* of the medulla oblongata forms the lower part of the floor of the fourth ventricle, but in its lower half it is directly continuous with the posterior aspect of the spinal cord. The dorsal white column of the spinal cord ends on the dorsal surface of the medulla oblongata just below the fourth ventricle in two poorly developed elevations, the *gracile* and the *cuneate tubercles*.

The **Pons** is immediately below the midbrain, and its convex anterior surface is related to the clivus (slope of the basi-occiput). On each side its transverse fibres group themselves into a bundle which enters the cerebellum to form its *middle peduncle*.

The *dorsal surface* of the pons forms the upper part of the floor of the fourth ventricle.

The large sensory and the small motor roots of the trigeminal nerve emerge from the lateral part of the front of the pons near its upper border. They run forwards and laterally to the apex of the petrous portion of the temporal bone, where they enter the *cavum trigeminale* of the dura mater (p. 280).

The abducent nerve emerges from the anterior surface of the pons at its lower border and close to the median plane (p. 331). The facial and the vestibulocochlear nerve also appear at the lower border, but they are situated more laterally, where the pons merges into the middle cerebellar peduncle. They run forwards and laterally together to enter the internal auditory meatus. (The superficial origins of these three cranial nerves at the same horizontal level may be due to downward enlargement of the ventral part of the pons in its evolution (p. 323).)

THE INTERNAL STRUCTURE OF THE MEDULLA OBLONGATA AND PONS

Medulla Oblongata. 1. A transverse section through the lower half of the closed portion of the medulla oblongata passes through

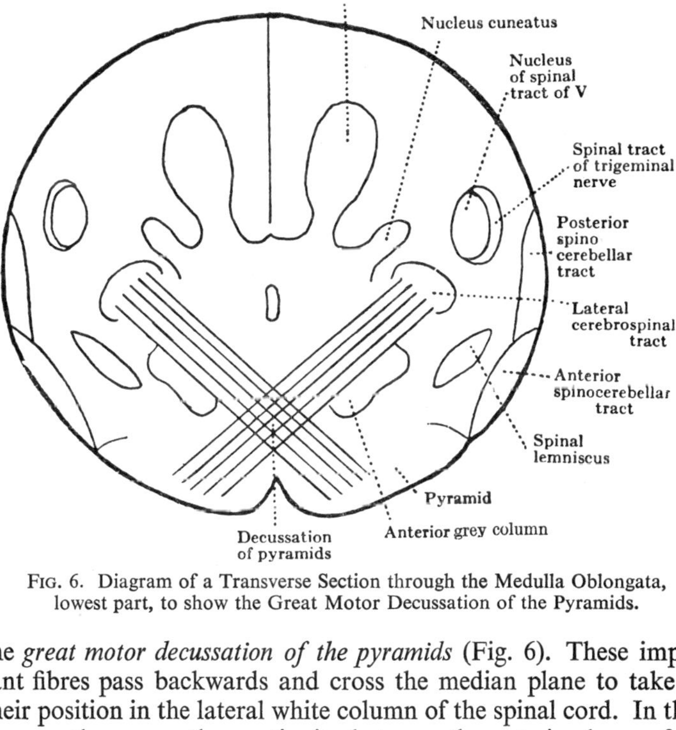

FIG. 6. Diagram of a Transverse Section through the Medulla Oblongata, lowest part, to show the Great Motor Decussation of the Pyramids.

the *great motor decussation of the pyramids* (Fig. 6). These important fibres pass backwards and cross the median plane to take up their position in the lateral white column of the spinal cord. In their passage they sever the continuity between the anterior horn of the grey matter of the spinal cord and the grey matter which surrounds the central canal. The upward continuations of the fasciculus gracilis and the fasciculus cuneatus lie posterior to the central grey matter, from which the lower ends of the *gracile and cuneate nuclei* project dorsally (Fig. 6, p. 315). Close to the surface and ventrolateral to the fasciculus cuneatus, the *nucleus of the spinal tract of the trigeminal*, with the spinal tract of the trigeminal nerve on its lateral aspect is easily discerned. The nucleus is continuous inferiorly with the substantia gelatinosa (p. 306). The area between it and the pyramid contains the *rubrospinal tract*, obscured by the corticospinal fibres, and the ascending *spinocerebellar tracts* and the *spinal lemniscus.*

2. A transverse section through the upper half of the "closed" portion of the medulla oblongta passes through the *great sensory decussation.* This decussation lies immediately behind the two *pyramids*, and intervenes between them and the central canal and its surrounding grey matter, which are therefore displaced dorsally as compared with the previous section. Behind the central grey matter the *gracile and cuneate nuclei* are conspicuous, and from their ventral aspects the *internal arcuate fibres* sweep forwards to take part in the great *sensory decussation* (Fig. 7). The *nucleus of the spinal tract* and the spinal tract of the trigeminal occupy the same positions as in the previous section. The area which lies between the sensory decussation and the lateral aspect of the medulla contains the *rubrospinal* and the ascending *spinocerebellar tracts* and the *spinal lemniscus*, but these tracts are crowded together and difficult to distinguish.

3. A transverse section through the upper half of the medulla oblongata passes across the lower part of the floor of the fourth ventricle. The two *pyramids*, lying one on each side of the median plane and separated by the anterior median fissure, occupy the anterior part of the section (Fig. 13, p. 335). Dorsolateral to the pyramid lies the *olivary nucleus.* It is a flask-shaped, crenated mass of grey matter, the mouth of which is directed medially, and it produces the surface elevation, termed the *olive.* The cells of the olivary nucleus give rise to fibres which stream medially across the median plane, and enter the inferior cerebellar peduncle of the opposite side, constituting the *olivocerebellar tract.* These fibres pass, for the most part, to the neocerebellum (p. 322). The sources of the afferent fibres are the spinal cord, the opposite disk, and possibly the cerebral cortex, red nucleus, thalamus, globus pallidus and reticular formation.

The *dorsal* and *medial accessory olivary nuclei* also are found at this level (Plate XXIII, p. 324). Both are phylogenetically ancient nuclei and they send fibres by the inferior cerebellar peduncle (p. 324) to the palæocerebellum. The functioning of the olivary complex is still obscure, although it may be inferred from their cerebellar connexions that they are concerned in some way with muscular co-ordination.

At this level the *medial lemniscus* forms an elongated tract on each side of the median plane, dorsal to the pyramid (Fig. 13, p. 335). It

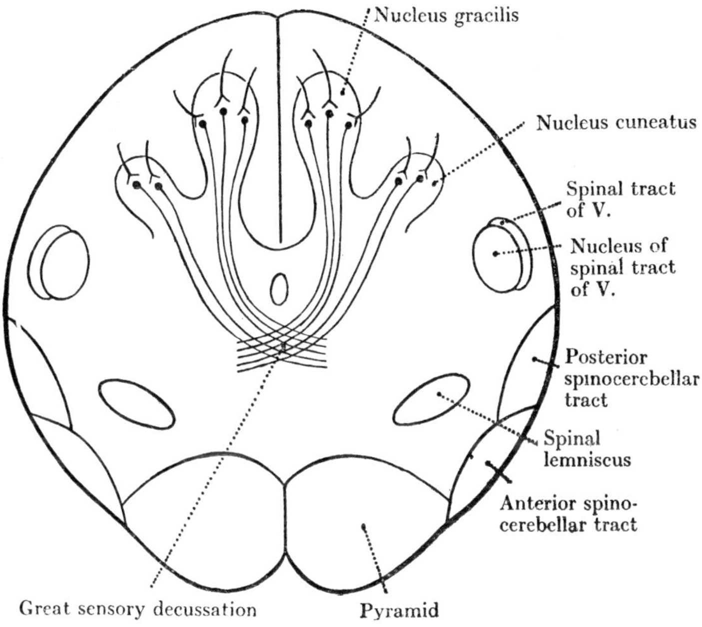

FIG. 7. Diagram of a Transverse Section through the Medulla Oblongata, lower part, showing the Great Sensory Decussation of the Medial Lemnisci. Observe fibres entering the Nucleus Cuneatus and Nucleus Gracilis from the corresponding fasciculi.

consists of fibres which are ascending from the sensory decussation to the thalamus. Dorsally, it is separated from the *hypoglossal nucleus* by the *medial longitudinal bundle* (p. 320).

The *dorsal nucleus of the vagus* lies immediately under the floor of the fourth ventricle, lateral to the hypoglossal nucleus. It is a mixed nucleus and contains general visceral efferent (parasympathetic) nerve cells, which innervate the muscle of the heart, stomach, etc., and general visceral afferent cells. The *tractus solitarius*, with the scattered cells which constitute its nucleus, lies ventrolateral to the vagal nucleus (Fig. 13). It is a special visceral afferent nucleus, concerned with the sense of taste and general visceral sensibility. It receives fibres from the seventh, ninth and tenth nerves. The *nucleus ambiguus* is situated more deeply in the reticular formation (Fig. 13) and lies dorsal to the spinal lemniscus. It is a branchial efferent nucleus and contributes motor fibres to the ninth and tenth nerves (pp. 334, 335) for the supply of the voluntary muscles which they innervate.

The extreme dorsolateral region of the section is occupied by the fibres of the inferior cerebellar peduncle (p. 324) as they ascend to reach the cerebellum. The *spinal tract of the trigeminal and its nucleus* lie on its ventromedial aspect (Fig. 13), and are traversed by the fibres of the vagus nerve. The *dorsal spinocerebellar tract*, as it enters the inferior cerebellar peduncle, intervenes between the spinal tract of the trigeminal and the surface of the medulla oblongata.

In the area between the olivary nucleus and the nucleus of the spinal tract of the trigeminal the *ventral spinocerebellar tract* lies near the surface, and the *spinal lemniscus* and the *rubrospinal tract* are situated more deeply. (The close topographical relationship of the spinal lemniscus to the nucleus ambiguus (Fig. 13) should be noted, as it accounts for the fact that a circumscribed vascular lesion in this situation may result in the curious combination of paralysis of the vocal fold and soft palate of the same side with loss of painful and thermal sensibility on the opposite side of the body.)

4. In a transverse section through the medulla oblongata immediately below the pons the *medial* and *inferior vestibular nuclei* appear on the medial side of the inferior cerebellar peduncle, but otherwise the picture shows little difference from the preceding section. All the nuclei of the vestibular and cochlear nerves are dealt with on pp. 332 to 334.

The Pons. 1. A transverse section across the lower part of the pons shows numerous differences from the upper part of the medulla oblongata. The section is divided into *basilar* (ventral) and *dorsal* portions by the transversely running fibres of the corpus trapezoideum (Figs. 8 and 9, pp. 319 and 321).

The *basilar portion* corresponds to the regions occupied by the pyramid and the olivary nucleus in the upper part of the medulla oblongata. The grey matter, however, does not form a single nuclear mass but is scattered throughout the whole field in numerous small patches, termed the *nuclei pontis*. The corticopontine fibres of the crus cerebri of the midbrain end in the nuclei pontis, the cells of which give origin to the *transverse fibres* of the pons. These fibres intersect the *corticospinal tracts* and break them up into a number of small bundles (Fig. 9). After crossing the median plane the transverse fibres of the pons enter the middle cerebellar peduncle and are finally distributed to the cerebellar hemisphere (neocerebellum). This cerebropontocerebellar pathway is the main connexion between the cerebral cortex and the cerebellum, and the acquisition of increasingly complex limb movements in the process

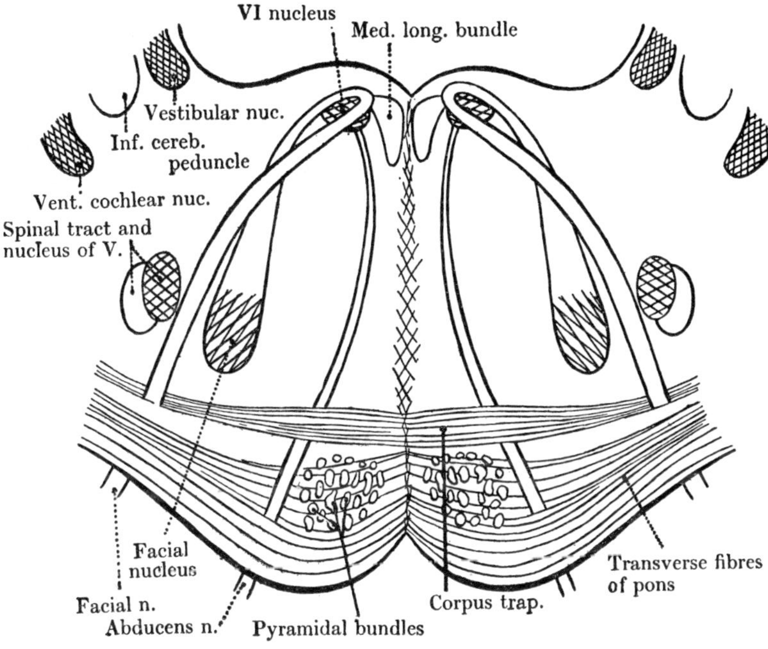

FIG. 8. Diagram of a Transverse Section through the lower part of the Pons. Note the unusual course taken by the fibres of the facial nerve after leaving the nucleus.

of evolution is to be correlated with the simultaneous expansion of the constituent parts of the pathway.

Extensive lesions of any part of the cerebropontocerebellar pathway are marked by pronounced cerebellar ataxia, and movements are accompanied by a rhythmical tremor which develops and increases as they proceed (intention tremor).

The fibres of the *corpus trapezoideum* intersect the *medial lemniscus*, which has undergone an alteration in position, and now lies with its long axis at right angles to the median raphe (Fig. 9). In the dorsal portion of the section, the *facial nucleus* lies dorsal to the lateral part of the medial lemniscus. The fibres of the facial nerve take a peculiar course in their passage from the nucleus to the surface of the pons (p. 332). As they approach the surface they lie between the facial nucleus and the upper end of the *nucleus of the spinal tract of the trigeminal nerve* (Fig. 8, p. 319).

The *medial longitudinal bundle* lies immediately under the floor of the fourth ventricle close to the median plane. To its lateral side, underlying the facial colliculus, lies the *abducens nucleus*, with the outgoing fibres of the facial nerve on its medial aspect (Fig. 10).

The bundle extends throughout the whole length of the brainstem, from the upper limit of the midbrain to the lower end of the medulla oblongata, where it becomes continuous with the anterior intersegmental tract of the spinal cord. Situated in the dorsal part of the tegmentum, close to the median plane, it is immediately ventral to the nuclei of the somatic efferent column (hypoglossal, abducens, trochlear and oculomotor nuclei) (Figs. 8, 9, 10, 11, and 13).

The medial longitudinal bundle receives a substantial contribution of fibres from the vestibular and cochlear nuclei (p. 334), which join it from the dorsal nucleus of the corpus trapezoideum and the nucleus of the lateral lemniscus (p. 333). Outgoing fibres leave the bundle and pass to the nuclei of the third, fourth, sixth and eleventh cranial nerves. It therefore acts as a link between the eighth nerve and these nuclei, enabling vestibular and auditory stimuli to influence the movements of the head and eyes.

The *medial vestibular nucleus* lies lateral to the abducens nucleus and in close relationship with the *inferior cerebellar peduncle*, which occupies the dorsolateral corner of the section. The upper end of the *lateral* and the lower end of the *superior vestibular nucleus* are also found at this level, together with the *dorsal and ventral cochlear nuclei*. They are dealt with on p. 332. The spinal tract of the trigeminal nerve with its nucleus is separated from the ventromedial aspect of the inferior cerebellar peduncle by the entering fibres of the vestibular nerve.

The *spinal lemniscus* and the *anterior spinocerebellar tracts* lie in the lateral part of the dorsal portion of the pons.

2. A transverse section through the pons at the point of entry of the sensory root of the trigeminal nerve shows many differences, which are confined to the dorsal portion. The nuclei of the abducens and facial nerves do not extend to this level, but the large *motor nucleus* and *superior sensory nucleus of the trigeminal nerve* (p. 330) are seen in the lateral part of the dorsal area (Fig. 9, p. 321).

The *superior cerebellar peduncle* (p. 323) lies dorsolateral to the motor nucleus of the trigeminal and is very superficially placed. It is here joined by the ventral spinocerebellar tract (p. 323).

The *corpus trapezoideum* and the *medial lemniscus* occupy the same position as they did in the last section, but the fibres of the former can now be traced into the *lateral lemniscus* (p. 332), which lies at the lateral extremity of the medial lemniscus.

The *formatio reticularis* is extensive and contains the *spinal lemniscus* in its lateral portion.

CEREBELLUM

The **Cerebellum** occupies the posterior cranial fossa, and is

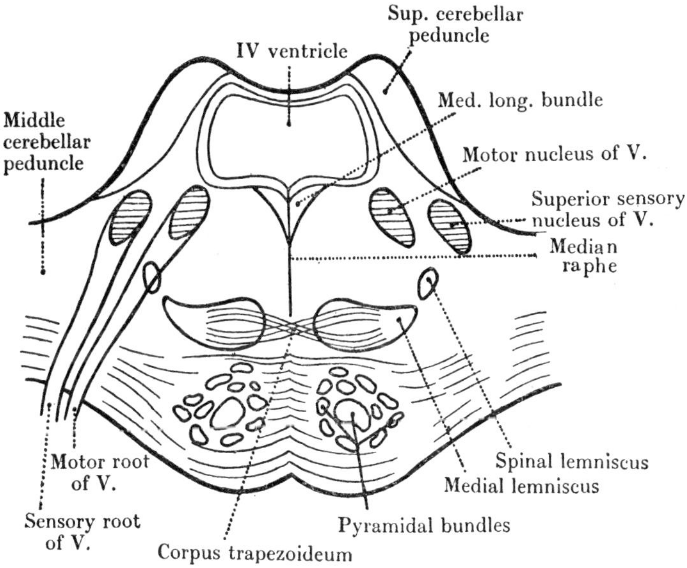

FIG. 9. Diagram of a Transverse Section through the upper part of the Pons, showing the Nuclei of the Trigeminal Nerve. (*After Cunningham.*)

therefore *intimately related to the sigmoid sinus and the tympanic antrum on each side*. Above, it is separated from the cerebral hemispheres by the tentorium cerebelli, and in front it is related to the pons and the medulla oblongata, from which it is separated by the fourth ventricle.

It is a great centre for the co-ordination of muscular movements. *All its activities are carried out without intruding themselves upon consciousness*.

The cerebellum consists of a median part, termed the *vermis*, and two hemispheres. On the *superior surface* the superior aspect of the vermis forms an elevated ridge, which is not marked off from the hemispheres. The inferior aspect vermis, on the other hand, is partially submerged and lies at the bottom of a deep groove, termed the *vallecula,* which lodges the falx cerebelli. Parallel grooves separate it from the two hemispheres.

The cortex of the cerebellum is folded by numerous parallel fissures, into the cerebellar *folia.* Each folium contains a lamina of white matter which gives off secondary laminæ, and these in turn may give off tertiary laminæ. All these laminæ are covered superficially by grey matter, and the resulting appearance of a paramedian section through a folium is termed the *arbor vitæ* of the cerebellum.

A small portion of the cerebellum, almost completely isolated from the rest, lies on the inferior aspect of the middle cerebellar peduncle close to the anterior border of the inferior aspect of the hemisphere. It is termed the *flocculus.* Oval in outline, its medial part is hidden by the lateral recess of the fourth ventricle and the rootlets of the glossopharyngeal and vagus nerves. It possesses a peduncle of white fibres, some of which gain the floor of the fourth ventricle, while others enter the inferior medullary velum, by which it is connected to the side of the most anterior subdivision of the inferior vermis—the *nodule.*

The flocculonodular lobe and the lingula are phylogenetically the oldest part of the cerebellum and constitute the *archicerebellum.* The hemispheres and the posterior parts of the vermis are a later formation in the evolution of the hindbrain. A wide V-shaped fissure, termed the *fissura prima,* crosses the upper surface of the cerebellum. Its apex is situated near the posterior end of the superior vermis and its limbs pass forwards and laterally to reach the antero-lateral borders. The area in front of this fissure constitutes the *anterior lobe*: the area behind the fissure, together with nearly the whole of the inferior surface, constitutes the *middle lobe*: the nodule and the flocculi constitute the *posterior lobe.* The anterior lobe, though later to evolve than the flocculonodular is itself phylogenetically older than the main cerebellar mass (neocerebellum). It is therefore referred to as the *palæocerebellum.*

A deep *horizontal fissure* cuts into the cerebellum along the margin which separates the upper from the lower aspect. Anteriorly, on each side, it widens to allow the middle cerebellar peduncle to gain the interior of the cerebellum. Despite its depth and extent this fissure has no morphological significance.

There are two features of the cerebellum which are especially noteworthy. In the first place the grey matter forms a layer of cortex, being placed on the surface and not centrally as in the spinal cord and brainstem. In this way the cerebellum resembles the cerebrum, and the arrangement can be associated with the enormous expansion which both have undergone in the process of evolution. In the second place, the cortex of the cerebellum, unlike the cortex of the cerebrum, shows no local differences in its minute structure, but is everywhere the same. This is evidence that there is no diversity of function in the cerebellum. While, in the cerebrum, certain definite areas are primarily associated not only with specific funtions but also with particular parts of the body, in the case of the cerebellum there is a much greater uniformity of function, and, although a degree of localization is present, in relation to both afferent and efferent connexions, this is on a wider scale—at least, insofar as available data indicate.

Within the central white core of the cerebellum subcortical collections of grey matter are found. Of these the largest and most important is the crenated *dentate nucleus*, which lies in the medial part of the hemisphere. To its medial side lie the nuclei emboli-formis, globosus and fastigii, which, like the dentate nucleus, are all closely related to the roof of the fourth ventricle. All these nuclei constitute cell-stations on the efferent pathway from the cerebellum.

The enormous size of the neocerebellum in mammals, and especially in man, is explained by the acquisition of the power to learn and carry out movements of great complexity, which demand perfect co-ordination of all the muscles involved. It is to be associated closely with (1) the concurrent expansion of the cerebrum and the basilar part of the pons and the establishment of a wealth of cerebrocerebellar connexions; and (2) the expansion of the olivary nuclei which project extensively to it.

Cerebellar Connexions. The cerebellum is linked up with the cerebrum, the brainstem and the spinal cord by numerous efferent and afferent tracts, which are collected into three great bundles on each side, termed the cerebellar peduncles.

The *Superior Cerebellar Peduncle* emerges from the upper part of the anterior cerebellar notch, and runs upwards and forwards lateral to the upper half of the roof of the fourth ventricle, to enter the lower part of the midbrain. It contains a very large percentage of *efferent* fibres. These arise in the dentate and in the roof nuclei, decussate in the lower part of the midbrain, and terminate partly in the red nucleus and partly in the thalamus of the opposite side. In addition, the superior peduncle contains one *afferent* tract, viz., the ventral spinocerebellar tract, the fibres of which are distributed to the cortex of the palæocerebellum.

The *Middle Cerebellar Peduncle* is formed by the transverse fibres of the pons (p. 319), and the vast majority of its fibres are *afferent* to the cerebellum. They represent cerebrocerebellar connexions, and are distributed therefore to the neocerebellum.

The *Inferior Cerebellar Peduncle* is formed in the medulla oblongata and includes a large number of tracts, for the most part *afferent* to the cerebellum. (1) The dorsal spinocerebellar tract from the spinal cord; distributed to the anterior portions of the vermis, *i.e.*, palæocerebellum. (2) The olivocerebellar tract from the lower and more recently acquired part of the olivary nucleus; distributed to the cortex of the hemisphere, *i.e.*, neocerebellum. (3) Fibres from the upper, older portion of the olivary nucleus and from the accessory olivary nuclei; distributed to the vermis, *i.e.*, palæocerebellum. (4) Vestibulocerebellar fibres from the vestibular nerve direct and from the vestibular nuclei; distributed to the archicerebellum. (5) External arcuate fibres from the cuneate nuclei of both sides; distributed to the neocerebellum. In addition to the afferent tracts, the inferior cerebellar peduncle contains *efferent* cerebellovestibular fibres, which arise in the dentate and roof nuclei and pass to the vestibular nuclei.

Fibres from the floccular peduncles travel direct to the vestibular nuclei and possibly to the nuclei of the oculomotor, trochlear, trigeminal and abducent nerves.

The **Fourth Ventricle** is situated between the cerebellum behind, and the upper part of the medulla oblongata and the lower part of the pons in front. Its upper angle becomes continuous with the aqueduct of the midbrain, and its lower angle with the central canal of the spinal cord. Each lateral angle is drawn out to form a tubular pouch, termed the *lateral recess;* it extends in a lateral direction, at first behind and then below the inferior cerebellar peduncle, and can be seen on the basal surface of the brain, where it overlies the medial part of the flocculus. Each lateral recess opens at its extremity into the subarachnoid space and a part of the choroid plexus of the fourth ventricle protrudes from the opening, which is termed the *foramen of the lateral recess.*

The *floor* of the fourth ventricle is diamond-shaped (rhombic) in outline, and is crossed at its widest point by the transversely running *striæ medullares* (auditory striæ, p. 333), which conveniently divide it into upper or pontine, and lower or medullary, portions. The latter is bounded on each side by the gracile tubercle, the cuneate tubercle and the inferior cerebellar peduncle. The floor is divided into right and left halves by a median groove. To the lateral side of the groove an elongated triangular elevation, placed with its apex directed downwards, overlies the nucleus of the twelfth nerve, and

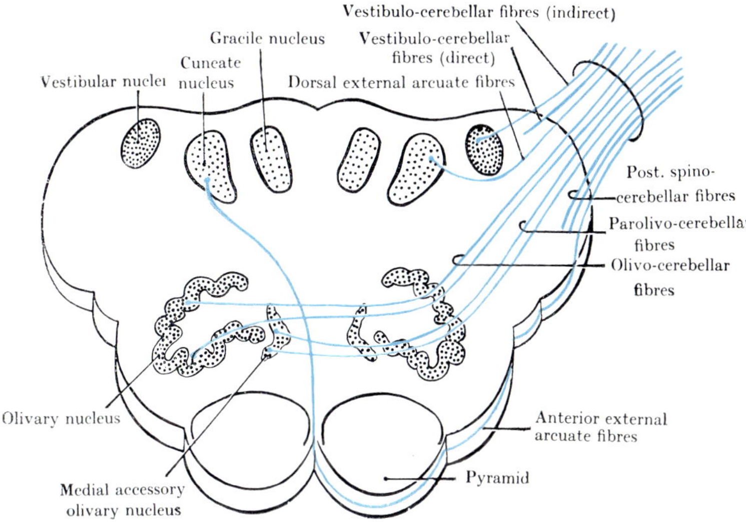

Diagram of a section through the Medulla Oblongata to show the constitution of the Inferior Cerebellar Peduncle.

To face p. 324

to the subthalamic region, and gives origin to the oculomotor and trochlear pairs of cranial nerves.

Its dorsal, or posterior, aspect is occupied by the *colliculi* (*corpora quadrigemina*), which are subdivided by a vertical and a transverse groove into a superior and an inferior pair. The *superior colliculi* are centres for *visual* reflexes (p. 338), and the *inferior* are lower *auditory* centres. Below, in the median plane, the groove between the inferior colliculi is continuous with the superior medullary velum, from which the trochlear nerves emerge. *This is the only one of the twelve cranial nerves to emerge from the dorsal aspect of the brainstem*, and it winds round the lateral aspect of the midbrain to gain the cisterna interpeduncularis. It then runs forwards below the third nerve, and enters the lateral wall of the cavernous sinus by piercing the dura mater near the point where the free and the attached borders of the tentorium cerebelli cross each other.

On the lateral aspect of the midbrain the *superior* and *inferior brachia* run upwards and forwards from the superior and inferior colliculi, respectively. They disappear from view near the pulvinar of the thalamus. The *medial geniculate body* (p. 357), which is a derivative of the diencephalon, forms a small oval elevation on the upper part of the lateral aspect of the midbrain. It hides the inferior brachium, and is partly obscured by the overhanging thalamus. The medial geniculate and the inferior colliculi constitute the *lower auditory centres.*

The ventral or anterior aspect of the midbrain is deeply notched in the median plane and the rope-like strand which projects forwards and limits the interpeduncular fossa on each side is termed the *cerebral peduncle.* It corresponds to the pyramid of the medulla oblongata but, in addition to the cerebrospinal fibres, it contains a large number of cerebropontine fibres, which terminate below in the nuclei pontis. The oculomotor nerve emerges from a groove on the medial side of the basis pedunculi.

THE INTERNAL STRUCTURE OF THE MIDBRAIN

On transverse section of the midbrain the *aqueduct* is easily recognisable, surrounded by the *central grey matter.* The region dorsal to it is termed the *tectum*, and consists of the grey and white matter of the colliculi. The region ventral to the aqueduct constitutes the cerebral peduncles, which are separated ventrally by a deep notch. The peduncles resemble the pons in structure; on each side a sheet of deeply pigmented grey matter, the *substantia nigra*, divides each peduncle into a *crus cerebri* in front and *tegmentum* behind. Owing to the notch referred to above, the crura are separated from each other, but the tegmentum is continued uninterruptedly across

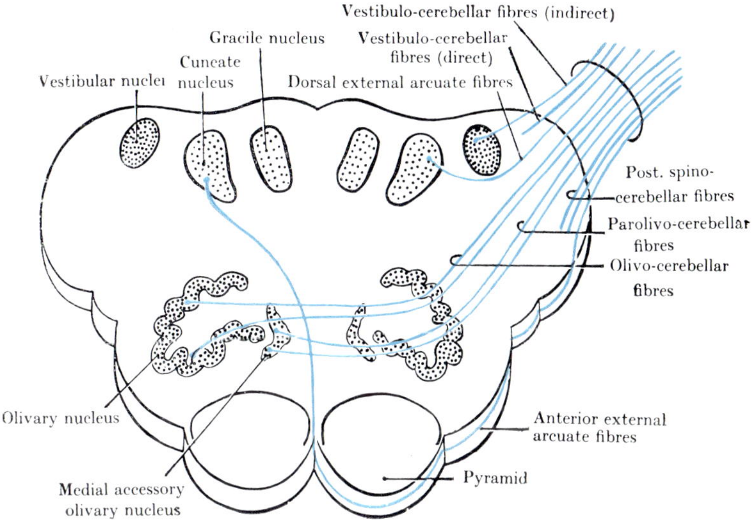

Diagram of a section through the Medulla Oblongata to show the constitution of the Inferior Cerebellar Peduncle.

is termed the *trigonum hypoglossi*. Lateral to the trigonum hypoglossi is the *trigonum vagi*, placed with its apex upwards and close to the striæ auditoriæ. It is usually slightly depressed, and it overlies the dorsal nucleus of the vagus. The lateral angle of the medullary portion of the floor is occupied by the *vestibular area*.

The *pontine portion* of the floor is marked by the upward continuation of the median groove, and lateral to it there is a small rounded elevation, which is continued upwards as a faint rounded ridge. These constitute respectively the *facial colliculus* and the *medial eminence*. The former overlies the nucleus of the sixth nerve. On each side this part of the floor is bounded by the superior cerebellar peduncle as it sweeps upwards and forwards from the cerebellum to the midbrain.

The *roof*, or posterior wall, of the fourth ventricle is drawn backwards towards the cerebellum. In its upper part it consists of the medial borders of the two superior cerebellar peduncles and a connecting sheet of white matter, termed the *superior medullary velum*. Its lower part is also divisible into two areas. The upper is occupied by the *inferior medullary velum* on each side and by the white matter on the upper surface of the root of the nodule in the median plane. Owing to the fact that the roof is drawn back into the cerebellum in a tent-like manner, this part of the cavity of the ventricle forms a recess with an upper wall, formed by the lower end of the superior medullary velum, and a lower wall, formed by the upper surface of the root of the nodule. On each side of the median plane the roof contains similar but wider recesses.

The lower half of the lower part of the roof consists of ependyma and pia mater in contact with each other and contains no nerve tissue. This part of the roof is pierced by the wide *median aperture*, which connects the interior of the ventricular system to the subarachnoid space, and so enables the cerebrospinal fluid to drain away into the latter. Two similar foramina are placed at the drawn-out lateral angles of the roof (*foramina of the lateral recesses*).

The thin, lower part of the roof is invaginated into the interior of the cavity by the *choroid plexus of the fourth ventricle*. This plexus is quite a distinct structure from the similarly named plexuses in the lateral and third ventricles, although its mode of formation is almost identical. A portion of the plexus is thrust out through the foramen of the lateral recess on each side, and can be seen from the anterior aspect of the brainstem immediately behind the emerging rootlets of the glossopharyngeal nerve and in front of the flocculus (p. 324).

The **Midbrain** (Mesencephalon) connects the pons and cerebellum to the subthalamic region, and gives origin to the oculomotor and trochlear pairs of cranial nerves.

Its dorsal, or posterior, aspect is occupied by the *colliculi* (*corpora quadrigemina*), which are subdivided by a vertical and a transverse groove into a superior and an inferior pair. The *superior colliculi* are centres for *visual* reflexes (p. 338), and the *inferior* are lower *auditory* centres. Below, in the median plane, the groove between the inferior colliculi is continuous with the superior medullary velum, from which the trochlear nerves emerge. *This is the only one of the twelve cranial nerves to emerge from the dorsal aspect of the brainstem*, and it winds round the lateral aspect of the midbrain to gain the cisterna interpeduncularis. It then runs forwards below the third nerve, and enters the lateral wall of the cavernous sinus by piercing the dura mater near the point where the free and the attached borders of the tentorium cerebelli cross each other.

On the lateral aspect of the midbrain the *superior* and *inferior brachia* run upwards and forwards from the superior and inferior colliculi, respectively. They disappear from view near the pulvinar of the thalamus. The *medial geniculate body* (p. 357), which is a derivative of the diencephalon, forms a small oval elevation on the upper part of the lateral aspect of the midbrain. It hides the inferior brachium, and is partly obscured by the overhanging thalamus. The medial geniculate and the inferior colliculi constitute the *lower auditory centres*.

The ventral or anterior aspect of the midbrain is deeply notched in the median plane and the rope-like strand which projects forwards and limits the interpeduncular fossa on each side is termed the *cerebral peduncle*. It corresponds to the pyramid of the medulla oblongata but, in addition to the cerebrospinal fibres, it contains a large number of cerebropontine fibres, which terminate below in the nuclei pontis. The oculomotor nerve emerges from a groove on the medial side of the basis pedunculi.

THE INTERNAL STRUCTURE OF THE MIDBRAIN

On transverse section of the midbrain the *aqueduct* is easily recognisable, surrounded by the *central grey matter*. The region dorsal to it is termed the *tectum*, and consists of the grey and white matter of the colliculi. The region ventral to the aqueduct constitutes the cerebral peduncles, which are separated ventrally by a deep notch. The peduncles resemble the pons in structure; on each side a sheet of deeply pigmented grey matter, the *substantia nigra*, divides each peduncle into a *crus cerebri* in front and *tegmentum* behind. Owing to the notch referred to above, the crura are separated from each other, but the tegmentum is continued uninterruptedly across the median plane. The tegmentum corresponds to the dorsal part of the pons and contains the upward continuation of the same tracts.

It is of benefit to examine two transverse sections, one through the inferior and the other through the superior colliculi.

1. *Section at the Level of the Inferior Colliculi.* The crus, which contains important descending tracts, is separated from the tegmentum by the substantia nigra. The *cerebrospinal tract* occupies the middle third of the crus and it is flanked medially by the *frontopontine* fibres, and laterally by the *temporo-* and *occipito-pontine fibres.* These three groups connect the cerebral cortex to the pons, and so with the cerebellum (p. 324). The *substantia nigra* is a mixed nucleus, which extends from the upper border of the pons into the subthalamic region. It receives afferent fibres from the motor cortex, corpus striatum, and red nucleus and some of its efferent fibres may reach ventral grey column cells in the spinal cord. It is regarded as a part of the extrapyramidal system and is concerned with muscle tone (p. 353).

The tegmentum of the midbrain contains the important ascending tracts and several nuclear masses of grey matter. The *medial lemniscus* ascends dorsal to the substantia nigra, and the *lateral lemniscus* stretches backwards from its lateral extremity (Fig. 10). The *trigeminal* and *spinal lemnisci* are associated with the lateral part of the medial lemniscus.

In the ventral part of the central grey matter the *motor nucleus of the trochlear nerve* lies close to the median plane and on the dorsal aspect of the *medial longitudinal bundle.* Lateral to the aqueduct are the *mesencephalic nuclei of the trigeminal nerve* (p. 331). The whole of the central portion of the tegmentum is occupied by the *decussation of the superior cerebellar peduncles* (Fig. 10), which continue upwards after crossing the median plane.

The grey matter of the inferior colliculus lies dorsal to the central grey matter and under the corresponding surface elevation. It receives many of the terminal fibres of the lateral lemniscus.

2. *Section at the Level of the Superior Colliculi.* As regards the position of the substantia nigra and the constituents of the cerebral peduncle there is but little difference from Section 1.

In the tegmentum the *medial* and *spinal lemnisci* occupy approximately the same positions as in Section 1, but the lateral lemniscus does not extend upwards to this level.

The *Red Nucleus* is an ovoid mass of grey matter which extends through the upper half of the midbrain into the subthalamic region. It lies dorsal to the medial part of the substantia nigra and medial to the medial lemniscus, and its upper end is dorso-medial to the subthalamic nucleus (p. 359). It is related superiorly to the thalamus and inferiorly to the ascending fibres of the superior cerebellar peduncle, by which it is surrounded. *Afferent* fibres reach the red nucleus from (1) the cerebellum, *viâ* the superior cerebellar peduncle; (2) the globus pallidus of the lentiform nucleus, *viâ* the striatorubral

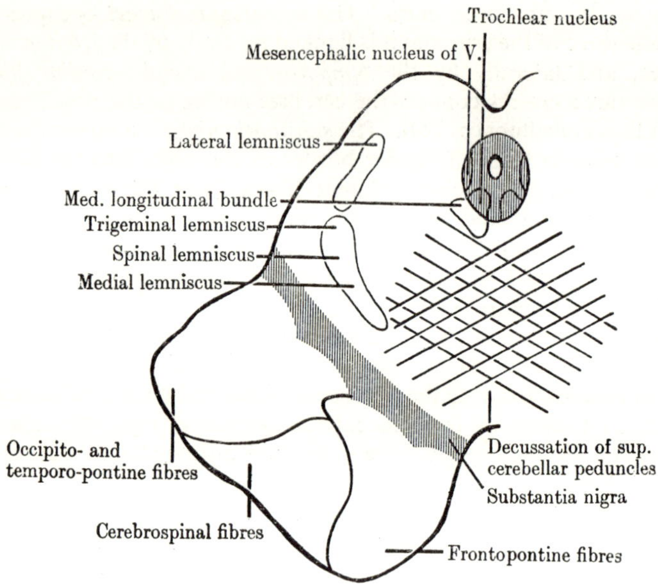

FIG. 10. Diagram of a Transverse Section through the right half of the Midbrain at the level of the Inferior Corpus Quadrigeminum.

pathway (p. 352); the subthalamic nucleus (p. 359); and (4) the cerebral cortex, though the existence of corticorubral connexions is still uncertain. *Efferent* fibres leave the red nucleus and pass (1) to the spinal cord, *viâ* the rubrospinal tract (p. 312); (2) to the grey matter of the reticular formation in the brainstem and possibly the spinal cord, *viâ* the rubroreticular tract (*vide infra*); (3) to the thalamus; and (4) and to the subthalamic nucleus.

It is generally believed that the red nucleus, through the rubrospinal, rubroreticular and perhaps other tracts, exercises an inhibitory influence on muscle tonus. (See also p. 352.)

The *rubroreticular tract* arises from the cells of the red nucleus, crosses the median plane immediately, and descends in the reticular formation of the brainstem.

The *oculomotor nucleus* is described in the following section.

The grey matter of the *superior colliculus* lies under the corresponding surface elevation. It receives afferent fibres from the spino-tectal tract, the visual cortex and the optic nerve. The efferent fibres form the tectospinal and the tectobulbar tracts, which curve forwards round the central grey matter and form the

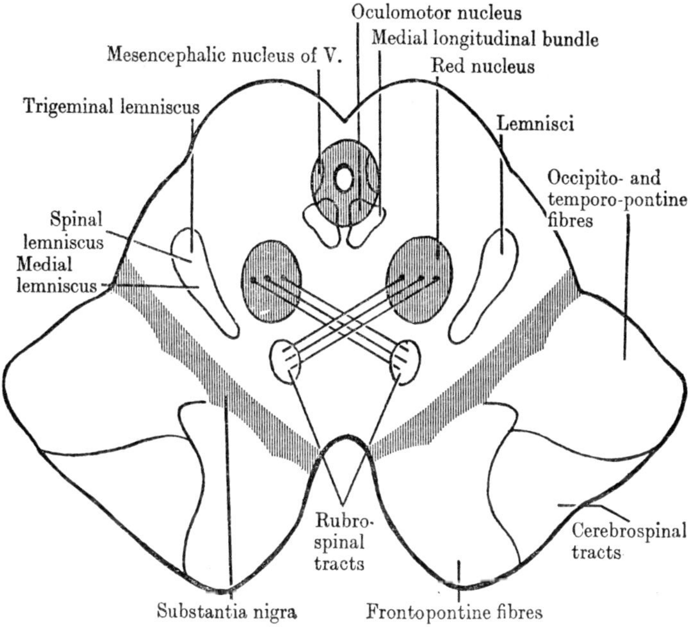

FIG. 11. Diagram of a Transverse Section through the Midbrain, at the level of the Superior Colliculi (*After Herrick.*)

dorsal tegmental decussation. They may connect the tectum to motor cells in the spinal cord and nuclei of the third, fourth, sixth and eleventh cranial nerves and are responsible for the reflex movements of the eyes, head and neck in response to visual stimuli. The fibres which form the afferent pathway from the retina for the *light reflex* end in the *pretectal nucleus*, a small collection of nerve cells lying deep to the supero-lateral part of the superior colliculus. Relayed there, the path passes to the accessory oculomotor (Edinger-Westphal) nucleus (p. 330) and thence to the oculomotor nerve.

THE CENTRAL CONNEXIONS OF CRANIAL NERVES III—X

The deep connexions of the olfactory nerve (pp. 337, 350) and the path of the visual fibres (p. 337) will be described later.

The **Oculomotor Nerve,** which supplies all the muscles of the orbit, with the exception of the superior oblique and the lateral rectus, arises from a nucleus which is situated in the ventral part of the grey matter surrounding the aqueduct of the midbrain on a level with the superior colliculus (Fig. 11). The medial longitudinal bundle lies ventral to the nucleus and, in all probability, constitutes the main channel for connexions between the oculomotor nucleus and the nuclei of the vestibular nerve. The nucleus may receive afferent fibres from the cerebrospinal tract of both sides, but this is unproven. Its outgoing fibres pass ventrally through the midbrain to emerge at the sulcus oculomotorius. It receives afferent fibres from the superior colliculus *viâ* the tectobulbar tract.

The oculomotor nucleus comprises a number of distinct cell-groups, which are associated with particular muscles. Perfect co-ordination of muscles plays an essential part in connexion with binocular vision. Thus, the superior oblique and the inferior rectus of both sides, in downward movements, the inferior oblique and the superior rectus of both sides, in upward movements, and the lateral rectus of one side and the opposite medial rectus, in side to side movements, must always exhibit perfect co-ordination, otherwise double vision will result. Nevertheless, it is most improbable that any movement does not involve all the muscles, since all must shorten or lengthen with any movement of the globe. The central control must therefore be highly complex.

The accessory nucleus, a paired small-celled nucleus placed immediately cranial to the oculomotor nucleus, gives origin to the preganglionic parasympathetic fibres which run in the oculomotor nerve to the ciliary ganglion where they are relayed to the ciliary muscle and the sphincter pupillæ, constituting the *efferent pathway for the light reflex*. (N.B. The majority of these fibres control the ciliaris and are therefore concerned with accommodation).

The **Trochlear Nerve,** which supplies the superior oblique muscle of the orbit (p. 275), arises from a nucleus which is practically continuous with the lowest cell-group in the nucleus of the oculomotor nerve. It occupies a similar position with reference to the central grey matter and the medial longitudinal bundle, but it lies on a level with the inferior colliculus (Fig. 10). The course of the outgoing fibres is peculiar. *They curve backwards and medially, decussate with the corresponding fibres of the opposite side in the superior medullary velum, and emerge from the dorsal aspect of the midbrain* below the inferior colliculus (p. 326).

The deep connexions of the **Trigeminal Nerve** are as follows.

(*a*) The *motor nucleus* is placed in the dorso-lateral part of the dorsal portion of the pons (Fig. 9, p. 321). It receives afferent fibres from the cerebrospinal tract both of the same and of the opposite side (Fig. 5, p. 313), and its outgoing fibres run forwards and laterally to reach the ventral surface of the pons, where they have already been examined (p. 314).

(*b*) The *superior sensory nucleus* lies in the dorsal part of the pons (Fig. 8), ventrolateral to the motor nucleus, and it is continuous below with the *nucleus of the spinal tract* of the trigeminal nerve, which extends downwards throughout the whole length of the medulla oblongata (Figs. 6, 7, 8) into the upper part of the spinal cord. The incoming fibres of the sensory root of the trigeminal divide into short ascending and longer descending branches. The former terminate in the superior nucleus, and the latter in the nucleus of the spinal tract, constituting the *spinal tract* of the trigeminal nerve (Fig. 7). It would appear that fibres conveying tactile and pressure stimuli terminate in the superior sensory nucleus, whereas those conveying painful and thermal stimuli end in the nucleus of the spinal tract. The upper end of the latter receives fibres from the mandibular nerve, while its lower end is associated with the ophthalmic nerve, and its intermediate part with the maxillary nerve.

(*c*) In addition, the trigeminal nerve possesses a *mesencephalic part*, which passes upwards in the lateral part of the pons and terminates in a nucleus placed in the lateral part of the central grey matter of the midbrain (Fig. 10, p. 328). Its fibres, though sensory, pass through the trigeminal ganglion without being interrupted and then travel in the sensory root of the nerve. They probably convey proprioceptive impulses from the muscles of mastication and, perhaps, also from the muscles of the orbit.

New fibres arise in the superior sensory nucleus and the nucleus of the spinal tract, and they cross to the opposite side. There to ascend as the *trigeminal lemniscus* to the thalamus.

The **Abducens Nerve** arises from a *motor nucleus* in the dorsal part of the pons. It is placed close to the median plane, beneath the floor of the fourth ventricle and dorsolateral to the medial longitudinal bundle (Fig. 8, p. 319). It will be seen that the position of this nucleus in the pons is very similar to that occupied by the trochlear and by the oculomotor nucleus in the midbrain and all three belong to the somatic efferent column.

The nucleus of the abducens receives afferent fibres from the cerebrospinal tract of both sides, and is brought into communication with the tectum by the tectobulbar tract and with the oculomotor and vestibular nuclei through the medial longitudinal bundle. The relation of the emerging fibres of the facial nerve to the sixth nucleus is described below.

The **Facial Nerve** arises from a *motor nucleus* which lies in the ventrolateral part of the dorsal portion of the pons, medial to the nucleus of the spinal tract of the trigeminal (Fig. 8, p. 319). It receives fibres from the cerebrospinal tract, principally of the opposite side, and its outgoing fibres have a peculiar course. They run at first dorsally and medially till they reach the abducens nucleus, where they curve medially between the nucleus and the floor of the fourth ventricle. Coming into relationship with the dorsal aspect of the medial longitudinal bundle, the fibres ascend on the medial aspect of the abducens nucleus and then curve laterally and forwards (Fig. 6, p. 315). Finally they retrace their course through the substance of the pons, and, passing between the facial nucleus and the nucleus of the spinal tract of the trigeminal, they emerge on the ventral surface of the pons near its lower border (p. 315).

Some of the outgoing fibres of the facial nerve are parasympathetic fibres. They arise from the *superior salivary nucleus* in the pons, and constitute the secretomotor fibres for the submandibular and sublingual salivary glands (p. 266). They leave the facial nerve in the chorda tympani, by which they are conveyed to the lingual nerve and the submandibular ganglion.

It should be noted that the abducens nucleus and the outgoing fibres of the facial nerve together raise the facial colliculus of the fourth ventricle (p. 325).

The fibres of the sensory part of the facial nerve arise in the ganglion of the nerve (p. 373) and run centrally to terminate in the upper part of the *nucleus* of the *tractus solitarius* (p. 317).

The **Vestibulocochlear (Auditory, Stato-acoustic) Nerve** consists of two quite distinct parts, viz., the cochlear division and the vestibular division.

The fibres of the **Cochlear Nerve,** which is the path for auditory impulses, arise in the spiral ganglion of the cochlea and run medially to enter the lower border of the pons, on the lateral side of the emerging facial nerve and separated from it by the vestibular nerve. Most of the fibres end in the *ventral* and *dorsal cochlear nuclei*, so called from their relation to the inferior cerebellar peduncle (Fig. 12).

From the *ventral cochlear nucleus* new fibres arise and run medially through the pons, forming the *corpus trapezoideum* (Fig. 12). After crossing the median plane, they ascend through the dorsal part of the pons and midbrain as the *lateral lemniscus*. The latter terminates in the inferior colliculus and medial geniculate body, which constitute the *lower auditory centres*.

From the *dorsal cochlear nucleus* most of the fibres sweep medially to the median plane. At the median plane they decussate with the corresponding fibres of the opposite side, and ultimately join the

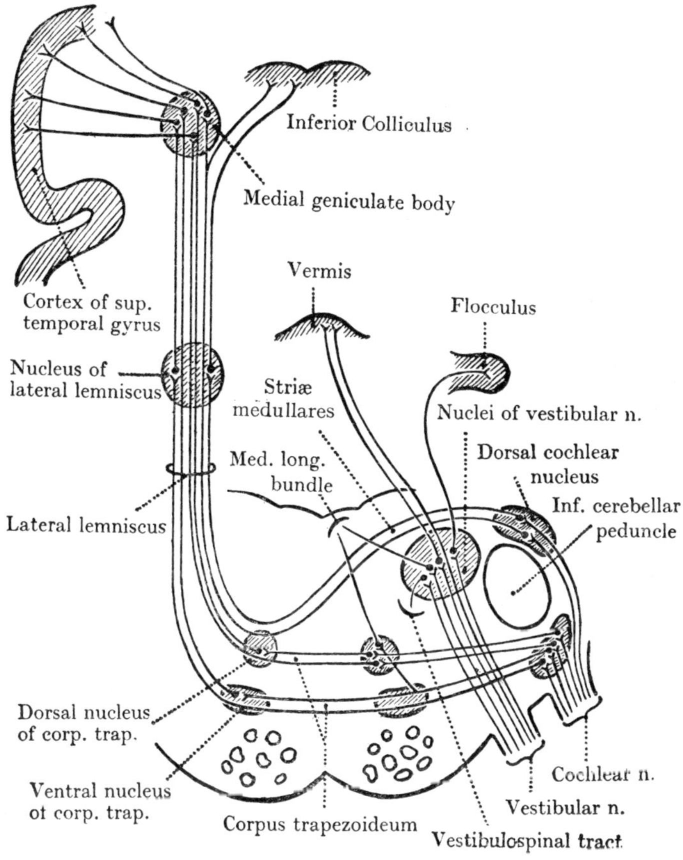

FIG. 12. Schematic representation of the connexions of the Vestibulocochlear Nerve (*After Morris.*) *N.B.*—The vestibular nuclei are shown as a single group.

lateral lemniscus. (N.B. These fibres are not those often still referred to as the auditory striæ of the fourth ventricle, *v.* p. 324).

Many of the fibres of the corpus trapezoideum and the lateral lemniscus have cell-stations in, or give collaterals to, the ventral and dorsal nuclei of the corpus trapezoideum and the nucleus of the lateral lemniscus (Fig. 12). From the dorsal nucleus of the corpus trapezoideum fibres pass to the medial longitudinal bundle and so gain access to the nuclei of the third, fourth and sixth cranial nerves.

By this means auditory impressions may produce reflex movements of the eyes.

The fibres of the **Vestibular Nerve** arise in the *vestibular ganglion*, which is placed on the nerve in the internal auditory meatus, and they enter the pons close to the medial side of the cochlear nerve. After passing dorsally, medial to the inferior cerebellar peduncle, they divide into ascending and descending branches.

Its fibres terminate in *the lateral vestibular nucleus*, which lies under the medial part of the auditory tubercle of the fourth ventricle (Fig. 12), and perhaps in other vestibular nuclei. Fibres from them, and also direct fibres of the vestibular nerve, reach the cortex of the palæocerebellum (p. 324).

Important connexions are established between the vestibular nuclei and the motor nuclei, especially of the third, fourth, sixth and eleventh cranial nerves through the medial longitudinal bundle, and equally important are the connexions established with the motor cells in the anterior column of the grey matter of the spinal cord through the *vestibulospinal tract* (Fig. 12). This tract (p. 312) starts from the large motor cells of the lateral vestibular nucleus, and its fibres run downwards through the same side of the brainstem and spinal cord. Through these connexions impulses arising in the membranous labyrinth can influence the movements of the eyes, head, neck and trunk.

Although, as set out above, the cochlear and vestibular nerves have quite different connexions, to a certain extent these connexions are shared. For example, cochlear nerve fibres can be traced into the lateral vestibular nucleus and fibres from the vestibular nuclei contribute to the corpus trapezoideum. Both divisions of the nerve, therefore, are capable of causing reflex movements of the eyes, head, neck and trunk.

The **Glossopharyngeal Nerve** is closely associated with the vagus nerve in its origin. The *motor fibres* arise from the upper end of the *nucleus ambiguus* (p. 318), which extends through the medulla oblongata dorsal to the olivary nucleus (Fig. 13). The *secretomotor fibres* arise from the *inferior salivary nucleus*, and leave the medulla in the glossopharyngeal nerve. They are destined for the parotid gland (p. 266). (The superior (p. 332) and inferior salivary nuclei are groups of small cells at the uppermost level of the dorsal vagal nucleus, just bellow the lower end of the facial nucleus. Their identity is not universally accepted.)

The *sensory fibres* terminate in the *nucleus of the tractus solitarius* (p. 317), which extends through the medulla oblongata, lying lateral to the dorsal nucleus of the vagus (Fig. 13).

The **Vagus Nerve** possesses *two motor nuclei.* Those motor fibres which innervate branchial muscle (*e.g.*, recurrent laryngeal) arise from the *nucleus ambiguus* below the glossopharyngeal. On the other hand, those fibres which innervate unstriped muscle (gastric, cardiac branches, etc.) arise from the *dorsal nucleus of the vagus*, which lies under the trigonum vagi of the fourth ventricle (p. 317).

The *sensory* fibres of the vagus terminate partly in the *nucleus of the tractus solitarius* and partly in the *dorsal nucleus*, which is a mixed nucleus.

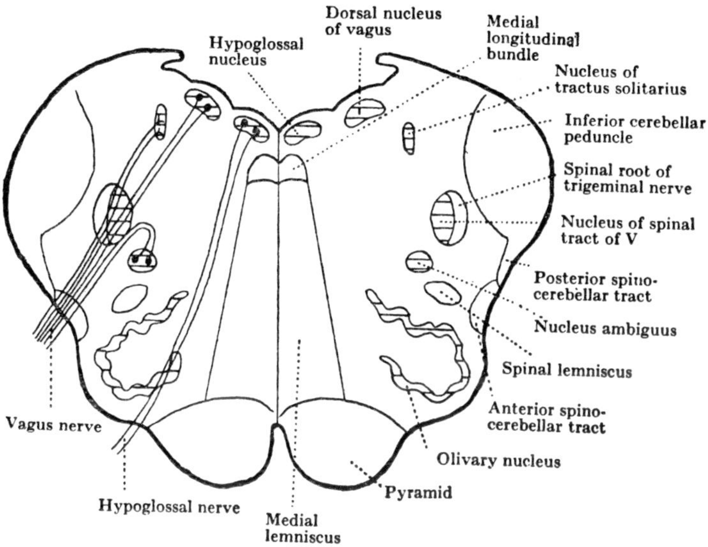

FIG. 13. Diagram of a Transverse Section through the Medulla Oblongata, upper part, showing the constitution of the Vagus Nerve on the right side. The Section passes through the lower part of the Floor of the Fourth Ventricle.

N.B.—Very little is known regarding the further pathways along which afferent visceral impressions pass after reaching the nucleus of the tractus solitarius and the dorsal nucleus of the vagus.

The **Accessory Nerve** contains *motor fibres* which arise from two separate nuclei: (*a*) The fibres which join the vagus and are distributed by it to striped muscle arise from the downward continuation of the *nucleus ambiguus.* (*b*) The branchial fibres which supply the sternomastoid and trapezius muscles arise from the *ventral grey column* of the spinal cord behind the upper five cervical nerves. They emerge from the lateral aspect of the spinal cord *midway between the anterior and posterior nerve roots*, and ascend through the foramen magnum to join the rest of the nerve at the jugular foramen. They also are considered to be branchial.

The **Hypoglossal Nerve** possesses a *motor nucleus* which is placed close to the median plane and immediately under the floor of the fourth ventricle (trigonum hypoglossi, p. 325). Its outgoing fibres run ventrally through the formatio reticularis, and reach the surface at the groove between the pyramid and the olive (Fig. 13), which is in line with the anterior roots of the spinal nerves. The nucleus belongs to the somatic efferent column.

THE CEREBRUM

The cerebrum is derived from the primitive forebrain, which becomes subdivided, at an early stage in development, into a cephalic portion, termed the *telencephalon*, and a caudal portion, termed the *diencephalon*. Two hollow diverticula grow out, one on each side, from the anterior part of the forebrain and their walls constitute the *pallium*. The diverticula become enormously expanded to form the cerebral hemispheres, but their contained cavities retain their communication with the median cavity of the forebrain vesicle and it persists as the *interventricular foramen*. The part of the forebrain which lies caudal to the foramen constitutes the diencephalon (pp. 355 et seq.). It remains relatively small and its cavity forms all but the anterior portion of the third ventricle. The thalamus develops in its lateral wall. The anterior part of the forebrain and the two diverticula constitute the telencephalon.

In lower vertebrates the pallium is almost entirely concerned with the appreciation and interpretation of olfactory impressions, but in higher forms other varieties of sensibility and higher motor centres become increasingly represented in it. As these areas of *neopallium* develop and expand, the olfactory areas, which constitute the *archipallium*, become relegated to the medial and inferior aspects of the hemisphere. In the course of evolution association areas, where sensory impressions coming from different sources can be correlated consciously, are laid down in the neopallium and provide a mechanism which enables the animal to benefit by past experience. In the human brain the archipallium has been reduced both relatively and actually, and its further expansion and elaboration of association areas has enabled man to derive benefit not only from his own past experience but also, through the process of education, from the experience of others. It is no exaggeration of their importance to attribute man's position in the animal kingdom to the size and potentialities of the association areas of the brain.

The **Inferior Surface of the Brain.** Before revising the sulci and gyri on the various surfaces of the hemisphere, the student should first review the inferior surface of the brain as a whole.

The *Interpeduncular Fossa* occupies the central region. It is bounded in front by the *optic chiasma*, antero-laterally by the optic tracts, and postero-laterally by the *cerebral peduncles*. In its anterior part lies the *infundibulum* (p. 359), which has been cut away from the *hypophysis cerebri*, and the flattened area in its immediate neighbourhood is termed the *tuber cinereum*.

The *Corpora Mamillaria* are two small, rounded, surface elevations which lie, one on each side of the median plane, in the posterior part of the interpeduncular fossa. They consist of two nuclei of grey matter and constitute cell-stations apparently on the efferent pathway from the rhinencephalon but probably concerned with visceral sensation. They receive afferent fibres from the anterior columns of the fornix (p. 349) and send efferent fibres to the thalamus (mamillothalamic tract) and to the tegmentum of the brainstem (mamillotegmental tract).

Behind the corpora mamillaria lies the *posterior perforated substance*, in the angle between the bases of the cerebral peduncles. It is pierced by the branches of the posterior cerebral arteries which supply the thalami. The structures in the interpeduncular fossa form constituent parts of the hypothalamus (p. 358).

The **Anterior Perforated Substance** lies lateral to the optic tract and chiasma and medial to the uncus. It is pierced by the central branches from the middle cerebral, which supply the internal capsule, the caudate nucleus and the putamen of the lentiform nucleus.

The **Olfactory Bulb** lies in contact with the orbital surface of the frontal lobe and, inferiorly, rests on the lateral part of the cribriform plate of the ethmoid, through which the olfactory nerves from the nasal mucous membrane (upper third) pass to enter its substance. The *olfactory tract* runs backwards from the bulb and ends by dividing into medial and lateral roots. The former passes medially and ends in the *induseum griseum* of the corpus callosum (pp. 346, 350). The lateral root runs laterally over the lateral part of the anterior perforated substance and then bends medially to terminate in the uncus. The area between the two diverging roots sometimes forms a small elevation, and is termed the *olfactory pyramid*. It is phylogenetically the oldest part of the cortex.

The Path of the Visual Fibres. When the optic nerves are traced backwards from the optic foramina they rapidly converge and are connected to one another to form an X-shaped field of fibres, termed the **Optic Chiasma,** which is the anterior boundary of the inter-peduncular fossa. Its upper surface is attached to the lamina

cortex exhibit a laminated arrangement, which is much more elaborate in the neopallium, where not less than six layers can be identified, than in the archipallium, where typically three layers are present.

Certain gyri are largely associated with particular functions, and these different functional areas show structural variations in their cortex. In certain regions, the differences are sufficiently marked to be recognisable by the naked eye, *e.g.*, the visual cortex, where the *visual stria* stands out prominently on section. It is seen as a thin whitish streak in the grey matter, and is due to the widening of a band of nerve fibres normally found in this situation but visible only with the aid of the microscope. These structural differences begin to develop in the cortex before the sulci make their appearance, and the sulci usually form in the marginal zones between different functional areas.

The introduction of the electroencephalograph has shown that changes in electrical potentials are constantly occurring in the cortex and that these changes are not limited to particular functional areas and are probably associated with similar changes in the subcortical collections of nerve cells. Under normal conditions in waking hours complex wave patterns of varying rhythms are elicited, but as yet little is known about their functional significance.

The *Longitudinal Fissure* separates the two cerebral hemispheres from each other, except in its central part, where the corpus callosum forms its floor. It contains the falx cerebri (p. 363), which projects into it from the cranial vault.

Position. The cerebral hemisphere lies upon the anterior and middle cranial fossæ. It is separated (1) from its fellow by the longitudinal fissure, into which a sickle-shaped fold of dura mater, termed the *falx cerebri*, is projected from the vault, and (2) from the cerebellum by a second fold of dura mater, termed the *tentorium cerebelli*. When the hemisphere is hardened *in situ*, its conformation corresponds to the walls of the space in which it lies. Thus, the *supero-lateral surface* is moulded to the cranial vault, the *medial surface* is flattened, and the *inferior surface* adapts itself to the irregularities of the floor of the anterior and middle cranial fossæ and to the upper surface of the tentorium.

Borders. An arched *supero-medial border* separates the supero-lateral from the medial surface, and abuts on the superior sagittal sinus. A curved *superciliary border* separates the supero-lateral surface from the inferior surface in the anterior cranial fossa. The *infero-lateral border* separates the supero-lateral surface from the inferior surface in the middle cranial fossa. In its posterior part this border abuts on the transverse sinus. A slight depression, often termed the *pre-occipital notch*, can be seen on this border about 2 inches or more in front of the occipital pole. Lastly, a short *infero-medial border* separates the posterior part of the medial surface from the inferior surface, and abuts on the straight sinus.

It is customary, for convenience in description, to divide the hemisphere into lobes, but this subdivision is purely arbitrary, and the lobes do not correspond accurately to the similarly named cranial bones or to any functional or evolutionary pattern.

The Frontal Lobe. On the lateral surface the frontal lobe is bounded *posteriorly* by the **Central Sulcus,** which separates it from the parietal lobe. This sulcus is of prime importance, *for the gyrus in front of it contains the motor cells through which are initiated the movements of the opposite side of the body.* It runs downwards and forwards across the lateral aspect from a little behind the mid-point of the supero-medial border, *and it is the only sulcus of any length on this surface which lies between two parallel and almost vertical convolutions.* The upper end of the central sulcus usually cuts the supero-medial border, but its lower end is separated from the posterior ramus of the lateral sulcus by a narrow bridge of cortex between the gyri which flank it.

Inferiorly, the posterior ramus of the lateral sulcus separates the frontal from the temporal lobe. It runs backwards and slightly upwards, and its posterior end bends sharply upwards into the parietal lobe. *Anteriorly,* it is continuous with the stem of the lateral sulcus, into which, when the brain is *in situ,* the sharp, free border of the lesser wing of the sphenoid projects.

Elsewhere the frontal lobe is bounded by the supero-medial and the superciliary borders.

The *precentral sulcus* lies parallel to, and a short distance in front of, the central sulcus. The *precentral gyrus* is situated between them. The cortex on its surface and lining the whole depth of the anterior wall of the sulcus is the motor area for movements of the opposite side of the body, and it should be carefully noted that in the cortex the body is represented in the inverted position, *i.e., the cells for the lower limb occupy the uppermost part of the convolution and extend over on to the medial surface. Below the lower limb, in order, come the trunk, the upper limb, the neck and the head.* These areas are not sharply marked off from one another, for there is both clinical and experimental evidence that there is considerable overlapping.

It must also be remembered that corresponding muscles of opposite sides of the body, *which are accustomed to work together,* are connected with the cortex of both cerebral hemispheres. For example, the movements of each half of the diaphragm, the movements of both eyes, etc., are represented bilaterally in the cerebral cortex. So it comes about that such movements are not obviously affected by unilateral lesions of the internal capsule.

The area immediately anterior to the precentral sulcus is related functionally to the motor area and is termed the *premotor area.* The successful performance of acts, which involve the execution of a series of movements in a definite order, is dependent on the integrity of the premotor area and its fibre connexions (p. 353).

The *superior* and *inferior frontal sulci* run forwards from the precentral sulcus and subdivide this area into *superior*, *middle*, and *inferior frontal gyri.* The middle frontal convolution is concerned with the movements of conjugate deviation of the eyes to the opposite side, which can be evoked from it.

The inferior frontal gyrus is indented by the *anterior horizontal* and *ascending rami of the lateral sulcus.* The cortex around these two limbs is known as *Broca's area*, and bears the same functional relation to the centres controlling the movements of the lips, tongue and vocal folds as the rest of the premotor area bears to the other parts of the motor cortex. They therefore constitute a motor speech centre. Broca's area consists of (1) a *pars orbitalis* below the horizontal ramus; (2) a *pars triangularis*, between the two rami; and (3) a *pars posterior*, behind the ascending ramus. It may be observed that the pars posterior is directly continuous with the cortex at the lower end of the precentral gyrus. Right-handed persons educate this region on the left side of the brain.

The anterior part of the frontal lobe is often known as a "silent area" of the brain, for clinical evidence shows that it may suffer very extensive damage often with little result, nor does stimulation produce observable effects. It receives numerous association fibres from the other sensory areas and determines the personal reactions of the individual in the light of past experience. It is therefore probably responsible for the higher control of conduct and behaviour. In addition, through its connexions with the medial nucleus of the thalamus, it may be regarded as exercising an influence over emotional or instinctive reactions to visceral stimuli (p. 360). The operation of "leucotomy," introduced of late years for the treatment of certain varieties of mental disease, aims at dividing the projection fibres proceeding to and from this area of the cortex.

Recent experimental work has shown that the activity of the motor and premotor cortex can be inhibited by stimulation of certain limited cortical areas which have been termed "suppressor areas" or "bands." Of these, one forms a narrow strip along the precentral sulcus and another an irregular strip at the junction of the premotor area and the anterior part of the frontal lobe. Similar bands have been found along the postcentral sulcus, in the anterior boundary of the occipital lobe and in the anterior part of the gyrus cinguli.

These areas or bands project on to the caudate nucleus, whence impulses reach the thalamus and are relayed back to the motor cortex. The inhibition of movements induced in this way is associated with the power of concentration and attention, which are usually regarded as functions of the anterior part of the frontal lobe, but the precise significance of these suppressor bands or strips is still not clear.

The **Parietal Lobe** is bounded in front by the central sulcus and above by the supero-medial border of the hemisphere. Posteriorly, it is demarcated from the occipital lobe by a line drawn from the parieto-occipital sulcus to the pre-occipital notch on the infero-lateral border. The *parieto-occipital sulcus* cuts the supero-medial border about 2 inches from the occipital pole. Inferiorly, the parietal lobe is limited by the horizontal part of the posterior ramus of the lateral sulcus, and a line drawn backwards from it to meet the posterior boundary. The limits of the parietal lobe on the supero-lateral aspect of the hemisphere are therefore very artificial.

The *postcentral sulcus*, which may be divided into upper and lower parts, lies parallel to, and a little behind, the central sulcus. The *postcentral gyrus* is placed between them. *It is a reception area for somesthetic sensibility*. Here and in the adjoining parietal region tactile, painful and other impressions are received, evaluated, localised and interpreted in the light of past experience. It should be noted that a disproportionately large area is associated with the hand of the opposite side. From the post-central salcus the *intra-parietal sulcus* runs backwards, nearly parallel to the supero-medial border, and may extend into the occipital lobe (*ramus occipitalis*). In this way a *superior parietal lobule* is demarcated from an *inferior parietal lobule*. Gross lesions of the latter produce the interesting and diagnostic sign of *astereognosis*, since it is in this region that visual and tactile impressions become associated. The inferior parietal lobule is cut into from below by the upturned ends of (1) the posterior ramus of the lateral sulcus, (2) the superior, and (3) the middle temporal sulci. Typically, the ends of these sulci are capped by arcuate gyri, termed the anterior, middle and posterior parts of the inferior parietal lobule. The anterior part lies under cover of the parietal eminence and can therefore be conveniently marked out on the surface. In and around the middle part, often termed the angular gyrus, on the left side there is an important sensory speech centre.

The whole of the parietal lobe behind the post-central sulcus and the adjoining parts of the occipital and temporal lobes constitute a large association area where visual, tactile and auditory impressions are correlated.

The **Temporal Lobe** is separated from the occipital lobe by the line drawn from the parieto-occipital sulcus to the pre-occipital notch, and from the frontal and parietal lobes by the posterior ramus of the lateral sulcus and its backward continuation.

The *superior temporal sulcus* runs parallel to the posterior ramus of the lateral sulcus, and its posterior extremity turns upwards into the parietal lobe, where it is surrounded by the middle part of the inferior parietal lobule. The *superior temporal gyrus* lies immediately above this sulcus. It contains the *auditory area*, which extends into the *transverse temporal gyrus* lying in the floor of the posterior ramus of the lateral sulcus behind the insula.

The *middle temporal gyrus* lies below the superior temporal sulcus and is bounded inferiorly by an interrupted sulcus, which is termed the *inferior temporal sulcus.*

The **Occipital Lobe** forms the posterior extremity of the supero-lateral surface of the cerebral hemisphere. Its boundaries have already been indicated. It is cut into above by the *intraparietal sulcus* (*ramus occipitalis*), and this sulcus separates the posterior part of the inferior parietal lobule from the arched gyrus which surrounds the end of the parieto-occipital sulcus.

The **Insula** is a submerged part of the cortex of the lateral aspect of the hemisphere. It lies at the bottom of the posterior ramus of the lateral sulcus, surrounded by a *circular sulcus*. The parts of the cortex which overlap it are termed the *opercula*, and these are four in number, viz., the temporal, the orbital, the frontal and the frontoparietal.

The Medial Surface of the Cerebral Hemisphere. The great white commissure, termed the *corpus callosum*, is a striking feature of this surface. In median sagittal sections of the brain the pointed rostrum, the anterior genu, the elongated body, and the rounded posterior end or splenium are easily recognised.

The *cingulate sulcus* begins below the rostrum, about midway between it and the margin of the hemisphere, and follows the curvature of the corpus callosum, separated from it by the *cingulate gyrus*. Opposite the splenium the cingulate sulcus turns upwards and cuts the supero-medial border of the hemisphere just behind the upper end of the central sulcus. The *medial frontal gyrus*, which lies above the sulcus, forms the medial surface of the frontal lobe, and immediately in front of the upper end of the central sulcus it contains the motor area for the movements of the toes, foot and ankle of the opposite side. This portion of the gyrus is termed the *paracentral lobule* and clinical evidence suggests strongly that it is also concerned with voluntary control of the defecation and micturition reflexes.

The *cingulate gyrus* is continued backwards round the splenium of the corpus callosum, and is separated from the parietal lobe by the interrupted *suprasplenial sulcus*.

The *precuneus* lies behind the upturned end of the cingulate sulcus and above the suprasplenial sulcus. It forms the medial surface of the parietal lobe, and is separated from the occipital lobe by the parieto-occipital sulcus, the upper end of which cuts the superomedial border of the hemisphere and appears on its supero-lateral surface.

The **Postcalcarine Sulcus** runs forwards from the occipital pole along, or just above, the short infero-medial border of the hemisphere. Anteriorly, it joins the parieto-occipital sulcus, and the two enclose a triangular area of cortex, termed the *cuneus*, which forms the medial surface of the occipital lobe. From the point of union of the two sulci *the calcarine sulcus* runs forwards on the inferior surface and cuts into the cingulate gyrus, so as to separate it, almost completely, from the hippocampal gyrus in front. The narrow part of the cingulate gyrus is termed the *isthmus*.

The visual cortex extends above and below the postcalcarine sulcus and below the calcarine sulcus (see also p. 338). It is this part of the cortex which is characterised by the presence of the visual stria (p. 339) and it is commonly termed the *striate area*.

The posterior end of the postcalcarine sulcus occasionally runs into the *lunate sulcus*, which is set at right angles to it. When present, it marks the posterior limit of the visual cortex.

The **Inferior Surface** of the hemisphere consists of an anterior part or orbital surface, forming the lower aspect of the frontal lobe, and a posterior part or tentorial surface, on which the temporal and occipital lobes appear.

The inferior surface of the frontal lobe rests on the floor of the anterior cranial fossa, and so is in relationship with the orbit, the frontal sinus and nasal cavity. It is bounded behind by the stem of the lateral sulcus.

The *Olfactory Tract* (p. 337), with the olfactory bulb at its anterior end, lies in contact with the medial part of this surface and hides the *olfactory sulcus*. The *gyrus rectus* intervenes between this sulcus and the longitudinal fissure. An H-shaped fissure, with medial, lateral and transverse limbs, indents the inferior surface of the frontal lobe lateral to the olfactory sulcus. Stimulation studies suggest that this part of the cortex is concerned in visceral control (vasomotor, respiratory, and gastric).

The *Tentorial Surface* lies on the floor of the middle cranial fossa and on the tentorium cerebelli, and is therefore related to the tympanum and the tympanic antrum. Its medial part is formed by the *hippocampal gyrus*, which is continuous posteriorly with the cingulate gyrus. The anterior end of this gyrus forms a distinct projection, termed the *uncus*, which receives incoming fibres from the olfactory tract, and is therefore concerned with olfactory impressions. It is separated from the temporal pole by the *rhinal sulcus*. The uncus and the adjoining part of the hippocampal gyrus constitute the *piriform area* of the rhinencephalon (p. 350). On its lateral side the hippocampal gyrus is bounded by the *collateral sulcus*, which begins near the occipital pole and runs forwards, nearly parallel to the calcarine sulcus. The *lingual gyrus*, which forms part of the visual area of the cortex, begins near the occipital pole and lies between the calcarine and the collateral sulci. Anteriorly, it becomes continuous with the hippocampal gyrus.

The *medial occipitotemporal gyrus* lies lateral to the lingual gyrus behind, and to the hippocampal gyrus in front. It is separated from the *lateral occipitotemporal gyrus* by the *occipitotemporal sulcus*.

The **White Substance of the Cerebrum** consists of medullated nerve fibres which, *like all other fibres in the central nervous system, are devoid of neurolemmal sheaths*. These fibres belong to three groups. (1) *Association fibres* run from one part of the cortex to another *in the same hemisphere*. They are therefore ipsilateral, and they vary greatly in length. (2) *Commissural fibres* cross from one hemisphere to the other, and so help to co-ordinate the activities of both. (3) *Projection fibres* run between the spinal cord, brainstem and cerebellum, on the one hand, and the cerebrum, on the other. They may be afferent to, or efferent from, the cerebrum.

(1) The *Short Association Fibres* lie immediately below the cortex and they connect adjoining gyri with one another. The *Long Association Fibres* tend to collect themselves into fasciculi, which can be readily demonstrated in the formalin-hardened brain, when the cortex and the short association fibres have been removed. They are, to a large extent, undeveloped in the area between the insula and the lentiform nucleus (p. 351). Several of these fasciculi are described, and one of them, termed the *Cingulum*, gives its name to the gyrus in which it lies. Commencing below the rostrum of the corpus callosum, the cingulum extends through the cingulate gyrus into the hippocampal gyrus. It gives off fibres and receives additions as it courses backwards, and it serves to bring the various parts of the cortex of the medial aspect of the hemisphere into association with one another and with adjoining cortical areas on the medial and inferior aspects of the hemisphere. Other long association fibres are also grouped together into bundles which, like the cingulum, are constantly receiving and giving off fibres throughout their whole length. Some of these fibres link together the various parts of the cortex which are concerned with the power of speech and the

comprehension of the written and the spoken word. Certain curious types of speech disorder (*e.g.*, word-blindness, with vision unimpaired; word-deafness, with hearing unimpaired) are perhaps attributable to lesions of one or other of the long association bundles.

(2) The *Commissures* of the cerebrum are three in number, viz.: the corpus callosum, which is very much the largest, the anterior commissure and the hippocampal commissure. All three develop in the lamina terminalis and for this reason. It is only in the region of the interventricular foramen that the hemispheres are connected to each other in the early stages of development and it is therefore in this situation that the commissural fibres must find their way across the median plane. The roof of the foramen is ependymal and the floor is occupied by the developing optic chiasma, so that the lamina terminalis is the only available route from one hemisphere to the other.

The earliest commissures to develop are associated with the sense of smell and are archipallial in origin. The anterior commissure, which connects the two olfactory bulbs and piriform areas, passes through the lower end of the lamina terminalis, and the hippocampal commissure, which connects the two hippocampal formations, traverses its upper end, *i.e.*, each takes the shortest course. At a later stage in development, neopallial fibres from the temporal cortex cross the median plane in the anterior commissure. The corpus callosum, which is a purely neopallial commissure, develops later, in the upper end of the lamina terminalis, and in its subsequent growth it curves backwards above the choroidal fissure. As it does so it invades the suprachoroidal part of the hippocampal formation, which it reduces to a thin vestigial layer, termed the *induseum griseum.*

The **Corpus Callosum** lies at the bottom of the longitudinal fissure and is placed nearer to the anterior than to the posterior end of the brain. The rostrum, genu, trunk and splenium of the corpus callosum have been seen already on the medial aspect of the hemisphere (p. 343).

The *Rostrum* is connected to the upper aspect of the optic chiasma by a thin sheet of grey matter, termed the *lamina terminalis* (p. 358). Its lower surface is covered by a thin layer of grey matter, the induseum griseum (pp. 337, 350) which is continued upwards on the genu and backwards on the upper surface of the trunk. The upper surface of the rostrum is attached to the septum pellucidum; its lower surface is related to the anterior cerebral vessels.

The *Genu* is the most anterior part of the corpus callosum, and from it the fibres curve forwards and medially into the frontal lobes, forming the *forceps minor.* The posterior (or deep) aspect gives attachment to the septum pellucidum in the median plane, and on each side forms the anterior limit of the lateral ventricle.

The *Trunk* of the corpus callosum lies at the bottom of the longitudinal fissure in the median plane, and on each side its fibres enter the medial surface of the hemisphere below the gyrus cinguli. *Inferiorly*, it gives attachment to the septum pellucidum in front, and it is closely related to the body of the fornix behind. On each side of the median plane it forms the roof of the lateral ventricle.

The *Splenium* overhangs the dorsal aspect of the midbrain. Below it the tela choroidea (p. 350) enters the transverse fissure of the cerebrum, and from between its layers the great cerebral vein passes backwards to join the straight sinus (p. 365). This vein intervenes between the splenium above, and the pineal body and the superior colliculi below. Traced *laterally*, the fibres of the splenium arch backwards and medially into the occipital lobe on each side, constituting the *forceps major*. These fibres cause a bulging of the medial wall of the posterior horn of the lateral ventricle, which is termed the *bulb of the posterior cornu*. Some of the fibres from the splenium and the posterior part of the trunk form the roof and lateral wall of the posterior horn and the lateral wall of the inferior horn of the lateral ventricle, as they pass laterally into the occipital and temporal lobes. They constitute the *tapetum*.

The **Anterior Commissure** is a small, rounded bundle of fibres, which crosses the median plane immediately in front of the anterior columns of the fornix and behind the upper end of the lamina terminalis. In this situation its posterior aspect can be seen in the anterior wall of the third ventricle. Traced laterally, it passes above the anterior perforated substance and below the corpus striatum, notching the inferior surface of the lentiform nucleus. Some of its fibres join the lateral root of the olfactory tract, but the remainder pass to the cortex of the temporal lobe.

The *Hippocampal Commissure* is described on p. 349.

(3) The *Projection Fibres, all of which traverse the internal capsule*, are described on p. 353.

The **Lateral Ventricle** is an elongated crescentic cavity in the cerebral hemisphere, and represents a diverticulum from the original neural tube. It is lined everywhere by a cubical or columnar ciliated epithelium, which is termed *ependyma*. The lateral ventricle communicates with the cavity of the third ventricle through the *interventricular foramen*. This opening is situated in the anterior part of the medial wall of the ventricle, *and is bounded in front by the anterior column of the fornix, and behind by the anterior end of the thalamus*. It serves, for descriptive purposes, as a dividing line between the anterior horn and the central part of the ventricle.

The *Anterior Horn* passes forwards into the frontal lobe, but its anterior extremity is $1\frac{1}{2}$ inches behind the frontal pole. The large convex head of the caudate nucleus forms the *lateral wall* of the cavity, and obscures the upper surface of the rostrum of the corpus callosum, which forms the *floor*.

The *medial wall* is formed by the septum pellucidum and the anterior column of the fornix. The *roof* is formed by the anterior part of the trunk of the corpus callosum and the *anterior wall* by its genu.

The *Central Part* of the lateral ventricle extends from the interventricular foramen backwards to the posterior end of the thalamus, where it becomes continuous with both the posterior and the inferior horns.

The *floor* contains a number of important structures. Its lateral part is occupied by the *body of the caudate nucleus*, which narrows rapidly as it passes backwards. This structure is separated from the thalamus by a groove which runs backwards and laterally from the interventricular foramen. On the medial side of this groove the floor is occupied by the upper surface of the *thalamus*, which is obscured in its medial part by the *body of the fornix*. It is partly hidden by the *choroid plexus*, which projects into the body of the ventricle through the slit-like interval between the free edge of the body of the fornix and the upper surface of the thalamus. This slit-like interval is the *choroidal fissure*, and through it the vessels of the choroid plexus invaginate the pia mater of the tela choroidea and the ependyma into the interior of the ventricle.

The *roof* is formed by the corpus callosum.

The *medial wall* varies in depth with the size of the septum pellucidum, but it is usually deficient posteriorly, where the floor (body of the fornix) and the roof (corpus callosum) come into apposition with each other.

The *Posterior Horn* curves backwards and medially into the occipital lobe. Its *roof* and *lateral wall* are formed by the tapetum of the corpus callosum, lateral to which lie the fibres of the optic radiation. Its medial wall shows two parallel elevations. The higher is caused by the forceps major, and is termed the *bulb of the posterior cornu*; the lower is produced by the calcarine sulcus, and is termed the *calcar avis*.

The *Inferior Horn* curves forwards, downwards and medially into the temporal lobe. Its *roof* is occupied by the *tail of the caudate nucleus* passing forwards to end in the *amygdaloid nucleus*, which produces an elevation in the anterior part of the roof. The *floor* shows a prominent elevation along its medial border. This is the *hippocampus*, and its anterior end is expanded and faintly furrowed to form the *pes hippocampi.* The cells of the hippocampus, which consists of grey matter, send their axons through its substance on to its upper surface, where they spread out as a thin layer of white matter, the *alveus.* The nerve fibres of the alveus converge on the medial border of the hippocampus, where they form a bundle, known as the *fimbria.* Only the free medial edge of the fimbria can be identified, as it runs backwards to become continuous with the posterior column of the fornix. In a freshly dissected brain the fimbria is hidden from view by the *choroid plexus* of the inferior horn. Lateral to the hippocampus, the collateral fissure forms a slight elevation known as the *eminentia collateralis.*

The *lateral wall* is formed by the tapetum. The *medial wall* is occupied by the lower part of the choroid fissure, through which the choroid plexus enters the inferior horn.

The **Septum Pellucidum (Lucidum)** is a vertical sheet, consisting of grey and white matter, which occupies the interval between the recurved rostrum and the anterior part of the trunk of the corpus callosum. Posteriorly, it is attached to the anterior columns and the body of the fornix, and it occupies the interval between that structure and the corpus callosum. It consists of two layers, with a slit-like cavity between them. As a whole, the septum pellucidum forms a partition between the anterior horns of the lateral ventricles.

The **Fornix** is made up partly of longitudinal, ipsilateral fibres, and partly of commissural fibres. It has long been considered to be purely olfactory in connexions, but there is much recent evidence to assign it a larger role in sensory and visceral functions.

It consists of a *Body,* narrow in front and expanded behind, which lies below the corpus callosum and is closely applied to it. *Inferiorly,* it lies on the tela choroidea and the epithelial roof of the third ventricle in the median plane and it extends laterally into the central part of the lateral ventricle, where it forms part of the floor. *Anteriorly,* the body divides into right and left anterior columns, and each of these rounded bundles turns downwards, forming the anterior boundary of the interventricular foramen. They sink into the lateral walls of the third ventricle as they descend to terminate in the corpora mamillaria, from which new fibres pass to the anterior nucleus of the thalamus, as the *mamillothalamic tract.*

Posteriorly, the body divides into two flattened posterior columns, which curve downwards behind the thalamus to gain the floor of the inferior horn. There each posterior column becomes continuous with the fimbria and the alveus. Some of the fibres of the posterior column of the fornix cross the median plane and constitute the *hippocampal commissure.*

The **Dentate Gyrus** is a narrow crenated strip of cortex which lies between the fimbria and hippocampal gyrus, deep in the groove between them. Anteriorly it can be traced into the uncus, and posteriorly it is continuous through the *splenial gyrus* with the induseum griseum (pp. 337, 346). Originally on the surface of the brain, it becomes buried by the overgrowth of the hippocampal gyrus. *It is regarded as a part of the olfactory cortex.*

At this stage it is apposite to summarise the parts of the brain which have been customarily grouped together as the *rhinencephalon* (Plate XXV). Incoming olfactory neurons have a cell-station in the olfactory bulb, and the second neurons run in the olfactory tract to the anterior perforated substance and the uncus. The further connexions of the olfactory pathway are uncertain in man, although the hippocampus, fornix, mamillothalamic tract, and the anterior nucleus of the thalamus have in the past been involved in the concept of a rhinencephalon, or "olfactory brain." The anterior nucleus is known to project extensively to the cingulate gyrus, and is now considered, together with the above "rhinencephalic" structures, to be concerned with autonomic (visceral) activities.

The **Tela Choroidea** is a two-layered fold of pia mater which intervenes between the body of the fornix above, and the upper surfaces of the two thalami and the third ventricle below. It is triangular in shape, and the pointed apex is placed at the interventricular foramen. The base lies below the splenium of the corpus callosum, and here the two constituent layers separate from each other. The upper layer passes on to the splenium; the lower layer descends over the dorsal aspect of the midbrain. The edges of the fold, containing the choroid plexuses, are invaginated into the lateral ventricle through the choroidal fissure, *i.e.*, the slit between the fornix and the thalamus. In the region of this narrow slit the medial wall of the cerebral hemisphere consists only of ependyma, and this is invaginated into the interior of the ventricle by the choroid plexus.

Posteriorly, the choroid plexus is continued down into the inferior horn, where it lies on the fimbria. This part of the plexus is invaginated into the interior of the inferior horn through the lower part of the choroidal fissure, which is bounded below by the fimbria and above by the tail of the caudate nucleus. Here again, the medial wall of the ventricle consists only of ependyma, which is carried into the interior as an investment for the choroid plexus. The lower and upper parts of the choroidal fissure are continuous with each other round the posterior end of the thalamus.

The *internal cerebral vein* is formed by the deep cerebral veins and drains the choroid plexus. The two internal cerebral veins run

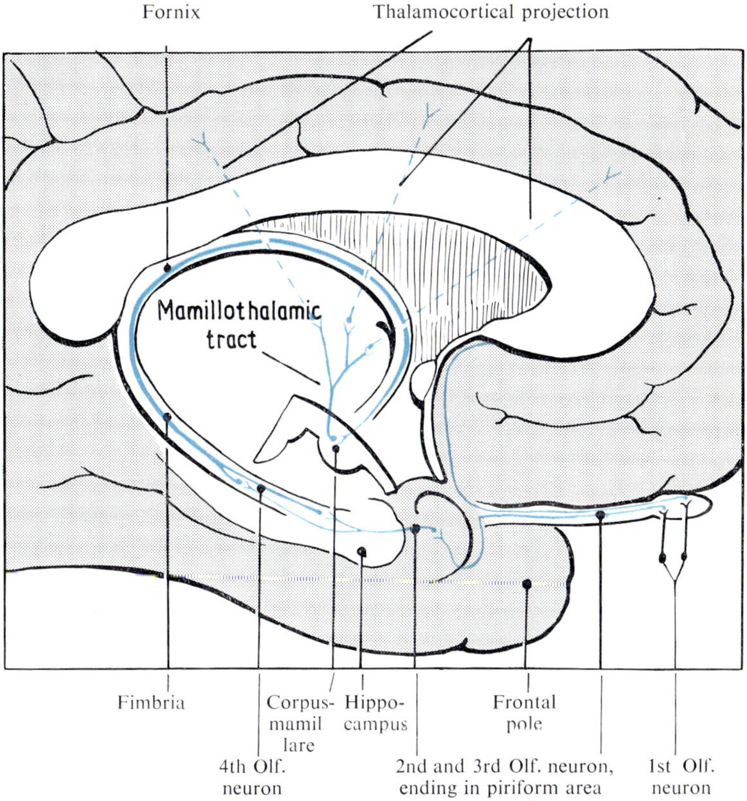

A Schema of the "Rhinencephalon."

The connexion from the piriform area (uncus) to the hippocampus, shown as 3rd "olfactory" neuron, can no longer be supported. The structures beyond the uncus, on this reputed olfactory pathway, are no longer regarded as olfactory in function. The "rhinencephalon" is shrinking.

To face p. 350

backwards between the two layers of the tela choroidea and, on emerging from its base, unite to form the *great cerebral vein*, which turns sharply upwards behind the splenium of the corpus callosum to join the inferior sagittal sinus and form the straight sinus (p. 365).

The **Basal Nuclei** are collections of grey matter found *within* the hemisphere. They comprise the corpus striatum (caudate and lentiform nuclei), the amygdaloid body (p. 348) and the claustrum.

The **Corpus Striatum** is situated lateral to the thalamus. It is almost completely divided by the internal capsule into the caudate nucleus and the lentiform nucleus. Below and in front, however, these two structures are directly continuous with each other, above the anterior perforated substance. The corpus striatum is a constituent of the extrapyramidal system (p. 353). (Strands of nerve cells, crossing the internal capsule, give this region a *striated* appearance.)

The **Caudate Nucleus,** like the thalamus, is partially exposed in the ventricular wall and partially buried in the hemisphere. It possesses a large rounded *head*, which forms the lateral wall of the anterior horn of the lateral ventricle. Inferiorly, the head becomes continuous with the grey matter of the anterior perforated substance, and also with the putamen of the lentiform nucleus. Laterally, the head is separated from the lentiform nucleus by the internal capsule.

The rapidly narrowing *body* of the caudate nucleus arches upwards as it passes backwards in the floor of the body of the lateral ventricle, and is separated from the thalamus by a well-marked groove. Its lateral aspect is closely related to the internal capsule.

The attenuated and recurved *tail* of the caudate nucleus runs forwards in the roof of the inferior horn and terminates in the amygdaloid nucleus.

The **Lentiform Nucleus** is completely embedded in the hemisphere. It consists of two portions, phylogenetically distinct, the putamen and the globus pallidus. They are separated by a whitish streak. best seen on coronal sections through the middle of the nucleus. The lateral portion is darker in colour and constitutes the *putamen*.

The *lateral aspect* of the nucleus is gently convex and is related to a thin covering of white fibres, termed the *external capsule*, which separates the nucleus from a thin sheet of grey matter, known as the *claustrum. The insula lies lateral to the claustrum and is practically co-extensive with it and with the lentiform nucleus.*

The *medial aspect* of the nucleus is related to the internal capsule. As seen in transverse section, this surface is also convex, and it projects medially to form the angle of the internal capsule.

Inferiorly, at its anterior end, the putamen of the lentiform nucleus becomes continuous with the caudate nucleus, and is deeply notched by the anterior commissure.

Despite the great size of the corpus striatum, its functions are not yet wholly understood. Its association with the great motor pathway is certain, exerting either a facilitatory or inhibitory influence. Phylogenetically the globus pallidus is the oldest part of the corpus striatum. There is evidence, both clinical and experimental, to show that the putamen and the caudate nucleus, which constitute the neo-striatum, exercise an inhibitory influence. *Afferent fibres* reach the caudate nucleus and putamen (and possibly the globus pallidus) from the thalamus, and connexions with the suppressor areas or bands (p. 341), have been demonstrated experimentally. Both the caudate nucleus and the putamen send numerous fibres to the globus pallidus, which is the source of most of the efferent fibres from the corpus striatum. These *efferent fibres* pass to the thalamus, the subthalamic nucleus, the substantia nigra and the red nucleus (striatorubral fibres). Clinical evidence shows that disease or injury of the caudate nucleus or of the putamen is associated with muscular tremors. (See also p. 354.)

The **Internal Capsule** is a broad bundle of nerve fibres, which almost completely divides the corpus striatum into its two parts, and which separates the thalamus from the lentiform nucleus. *It contains all the fibres which run between the cerebral cortex and the midbrain or parts below it*, and, in addition, most of the fibres which run from the thalamus and the basal nuclei to the cortex and from the thalamus and the basal nuclei to the midbrain or parts below it. The internal capsule thus includes almost all the important projection fibres of the cerebrum and connexions between the basal ganglia.

Superiorly, the fibres of the internal capsule, rapidly diverging, intersect the fibres of the corpus callosum and form the *corona radiata*. *Inferiorly*, rapidly converging, they pass into the cerebral peduncle of the midbrain, and, as they do so, they are crossed laterally by the optic tract. This continuity can be seen in coronal sections. *Laterally*, the capsule is related to the lentiform nucleus. *Medially*, it is related to the caudate nucleus and the thalamus.

As seen in transverse section, the capsule accommodates itself to the shape of the nuclei between which it lies, so that it is bent into a shorter anterior limb, a genu, and a longer posterior limb. The *anterior limb* is occupied by frontopontine, thalamocortical, and corticothalamic fibres.

The *Motor Fibres* from the precentral gyrus *occupy the genu and the anterior half of the posterior limb.* The fibres for the face, mouth, lips, etc., lie at the genu. Next in order come the fibres for the neck, upper limbs, trunk and lower limbs.

Behind the *motor fibres* lie the fibres of the *auditory radiation*, *i.e.*, the fibres connecting the lower auditory centres in the midbrain to the auditory cortex. Still more posteriorly the internal capsule is occupied by the fibres of the *optic radiation*, as they leave the lateral geniculate body on their way to the visual cortex.

The third neuron (thalamocortical) fibres of the exteroceptive and proprioceptive pathways to the postcentral gyrus are found throughout the posterior limb, intermingled with descending temporopontine and occipitopontine fibres.

The Extrapyramidal System. Reference has already been made to the relationship existing between voluntary movements and the performance of skilled acts, and it should be clear that complex skilled acts, which have a value transcending that of discrete movements as such, must imply perfect co-ordination between the activities of the motor and premotor areas of the cortex (p. 340) and, indeed, of much besides.

The descending pathway from the motor cortex to the spinal cord is the lateral corticospinal tract (p. 311), the fibres of which arise in the precentral gyrus and descend, uninterruptedly, to the spinal cord, where at various levels they terminate by establishing contacts with the cells of the ventral grey column. A corresponding but polysynaptic pathway begins in the premotor cortex, descends through the internal capsule, establishes connexions with the corpus striatum, thalamus, red nucleus and the substantia nigra, and is continued to a number of subsidiary collections of grey matter in the subthalamic region and the brainstem.

In addition to the motor cortex, the premotor cortex and its associated subcortical collections of grey matter both have a part to play in the intricate combinations of voluntary movements which comprise any skilled act. Both the corpus striatum and the substantia nigra come under the direct influence of the premotor cortex, and they in turn are linked with each other and with the other subcortical centres enumerated above by connecting pathways, all of which may not yet have been fully determined. Finally, the rubrospinal, reticulospinal, olivospinal and vestibulospinal tracts, which descend from the brainstem to the spinal cord, enable all these nerve cell groups to influence the final common motor path (lower motor neurons).

To distinguish these accessory motor pathways from the main (pyramidal) system, they have long been grouped together under the heading of "*Extrapyramidal System.*"

The extrapyramidal fibres from the cortex accompany the pyramidal fibres through the internal capsule, so that extensive lesions in this situation cut off the influence of both the motor and the premotor cortex. In such cases all the movements of the contralateral limbs are paralysed and the muscles are spastic or hypertonic.

On the other hand, below the internal capsule the paths of the pyramidal and extrapyramidal systems separate. The corticospinal fibres are more ventral position in the brainstem, descending through the cerebral peduncle (p. 326), the ventral pons and the pyramid of the medulla oblongata, before they decussate to form the lateral corticospinal tract (p. 311). The extrapyramidal fibres are placed more dorsally and descend, with relays through the tegmentum of the midbrain, and the reticular formation of the pons and the medulla oblongata. It is uncertain whether the reticulospinal fibres descend through a series of relays in the intersegmental tracts or whether they descend, uninterrupted, amongst the fibres of the lateral corticospinal tract, as some believe. (Note the overlap between extrapyramidal and reticular systems.)

In cases where lesions affect the pyramid only, the extrapyramidal system escapes. The muscles of the contralateral limbs are paralysed, although some movements may be retained, but the paralysis is flaccid or hypotonic.

The analysis of any skilled act will show that the orderly series of movements which are essential for its performance are often synchronous with arrest of movement in related parts of the body as well as with maintenance of posture. For example, a blow with a tool, weapon, or instrument, necessitates the combination of a secure grip with the synchronous appropriate movements of the trunk, shoulder, arm and forearm. At the same time, the perfect balance of the body must be maintained throughout. It would appear therefore that the performance of a skilled act demands the simultaneous and perfectly integrated activities of both the pyramidal and the extrapyramidal systems in order that it may be carried out successfully. The details of the process defy analysis, but that both the pyramidal and the extrapyramidal systems are concerned in the successful performance of all skilled acts has been established.

It must be borne in mind that the cerebellum and its pathways also play an essential part in the co-ordination of all types of movement initiated at cortical level.

The Reticular Formation. In both the brain and spinal cord there are, in addition to the long ascending and descending tracts, large numbers of neurons which make shorter connexions within the central nervous system. Their axons run not only for short distances in the axis of the nervous system but also subserve horizontal interconnexions. Large numbers of such cells are gathered deeply within the lateral white column of the cord, and in a corresponding position throughout the brainstem. These cells show an arrangement like that of the most primitive nerve nets, and the appearance of the fields in which they lie has prompted the term—*formatio reticularis*. (Among this somewhat diffuse arrangement certain brainstem groups of cells may be noted. These include the red nucleus, inferior olive, the tegmental reticular nuclei of the pons and the lateral reticular nucleus of the medulla. The reticular formation also displays cerebellar connexions. Note that there is some overlap between nuclei in the extrapyramidal and reticular systems.)

While the reticular formation has thus been known, in the anatomical sense, for more than half a century, it is only recently that any clear views of its functioning have been formulated. Stimulation of the reticular formation of the brainstem has been shown to be capable of changing the electroencephalogram of anæsthetised experimental animals from the sleeping to the wakeful pattern. This finding has led to the concept of an "arousal centre" in the brainstem, but this has not yet been satisfactorily equated with known anatomical structures. Inhibitor zones have also been described.

It has been known for a long time that long ascending tracts give off collaterals to brainstem nuclei, and that some of their fibres may actually terminate there. There is thus a polysynaptic pathway *viâ* the brainstem to the cerebrum and even its cortex. Similar polysynaptic pathways are described, involving the basal ganglia, and such masses of cells as the subthalamic, red, and olivary nuclei. It is not entirely clear how far these descending polysynaptic paths are to be differentiated from the extrapyramidal system.

Though it is not yet possible to give a clear picture of the precise part taken by the reticular formation in natural activity, these new concepts have at least the virtue of reminding us that the brain consists of more than a cortex. In sum, the reticular formation exerts (*a*) a stimulating effect on the cortex, (*b*) both excitatory and inhibitory influences over phasic and tonic muscular control, and (*c*) a modifying effect upon sensory signals. It should, however, be remembered that both in consciousness and motor activity all parts of the central nervous system act together as a continuum.

THE THALAMI AND THE THIRD VENTRICLE

These structures can only be studied comprehensively from prepared specimens, as otherwise the student can rarely have sufficient material for the purpose. He requires (1) a brain dissected to show the floor of the ventricles; (2) a similar dissection, with the corpus callosum, fornix and tela choroidea removed; (3) a median sagittal section of the brain; (4) a series of coronal sections; (5) a series of tranverse sections; and (6) a dissection showing the midbrain, thalami, and corpora striata, the cortex, etc., having been removed. With access to this material—and such specimens should be found in every anatomical museum—the student can rapidly revise the extent, position and relations of the thalamus and the other structures derived from the diencephalon (p. 304).

The **Thalamus** (p. 348) is a large mass of nerve cells, which is situated immediately above the midbrain and projects beyond it, both in front and behind. Its *anterior end* is narrow and rounded, and *forms the posterior boundary of the interventricular foramen.* It contains the anterior nucleus of the thalamus.

The *posterior end* of the thalamus is expanded, and the enlarged medial part of it constitutes the *pulvinar*, while a small elevation on the under aspect of its lateral portion is termed the *lateral geniculate body* (p. 357).

The *upper surface* of the thalamus can be divided into an extraventricular medial portion, covered by the tela choroidea and the fornix, and an intraventricular lateral portion, which lies in the floor of the central part of the lateral ventricle, covered by ependyma, and partly hidden by the choroid plexus.

The *medial surface* of the thalamus forms the lateral wall of the third ventricle and is connected to its fellow by the *connexus interthalamicus*, which represents a secondary adhesion. The *lateral surface* of the thalamus is related above to the caudate nucleus and below to the internal capsule, which separates it completely from the lentiform nucleus.

Inferiorly, the thalamus is continuous, through the subthalamic region, with the cerebral peduncle of the midbrain.

The thalamus constitutes the last cell-station on the sensory path to the cortex. It is divided into anterior, medial and lateral parts or regions; the last-named has several subdivisions. The *anterior* region receives its afferent fibres from the mamillothalamic tract (p. 337). It sends its efferent fibres to the cingulate gyrus (Plate XXVI). The *medial* part receives its afferent fibres from the nuclei of the hypothalamus (p. 359) and is regarded, therefore, as being concerned chiefly with visceral impressions. It has a two-way connexion with the frontal pole. The *lateral* part receives *afferent fibres* from the following sources. (1) Most of the fibres of the medial lemniscus (conscious proprioceptive, tactile and pressure

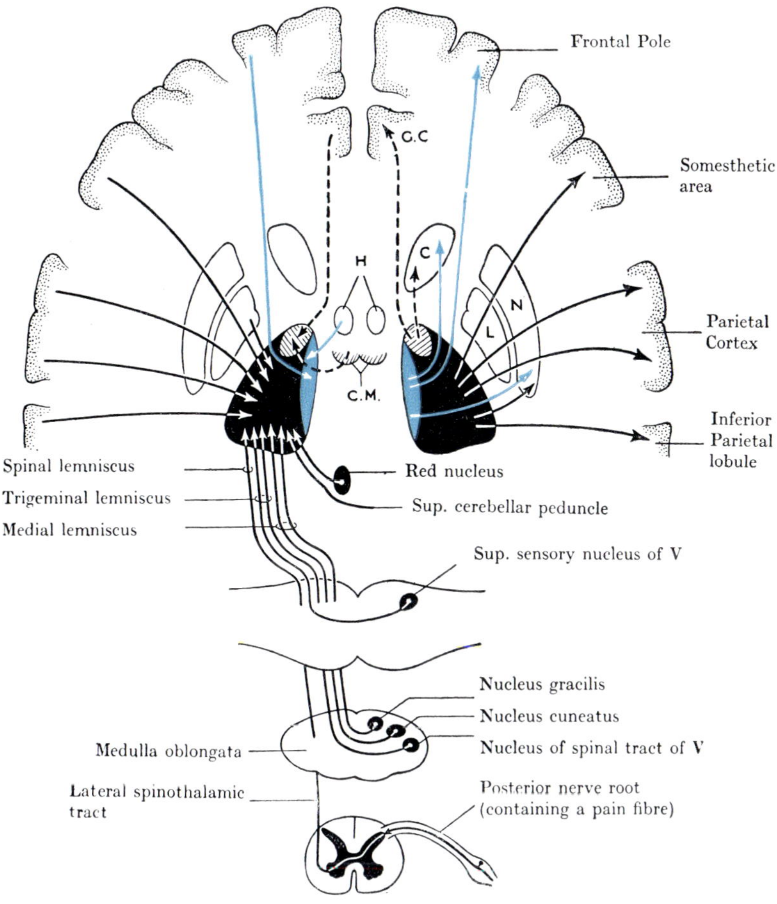

The Connexions of the Thalamus.

The anterior nucleus is stripped and its connexions are shown by interrupted arrows. The medial nucleus is shown in blue and its connexions by blue arrows. The lateral nucleus (not shown subdivided) is in solid black and its connexions are indicated by black arrows.

C.M. = Corpora mamillaria. C. = Caudate nucleus. G.C. = Gyrus cinguli. H. = Hypothalamic nuclei. L.N. = Lentiform nucleus.

sensibility). (2) The spinal and trigeminal lemnisci (painful and thermal sensibility). (3) Corticothalamic fibres, which enable the cortex to influence thalamic responses. (4) The superior cerebellar peduncle. The source from which the pulvinar receives afferent fibres has not yet been determined, but it sends efferent fibres to the inferior parietal lobule (p. 342). Taken as a whole, the thalamus sends *efferent* fibres, *viâ* the internal capsule, to all parts of the cerebral cortex, but *especially to the postcentral gyrus.* In addition, it sends fibres to the corpus striatum and to the subthalamic nucleus. Almost all the thalamus receives projection fibres from many parts of the cortex, a connexion which has been regarded for many years as inhibitory in function, though it is now considered to exercise a potentiating or stimulating influence.

The **Geniculate Bodies** constitute the metathalamus, and are derived, like the thalamus, from the lateral wall of the diencephalon. The *Medial Geniculate Body* is a small oval elevation, placed in the groove between the upper end of the lateral aspect of the midbrain and the overhanging pulvinar of the thalamus. It receives *afferent fibres* from the lateral lemniscus and the inferior colliculus *viâ* the inferior brachium, and sends *efferent fibres, viâ* the posterior limb of the internal capsule, to the superior temporal gyrus. *It functions as a relay on the auditory pathway.*

The *Lateral Geniculate Body* (p. 338) is a somewhat oval elevation on the under aspect of the lateral part of the posterior end of the thalamus. It receives *afferent fibres* from the lateral root of the optic tract and sends its *efferent fibres* through the optic radiation to the striate area of the occipital cortex (p. 344). *It constitutes the only synaptic interruption on the pathway from the retina to the visual cortex.*

Sections through the lateral geniculate body show that its constituent nerve cells is arranged in six laminæ, of which three are connected with a half retina of each eye. This arrangement has been held to be associated with the trichromatic nature of colour vision, but the view has received no satisfactory proof.

The **Third Ventricle** represents the lumen of the cephalic end of the primitive neural tube. It lies between the two thalami, forming a deep cleft, which communicates in front with the lateral ventricles through the interventricular foramina, and behind with the aqueduct of the midbrain, *i.e.*, the lumen of the mesencephalic portion of the neural tube.

The *roof* consists of ependyma, which is invaginated into the interior by the choroid plexus of the third ventricle. Superiorly it is related to the tela chorioidea with the contained internal cerebral veins, and to the fornix and corpus callosum. The *floor* consists of the optic chiasma, the infundibulum, the tuber cinereum, the corpora mamillaria, the posterior perforated substance and the grooved upper surface of the cerebral peduncles.

The *anterior wall* is formed by the lamina terminalis, across which the *anterior commissure* runs as a rounded bundle of fibres in front of the anterior columns of the fornix. At the junction of the floor and the anterior wall the *optic recess* passes for a short distance above the optic chiasma. The *posterior wall* is shallow. Below, it is occupied by the upper opening of the aqueduct of the midbrain, above which the posterior commissure crosses the ventricle. The stalk of the pineal body, into which the pineal recess burrows backwards, lies above the posterior commissure.

The *lateral wall* is marked by a shallow sulcus, which curves upwards and forwards from the aqueduct of the midbrain to the interventricular foramen and is termed the *hypothalamic sulcus.* Above this sulcus the lateral wall is formed by the medial surface of the thalamus, which is fused to the opposite wall over an area of variable extent, termed the *connexus interthalamicus.* Below the sulcus the lateral wall is formed by the hypothalamus (*vide infra*).

The **Pineal Body,** which is connected to the posterior wall of the third ventricle, lies in contact below with the superior corpora quadrigemina, and above with the great cerebral vein, as it passes backwards from the tela choroidea to join the straight sinus. The *stalk* of the pineal body is penetrated by the pineal recess, which subdivides it into upper and lower parts. The lower part curves downwards, covering the posterior commissure. It has been reputed to be a ductless gland but this has not been clearly demonstrated. Recent experimental studies suggest, nevertheless, that the pineal may exert an influence on sexual maturation in males, and that it produces a substance, melatonin, capable of causing aggregation of pigment granules in melanocytes. It becomes fibrosed and usually contains calcareous deposits in early adult life.

The **Posterior Commissure** is a small bundle of fibres which crosses the third ventricle immediately above the upper end of the aqueduct of the midbrain. It is intimately related to the lower part of the stalk of the pineal body, which clothes its anterior aspect.

The **Hypothalamus** comprises (*a*) the subthalamic tegmental region, (*b*) the structures which form the floor of the third ventricle, and (*c*) the structures which lie in the lateral wall of the third ventricle below and in front of the hypothalamic sulcus.

The *Subthalamic Region* lies immediately below the thalamus and connects it to the tegmental portion of the midbrain. It contains the uppermost parts of the red nucleus and the substantia nigra, and is traversed by the medial, the spinal and the trigeminal lemnisci, as they ascend to reach the thalamus. In addition, it contains a small group of motor cells, termed the *subthalamic nucleus*, which is a constituent part of the extrapyramidal and reticular systems (pp. 353, 354). Shaped like a biconvex lens, the subthalamic nucleus lies ventrolateral to the upper end of the red nucleus and dorsal to the upper end of the substantia nigra.

The optic chiasma is described on p. 337.

The *tuber cinereum* is a somewhat triangular field between the optic chiasma in front, and the corpora mamillaria behind. Its inferior surface, which is covered by the tuberal portion of the hypophysis cerebri—a thin layer—gives attachment to the infundibulum of the hypophysis.

The **Hypophysis Cerebri** is a small ductless gland which occupies the hypophyseal fossa of the sphenoid. It is related, on each side, to the cavernous sinus and its contents (p. 279) and, below, to the sphenoidal sinus. Above, it is roofed in by the *diaphragma sellæ*, a circular fold of dura mater with a central aperture through which the infundibulum connects the posterior lobe of the gland to the tuber cinereum. Anteriorly the diaphragma sellæ separates the anterior lobe of the gland from the optic chiasma.

The two lobes of the hypophysis differ in their development and in their structure. The *anterior lobe* arises as a hollow outgrowth from the ectodermal roof of the primitive mouth, immediately ventral to the buccopharyngeal membrane. The connexion with the mouth is soon lost, but the cavity of the outgrowth persists in the adult as a cleft which separates the lobe into a thicker, anterior part, and a thinner, posterior part. The anterior lobe grows backwards round each side of the posterior lobe and its anterior part extends upwards to surround the infundibulum and to cover the tuber cinereum with a thin layer, termed the tuberal part of the gland. The anterior part is very vascular and consists of granular epithelial cells grouped between trabeculæ. The posterior part of the anterior lobe fuses with the anterior part of the posterior lobe and forms the *middle part* (*pars intermedia*) of the gland. It contains few blood-vessels, and small masses of colloid material are found amongst its finely granular cells.

The *posterior lobe*, which arises as a hollow downgrowth from the floor of the diencephalon, contains no nerve-cells, but numerous neuroglial cells and fibres. Collections of colloid material are usually present. It receives numerous nerve fibres from the supra-optic nucleus of the hypothalamus, and is responsible for the secretion of pituitrin.

The secretion of the anterior lobe exercises an important influence on growth, including growth of bone. Further, it includes the follicle-stimulating hormone (FSH) and luteinizing hormone (LH), which stimulate the production of œstrin and progesterone by the ovaries, prolactin, which stimulates the initial secretion of milk, and a secretion which stimulates the thyroid gland.

The *corpora mamillaria* and the *posterior perforated substance* are described on p. 337.

Nuclei of the Hypothalamus. A number of nuclei, believed to play an important part in controlling and regulating visceral activities, are identifiable in the floor of the third ventricle and in its lateral wall below the hypothalamic sulcus. Some of them send efferent fibres to the medial nucleus of the thalamus.

The *supra-optic nucleus,* which straddles the ventricular surface of the optic chiasma, sends efferent fibres along the infundibulum to the posterior lobe of the hypophysis cerebri. Together with other nuclei (tuberal and paraventricular) it is associated with secretion of antidiuretic hormone and control of water balance in the body.

The *posterior hypothalamic nucleus* lies in the lateral wall of the third ventricle immediately above the mamillary body, while the *lateral hypothalamic nucleus* lies in front of this.

In general the anterior part of the hypothalamus appears to be associated with parasympathetic functions and the posterior part with the sympathetic.

Centres associated with temperature regulation and the sleep mechanism have also been inferred from experimental evidence.

THE MENINGES

The brain and spinal cord are surrounded by three membranes, or meninges, viz., the *pia mater*, the *arachnoid mater* and the *dura mater*.

The **Pia Mater** is the innermost. It is adherent to the surface of the brain and is carried into all the sulci by the branches of the cerebral arteries. A double fold of pia mater constitutes the tela choroidea (p. 350). Over the lower part of the roof of the fourth ventricle this membrane is in direct contact with the ependyma, and it is invaginated into the interior of the ventricle by the choroid plexus. In this situation it is pierced by the median aperture of the fourth ventricle (p. 325).

In the vertebral canal it is adherent to the spinal cord and dips into the anterior median fissure. Along the lateral aspect of the cord, from the foramen magnum to the first lumbar vertebra, the pia mater is attached to the dura by a thin membrane, termed the *ligamentum denticulatum.* The denticulated lateral border of this ligament is attached to the dura in the intervals between the spinal nerves and therefore does not form a complete partition. *The roots of the first lumbar nerve lie below the lowest denticulation.* Inferiorly, the pia mater terminates on the filum terminale (p. 305).

The **Arachnoid Mater,** a weblike membrane, is situated between the pia and the dura, bridging over the various sulci on the surface of the brain; but it is carried into the longitudinal fissure by the falx cerebri. It is everywhere closely applied to the dura mater.

Over the convolutions the arachnoid and pia are closer to each other than at the sulci, and in certain other regions but everywhere the two are separated by the *subarachnoid space.* This space contains cerebrospinal fluid, and is crossed by a reticulum of fine fibres which connect the two membranes. In certain situations this network is much reduced, and the two membranes are more widely separated to form the subarachnoid *cisternæ.*

The *Cisterna Cerebellomedullaris* (*C. Magna*) lies between the under surface of the cerebellum and the lower part of the roof of the fourth ventricle. *It is into this cisterna that the cerebrospinal fluid passes directly from the ventricle through the median aperture* (p. 325).

The *Cisterna Pontis* lies in front of the pons and medulla oblongata. It is traversed by the roots of the lower eight cranial nerves. It is into the lower part of this cisterna that the foramina of the lateral recesses of the fourth ventricle open.

The *Cisterna Interpeduncularis* lies in the interpeduncular fossa and has offshoots in the lateral sulcus and the longitudinal fissure. It is traversed by the third and fourth cranial nerves.

These cisternæ communicate freely with one another, being completely continuous with the general subarachnoid space.

The *Arachnoid Granulations* are best marked in old age, and they frequently give rise to pitting of the parietal bones. They are enlargements of the *arachnoid villi,* which grow into the lumen of the superior sagittal sinus and the adjoining venous lacunæ (p. 364), invaginating the arachnoid into them. *They serve as the channels for the return of the cerebrospinal fluid to the blood stream.*

In the *Vertebral Canal* the arachnoid mater forms a very loose investment for the spinal cord and the cauda equina, *and it ends below at the second sacral vertebra.* In the cervical region it is connected to the pia mater by an incomplete posterior median septum. The spinal subarachnoid space is continuous above with the cisterna cerebellomedullaris and the cisterna pontis, and contains cerebrospinal fluid.

The *Cerebrospinal fluid* is secreted by the vessels of the choroid plexuses into the interior of the lateral, third and fourth ventricles. It passes out through the opening in the lower part of the roof of the fourth ventricle into the cisterna cerebellomedullaris and the lower part of the cisterna pontis. From there it circulates both upwards and downwards in the subarachnoid space. It flows through the gap in the tentorium cerebelli (p. 363) and then forwards over the base of the brain. It ascends over the medial and lateral surfaces of the hemispheres, accompanying the larger blood vessels and following the larger sulci. Small ramifications of the subarachnoid space form perivascular channels around the small vessels which penetrate the cortex and so bring the cerebrospinal fluid into intimate relation with the cortical nerve cells. Finally the fluid passes into the blind extensions of the space present in the arachnoid villi and returns to the blood stream.

The cerebrospinal fluid descends into the spinal subarachnoid space, largely by a process of diffusion aided by alterations of posture. Recently, arachnoid villi have been described in connexion with the veins of the spinal cord and these are regarded as offering an additional means for the return of the fluid to the blood stream.

The cerebrospinal fluid takes the place of lymph throughout the whole of the central nervous system, which is devoid of lymphatic vessels, and is regarded as the principal medium for the removal of the waste products of nerve cell activity. In addition, however, it provides an important means of protection for the delicate structure of the brain and spinal cord, acting as an efficient buffer to minimize the effects of blows and shocks.

The **Dura Mater** is a fibrous membrane, its outer aspect inseparably blended with, and in effect forming, the *endoperiosteum* of the skull. It is adherent to the bone except where it takes part in the formation of such folds as the falx cerebri and the tentorium cerebelli. Further, at the margins of the foramen magnum and the other foramina in the skull, it becomes continuous with the periosteum on the outside of the skull. Although very firmly adherent over the base of the skull, the endoperiosteum can be stripped off from the vault without much difficulty.

Within the vertebral canal the dura mater forms a loose envelope outside the arachnoid mater. Although firmly connected to the second and third cervical vertebræ, elsewhere it is not intimately associated with the periosteum. Inferiorly, it ends on the filum terminale below the second sacral vertebra.

The *Subdural Space* lies between the dura and the arachnoid mater. In life it is a capillary interval which contains the subdural fluid.

The *Extradural Space* is restricted to the vertebral canal and lies between the spinal dura mater and the ligaments and periosteum lining the canal. It contains a little loose fat and areolar tissue and a venous plexus, and it extends laterally for a short distance along the spinal nerves. Local anæsthetics injected in the neighbourhood of one spinal nerve may spread upwards or downwards to involve neighbouring spinal nerves or they may spread across the median plane to affect the corresponding nerves of the opposite side. In each case the spread occurs through the extradural space, which is known to some clinicians as the *epidural space*.

The pia and arachnoid mater are developed from cells derived from the neural crest and are therefore ectodermal in origin, but the dura mater is developed from mesoderm.

The **Falx Cerebri** is a sickle-shaped fold of dura mater which occupies the longitudinal fissure. Narrow in front, where it is attached to the *crista galli* of the ethmoid bone, the falx becomes deeper as it is traced backwards.

It contains the inferior sagittal sinus in its lower border and the superior sagittal sinus in its upper border, and it shares with the tentorium in supporting the straight sinus.

The **Tentorium Cerebelli** forms a partition between the cerebellum and the posterior parts of the cerebral hemispheres. Like the falx, it consists of fibrous tissue, covered on both surfaces by a layer of mesothelium. Anteriorly it leaves a wide gap—the tentorial notch —for the passage of the midbrain, so that it possesses an inner, or free border and an outer, or attached border. On each side the latter is attached to the margins of the groove for the transverse sinus on the occipital bone, to the margins of the groove for the superior petrosal sinus on the petrous portion of the temporal bone, and finally to the posterior clinoid process of the sphenoid. The free border runs forwards to the anterior clinoid process, and after crossing the attached border forms a ridge on the upper wall of the cavernous sinus. The oculomotor and trochlear nerves pierce the dura mater on the medial side of this ridge, just in front of the point where the free and attached borders of the tentorium cross each other.

In the median plane the upper layer of the tentorium becomes continuous with the falx cerebri, and in this situation the straight sinus runs backwards to the *confluence of the sinuses*.

The *Falx Cerebelli* is a less prominent fold, precisely similar in construction to the falx cerebri, which projects slightly into the gap between the two cerebellar hemispheres inferiorly.

The arrangement of the cranial and spinal nerves, as they pierce the meninges, requires further mention. As they leave the surface of the brain the cranial nerves carry fine coverings of the pia and the arachnoid mater with them, and they acquire a further investment from the dura mater. It must be noted, however, that the third, fourth, fifth and sixth nerves pierce the inner aspect of the dura at some distance from the point at which they make their exits from the cranial cavity. In this part of their course they lie within the thickness of the dura mater. The manner in which the roots of the fifth nerve are related to the dura mater is described on p. 380. The trigeminal ganglion is placed on the sensory root as it lies in the cavum trigeminale on the apex of the petrous part of the temporal bone.

As the vagus and accessory nerves pierce the dura over the jugular foramen they acquire a common sheath. On the other hand, the hypoglossal nerve pierces the dura in two parts, each of which receives a separate sheath, but the two unite in the anterior condylar canal.

The spinal nerve roots not only gain separate sheaths of pia and arachnoid mater, but they pierce the dura mater at separate points, and it is not until the ganglion on the posterior nerve root is reached that the two sheaths unite.

The intracranial **Venous Blood Sinuses** receive tributaries from the various parts of the brain, from the diploe, from the orbit and the internal ear. *Unlike the other veins in the body, their walls consist of a single layer of endothelium closely applied to the unyielding dura mater. As a result, there is no tendency for them to collapse when they are opened*, and hæmorrhage can only be controlled by pressure.

The **Superior Sagittal Sinus** begins at the foramen cæcum, in front of the crista galli, where it may, occasionally, communicate with the veins of the nasal mucous membrane. It runs upwards and backwards in the upper border of the falx cerebri, grooving the vault of the skull and invaded by arachnoid villi and granulations (p. 361). At the internal occipital protuberance it lies a little to one side (usually the right) of the median plane and forms a dilatation, termed the *confluens sinuum*—confluence of the sinuses—which communicates with the transverse sinus of the opposite side. At this point the sinus bends sharply to the right (sometimes to the left) and becomes continuous with the transverse sinus. In its course it is joined by the superior cerebral veins, which run forwards and medially on the lateral surface of the hemisphere (against the direction of flow in the sinus).

Two or three irregularly shaped *venous lacunæ* communicate with each side of the sinus by small openings. It is in these lacunæ that the meningeal and diploic veins terminate and numerous arachnoid villi and granulations project into their interior.

The **Inferior Sagittal Sinus** runs backwards in the lower border of the falx cerebri, and at the free margin of the tentorium cerebelli unites with the *great cerebral vein* (p. 351) to form the straight sinus.

The **Straight Sinus,** formed in this way, runs backwards along the line of attachment of the falx cerebri to the tentorium. At the internal occipital protuberance it bends sharply to the left (sometimes to the right) to form the transverse sinus.

The **Transverse Sinus** begins at the internal occipital protuberance. It is a paired structure, and one of them, usually the right, is continuous with the superior sagittal sinus, and the other is continuous with the straight sinus. It runs laterally in the attached border of the tentorium, grooving the occipital bone and the postero-inferior angle of the parietal bone, where it bends downwards and medially to become the sigmoid sinus.

The transverse sinus is joined by (1) the superior petrosal sinus; (2) some of the inferior cerebral veins; and (3) cerebellar veins.

The **Sigmoid Sinus** runs downwards and medially, grooving the mastoid portion of the temporal bone. *In this part of its course it forms an important postero-medial relation of the tympanic antrum* (p. 372). Below it passes forwards, grooving the jugular process of the occipital bone, and reaches the jugular foramen, where it turns downwards to become the internal jugular vein. It receives a number of cerebellar veins and communicates with veins outside the skull through the mastoid and the condylar foramina.

In suppurative conditions of the tympanic cavity or tympanic antrum the sigmoid sinus may become the site of a septic thrombus, and through its cerebellar tributaries may give rise to a cerebellar abscess.

The cavernous and petrosal sinuses are described on p. 279.

The **Cerebral Arteries** are derived from two sources, viz., the internal carotid and the vertebral arteries (Plate XXI, p. 160).

The **Internal Carotid Artery** leaves the cavernous sinus medial to the anterior clinoid process of the sphenoid bone, where it pierces the dura mater and the arachnoid mater, then giving off the opthalmic artery (p. 276). In the subarachnoid space it gives off the posterior communicating artery to join the posterior cerebral, and, after giving origin to the anterior choroid artery, it terminates below the anterior perforated substance by dividing into the anterior and middle cerebral arteries. Of these the latter is the larger vessel, and is nearly in direct line with the main trunk. As a result, small emboli which pass up the internal carotid are almost invariably carried into the middle cerebral artery, and become arrested in one or other of its smaller branches.

The *posterior communicating artery* gives off a number of small central branches, which pierce the posterior perforated substance to supply the medial part of the thalamus. The *anterior choroidal artery* supplies the optic tract, the lateral geniculate body and the optic radiation and then enters the inferior horn of the ventricle through the choroidal fissure to supply the choroid plexus.

The **Anterior Cerebral Artery** runs medially from the internal carotid artery to reach the longitudinal fissure of the cerebrum. It then bends sharply forwards, coming into close relationship with its fellow of the opposite side, to which it is connected by the short *anterior communicating artery*. In the rest of its course this artery is closely related to the corpus callosum, at first lying below the rostrum, then curving upwards round the genu, and finally passing backwards above its main mass, or trunk.

It supplies *cortical branches* to the whole of the medial surface of the hemisphere, as far back as the parieto-occipital sulcus, *but it does not reach the cuneus.* In addition its branches emerge from the longitudinal fissure and supply a strip of cortex, about 1 inch wide, on the adjoining lateral and orbital surfaces.

It will be clear therefore that the upper end of the motor area, i.e., the centre for the lower limb, is supplied by the anterior cerebral artery.

Central branches supply the corpus callosum and the head of the caudate nucleus.

The **Middle Cerebral Artery** runs laterally from the internal carotid in the stem of the lateral sulcus. It is then continued backwards across the surface of the insula in the posterior ramus of the sulcus.

Cortical branches emerge from the lips of the lateral sulcus and supply the whole of the lateral surface of the hemisphere, except (1) the narrow strip supplied by the anterior cerebral artery, and (2) the occipital lobe and a narrow strip along the infero-lateral border of the hemisphere, which are supplied by the posterior cerebral artery. In addition, the middle cerebral supplies the temporal pole, the insula, and the lateral part of the orbital surface of the frontal lobe.

It will be seen that this artery is responsible for the blood supply of (1) the whole of the motor area except its upper part, and (2) the areas associated with speech and hearing.

Central branches enter the brain at the anterior perforated substance to supply the putamen, the head of the caudate nucleus, and the anterior limb of the internal capsule. One of these arteries is known as "the artery of cerebral hæmorrhage," and hæmorrhage from this vessel, unless very limited in extent, at once causes pressure on the motor fibres in the internal capsule and produces hemiplegia, *i.e.*, paralysis of the muscles of the opposite side of the body.

The **Vertebral Artery** pierces the dura mater and arachnoid mater of the lateral mass of the atlas (p. 283) and enters the skull through the foramen magnum. It runs upwards, forwards and medially on the medulla oblongata, and at the lower border of the pons it unites with its fellow of the opposite side to form the *basilar artery*. It supplies branches to the medulla oblongata, the cerebellum and the spinal cord. Of these the most important is the *posterior inferior cerebellar artery*, which supplies the dentate nucleus of the cerebellum and an area of the medulla oblongata, dorsal to the olivary nucleus and including the spinal lemniscus, the nucleus ambiguus and the nucleus of the spinal tract of the trigeminal nerve (p. 318).

The **Basilar Artery** ascends in the median plane in front of the pons, and ends at its upper border by dividing into the two posterior cerebral arteries. It supplies branches to the pons, the internal ear and the cerebellum.

The **Posterior Cerebral Artery** curves backwards round the midbrain, passes above the tentorium and ends by supplying the occipital lobe.

Cortical branches supply the inferior surface of the hemisphere behind the temporal pole, and in addition the medial and lateral surfaces of the occipital lobe. *The posterior cerebral artery supplies, therefore, the whole of the visual cortex.*

Central branches enter the brain at the posterior perforated substance and supply the midbrain, the subthalamic region, the thalamus and the corpus mamillare. Others arise from the main trunk after it has curved round the midbrain and supply the posterior part of the thalamus, the colliculi, the pineal, and medial geniculate bodies. Small *posterior choroidal arteries*, three or four in number, enter the choroidal and transverse fissures to supply the choroid plexuses, and one of them helps the anterior choroidal artery to supply the lateral geniculate body.

The **Circulus Arteriosus** lies in the cisterna interpeduncularis in the neighbourhood of the interpeduncular space. The anterior communicating, the anterior cerebral, the internal carotid, the posterior communicating, the posterior cerebral and the basilar arteries all take part in its formation. The "circle" so formed lies above the optic chiasma in front, the cavernous sinus on each side, and the dorsum sellæ behind. Within it lie, from before backwards, the stalk of the hypophysis, the tuber cinereum, the corpora mamillaria and the posterior perforated substance. The cortical branches of the cerebral arteries anastomose with one another before, but not after, they enter the brain. The central branches are end-arteries, *i.e.*, they do not anastomose with neighbouring vessels, although their capillaries do.

The **Meningeal Vessels** lie within the dura mater, in close contact with the bone which they chiefly supply, despite their name. The veins, like the intracranial blood sinuses, have very thin walls, and are therefore easily injured.

The **Middle Meningeal Artery** (p. 264) enters the middle cranial fossa through the foramen spinosum and runs laterally, forwards and upwards on the greater wing of the sphenoid, where it divides into anterior and posterior branches.

The *anterior branch* runs upwards, grooving or tunnelling the upper part of the greater wing and then grooving the anterior part of the parietal bone. *Its course lies parallel to, and a little in front of, the central sulcus. The artery is therefore closely related to the motor area of the cortex*, and when it, or its accompanying veins, are injured—an accident, by no means uncommon, as the result of falls or blows on the head—the extravasated blood exerts pressure on the motor area, with resulting loss of power in groups of muscles of the opposite side of the body.

The *posterior branch* runs backwards, grooving the squamous portion of the temporal bone. Its course lies over, or near, the superior temporal sulcus. Injury of this branch is less common than injury of the anterior branch, but when it occurs the resultant hæmorrhage presses on the adjoining auditory centres in the superior temporal gyrus, causing unilateral deafness.

VESTIBULOCOCHLEAR APPARATUS

The **Auricle** (External Ear) possesses a framework of elastic fibrocartilage which gives it a characteristic form. The rim is termed the *helix*. Below and in front the *tragus* forms a backward projection, commonly semilunar in shape, which obscures the surface opening of the external auditory meatus. The *incisura intertragica* is a notch which bounds the tragus inferiorly and separates it from the *antitragus*. The *lobule* is the most dependent part of the auricle, and is devoid of cartilage. The *antihelix* forms a curved ridge, which constitutes the posterior boundary of the deep depression of the *concha*. The latter leads forwards to the external auditory meatus.

The skin covering the auricle receives its nerve supply from (1) the auriculotemporal nerve (the tragus and a small area adjoining); (2) the great auricular nerve (both surfaces); (3) the lesser occipital nerve (medial surface, upper part).

The **External Auditory Meatus** leads from the bottom of the concha to the tympanic membrane, and is about 1 inch long. In its lateral part the walls are supported by cartilage, and the cuticular lining is provided with fine hairs and sebaceous and ceruminous glands. In its medial part the walls are body, and the skin is closely adherent to the periosteum.

The meatus is at first directed upwards, forwards and medially, but, as can readily be confirmed in the reader's own ear, it soon bends backwards and medially. At the junction of the cartilaginous with the osseous part the meatus makes a second bend, and then runs forwards, medially and slightly downwards to the tympanic membrane. The narrowest part of the meatus lies 5 mm. from the membrane and is frequently referred to as the *isthmus.*

The *Nerve Supply* of the cuticular lining of the meatus and tympanic membrane is derived from two sources, viz. (1) the *auriculotemporal nerve* (p. 266), and (2) the *auricular branch of the vagus.* The latter supplies only a small portion of the floor and posterior wall of the deep part of the meatus and the adjoining part of the tympanic membrane.

The external auditory meatus represents the deepened dorsal end of the first visceral cleft. Tubercles appear at the dorsal ends of the first and second arches; they surround the dorsal end of the first cleft and are later modified to form the auricle.

The **Tympanic Membrane** is set very obliquely, so that its outer surface looks downwards and forwards as well as laterally. As a result, the floor and anterior wall of the meatus are longer than the roof and posterior wall. The membrane is concave laterally, and the point of deepest concavity, which is termed the *umbo*, corresponds to the tip of the handle of the malleus. When the membrane is examined by reflected light, the antero-inferior quadrant is always strongly illuminated, and is known clinically as "the cone of light." The apex of the cone lies at the umbo, and from this point the shadow thrown by the handle of the malleus may be traced upwards and forwards to a small whitish area, which corresponds to the lateral process of the malleus (p. 371). The anterior and posterior malleolar folds pass from the lateral process of the malleus to the extremities of the tympanic notch (p. 371). They form the lower limit of the small *flaccid part* of the membrane.

The **Tympanic Cavity** (Middle Ear) is an air-space in the petrous portion of the temporal bone containing the auditory ossicles. It is a narrow, oblique, slit-like cavity, having its vertical axis roughly parallel to the plane of the tympanic membrane.

The auditory (pharyngotympanic) tube opens on its anterior wall, and the aditus to the tympanic antrum on the upper part of its posterior wall. The tympanic cavity, therefore, communicates with the nasopharynx in front and with the tympanic antrum behind.

The *Roof* of the cavity is formed by the *tegmen tympani*, a thin plate of bone which separates it from the middle cranial fossa and the temporal lobe of the brain.

The *Floor* is thin centrally and intervenes between the middle ear and the superior bulb of the internal jugular vein.

The *Anterior Wall* opens directly into the auditory tube. Above the tube is a small canal which lodges the tensor tympani muscle, whilst the bone to its medial side constitutes the lateral wall of the carotid canal.

The *Posterior Wall* presents, *in its upper part*, the aditus leading into the tympanic antrum. At a lower level there is a small conical projection, termed the *pyramid*, from which emerges the tendon of the stapedius muscle.

The *Lateral Wall* is formed to a very large extent by the *tympanic membrane*, which does not, however, reach to the roof of the cavity. Consequently, the upper part of the lateral wall is formed by the squamous part of the temporal bone.

The *Medial Wall* separates the tympanic cavity from the labyrinth. It shows a well-marked, rounded projection, termed the *promontory*, which is formed by the first turn of the cochlea. The *fenestra vestibuli* (*ovalis*), occupied in life by the base of the stapes, lies above the posterior part of the promontory. Below the posterior end of the promontory a small depression leads to the *fenestra cochleæ* (*rotunda*), which is closed in the recent state by the *secondary tympanic membrane*. A rounded ridge, produced by the facial nerve in its bony canal, arches backwards on the medial wall above the promontory and the fenestra vestibuli. *Posteriorly it turns downwards in the medial wall of the aditus.*

The part of the middle ear which lies above the level of the tympanic membrane is termed the *epitympanic recess*, and the whole cavity and its offsets and its contents are lined by mucous membrane continuous, through the auditory tube, with the lining membrane of the nasal pharynx.

The **Tympanic Membrane** (p. 369) consists of (1) an outer, cuticular layer; (2) an inner, mucous layer; and (3) an intermediate fibrous layer containing a majority of radiating fibres, which pass from the umbo to the periphery. Except for its upper part, the circumference of the membrane is thickened and fits into a groove in the bone. The gap in the upper part of the groove is termed the *tympanic notch.* The greater portion of the tympanic membrane is held taut during life by the tonus of the tensor tympani muscle. The upper portion, which is attached to the tympanic notch, is referred to as the *pars flaccida.* It should be noted that pain is the only sensation that can be aroused from the membrane, and it is not surprising to find that only free nerve endings are present in its outer covering of modified skin.

The *Tympanic Ossicles* are three in number. (1) The *Malleus* is the largest and is connected to the tympanic membrane. Its rounded head lies in the epitympanic recess, and is connected to the rest of the bone by a constricted neck. It articulates with the incus by means of a notched facet placed obliquely on its posterior aspect. Below the neck the *handle* or *manubrium* passes downwards and backwards, closely attached in its whole extent to the tympanic membrane. The lateral process is a small elevation which projects from the lateral aspect of the upper end of the manubrium. It impinges on the membrane, and may be identified on otoscopic examination.

(2) The *Incus*, shaped like a two-fanged tooth, possesses a body, which lies posterior and medial to the head of the malleus, with which it articulates. Its two processes are widely divergent. The short process passes backwards and is attached to the posterior wall of the middle ear, while the long process lies parallel with the handle of the malleus and postero-medial to it. Its lower end is bent medially and tipped with cartilage to articulate with the head of the stapes. The shadow of the long process can sometimes be seen in the posterior part of the membrane on otoscopic examination.

(3) The *Stapes* possesses a head, for articulation with the incus, and a neck, which is connected by anterior and posterior limbs to an oval base. The latter is firmly held in place in the fenestra vestibuli by an annular ligament.

The *Tensor Tympani Muscle* lies in a small canal above the auditory tube, from the cartilage of which it takes origin. Its tendon emerges from the posterior end of the muscle and, bending at right angles round a bony pulley, runs laterally across the cavity of the middle ear to be inserted into the medial side of the manubrium of the malleus close to the neck of the bone.

Its *Nerve Supply* is derived from the mandibular nerve (p. 265).

The *Stapedius Muscle* arises *within* the posterior wall of the middle ear and its tendon emerges from its canal on the summit of the pyramid. It runs forwards to be inserted into the posterior aspect of the neck of the stapes.

Its *Nerve Supply* is derived from the facial nerve, which lies close behind the muscle, in its downward passage to the stylomastoid foramen.

Actions. Both the stapedius, which draws the neck of the stapes backwards, tilting the anterior part of the footplate laterally, and the tensor tympani have the effect of damping down the intensity of high-pitched notes.

The **Tympanic Antrum** lies in the posterior part of the petrous portion of the temporal bone, and is about the size of a small pea. *Superiorly*, it is roofed in by a backward continuation of the tegmen tympani, and is therefore related to the middle cranial fossa and the temporal lobe of the brain. Its *anterior wall* shows an opening in its upper part, which communicates with the epitympanic recess through the aditus. Its *posterior wall* separates the antrum from the sigmoid sinus and the cerebellar hemisphere. The *lateral wall*, which is formed by the squamous part of the temporal bone, is at least $\frac{1}{2}$-inch thick in the adult (p. 390).

Numerous air-cells open out of the antrum and out of one another, and burrow into the mastoid process (Plate XXVII, p. 386). They are all lined by mucoperiosteum and they all communicate, directly or indirectly, with the antrum.

At birth the tympanic antrum has reached its adult size, but its lateral wall is only 1–4 mm. thick. *The mastoid process does not form a definite projection until towards the end of the second year.* At the same time, it must be remembered that the tympanic part of the temporal bone simply forms an incomplete ring in the newly-born child. *As a result, the facial nerve, as it emerges from the stylomastoid foramen, is very much more superficial in the young child than it is in the adult.*

At birth the tympanic cavity, its contained ossicles and the tympanic membrane have all completed their growth.

The **Auditory (Pharyngotympanic) Tube** leads from the tympanic cavity downwards, forwards and medially into the nasopharynx. Its posterior third ($\frac{1}{2}$-inch long) is bony and lies anterolateral to the carotid canal. Its anterior two-thirds (1 inch long) partly cartilaginous and partly fibrous, becomes deeper as it runs forwards to the pharynx. This part of the tube is closely applied to the inferior aspect of the skull and lies in a narrow groove between the greater wing of the sphenoid and the petrous part of the temporal bone.

Laterally it is related to the tensor veli palatini muscle, which separates it from the mandibular nerve and the middle meningeal artery. It enters the nasopharynx by passing over the curved upper border of the superior constrictor muscle (p. 289), at the posterior border of the medial pterygoid plate.

The Intrapetrous Part of the Facial Nerve. The facial nerve and its sensory root accompany the auditory nerve into the internal auditory meatus. At the bottom of the meatus it enters the facial canal, which runs laterally above the vestibule of the labyrinth until the medial wall of the tympanic cavity is reached. It then bends at right angles and runs backwards on the medial wall, above the promontory and the fenestra vestibuli. At the medial wall of the aditus to the tympanic antrum the canal curves downwards, and eventually opens on the inferior surface of the temporal bone at the stylomastoid foramen.

In the first part of its course the facial nerve and its sensory root run side by side. At the bend or *geniculum*, however, the *geniculate ganglion of the facial nerve* is situated, and in it the sensory root ends. As it runs backwards, the facial nerve is separated from the middle ear and the aditus to the tympanic antrum only by a *very thin plate of bone*, and in the latter situation it is related superiorly to the ampulla of the lateral semicircular canal. In the descending part of its course the facial nerve gives off a small branch to the stapedius muscle, and also gives origin to the *chorda tympani*.

The **Chorda Tympani** passes forwards through the bone and emerges on the posterior wall of the tympanic cavity. It then crosses the upper part of the tympanic membrane and the handle of the malleus, covered on its medial side by the mucous membrane of the middle ear. At the anterior border of the tympanic membrane the nerve enters a minute canal, which conducts it to the exterior of the skull at the petrotympanic fissure. Its subsequent union with, and distribution in, the lingual nerve are described on p. 266. Traced centrally, the afferent fibres of the chorda tympani end in cells of the geniculate ganglion (i.e. they are elongated dendrites), and the centrally running axons of those cells constitute the sensory root (p. 332) of the facial nerve.

The tympanic cavity and the auditory tube are developed from the tubotympanic recess, which is formed from the first pharyngeal pouch and, as it expands, involves portions of the second arch and pouch. A part of the endoderm lining the recess remains in close relationship with the ectoderm of the dorsal end of the first visceral cleft and participates in the formation of the tympanic membrane. The tympanic cavity represents the expanded blind end of the recess and its connexion with the pharynx persists as the pharyngotympanic tube. The malleus and incus are derived from the dorsal end of Meckel's cartilage and the stapes from the dorsal end of the cartilage of the second arch. They lie at first in immediate proximity to the tubotympanic recess, and later invaginate its lining epithelium and appear in the cavity of the middle ear. The facial nerve is the nerve of the second arch and its chorda tympani branch is distributed to the caudal border of the first arch. Its passage across the tympanic membrane in the adult represents its passage from the second to the first arch in the embryo.

THE LABYRINTH OR INTERNAL EAR

The internal ear, or labyrinth, is situated in the petrous part of the temporal bone, medial to the middle ear. It is a complex, closed, membranous sac with several diverticula, surrounded, though not closely, by dense ivory-like bone, in conformity with the shape of the contained membranous structures and thus constituting a *bony labyrinth*.

The **Cochlea** consists of a central column, known as the *modiolus*, around which a hollow tube makes two-and-a-half spiral turns. The whole is shaped like a cone, the apex being directed forwards and laterally, and the base backwards and medially, the latter forming part of the floor of the internal auditory meatus. A spiral ledge of bone projects from the modiolus and subdivides the cochlea into a *scala vestibuli* above and a *scala tympani* below.

Posteriorly the cochlea opens into the *bony vestibule*, which lodges the membranous saccule and utricle. The openings of the fenestra vestibuli and the fenestra cochleæ, already described in connexion with the middle ear, are placed on its lateral wall.

The **Semicircular Canals**, which contain the membranous semicircular ducts, open into the posterior part of the vestibule. The *superior semicircular canal* lies in a plane at right angles to the long axis of the petrous part of the temporal bone, while the *lateral canal* is set in a horizontal plane and the *posterior canal* parallel to the long axis of the bone. The anterior part of the lateral semicircular canal lies in the medial wall of the aditus to the tympanic antrum immediately above the canal containing the facial nerve (p. 375).

The **Membranous Labyrinth** is much smaller than the space in which it lies, and the interval between it and the bone is filled by a fluid termed *perilymph*. The epithelium of the membranous duct of the cochlea is highly specialised and constitutes the *spiral organ* (of Corti), which is the essential part of the organ of hearing. An elongated *spiral ganglion* is lodged in a canal which winds round the modiolus in the base of the spiral lamina. The peripheral branches from this ganglion pass to the organ of Corti, while its central branches leave the bone through foramina at the bottom of the internal auditory meatus and constitute the cochlear part of the auditory nerve. Posteriorly the duct of the cochlea opens by the narrow *ductus reuniens* into the *saccule*, which lies in the vestibule.

The *Semicircular Ducts* are each ampullated at one extremity, and there also the epithelium is highly specialised. They open into the *utricle*, which lies in the posterior part of the vestibule, and both the utricle and the semicircular ducts are innervated by branches of the vestibular nerve.

The utricle and the saccule are only indirectly connected to each other. A narrow duct, termed the *ductus endolymphaticus*, leaves the posterior end of the saccule and is joined by the *ductus utriculo-saccularis* from the utricle. It then passes on to end in a small blind dilatation, named the *saccus endolymphaticus*, which projects through the aqueduct of the vestibule and lies in the dura mater, on the posterior surface of the petrous part of the temporal bone. The three form a continuous Y-shaped cavity.

The various parts of the membranous labyrinth, therefore, all communicate with one another, and they contain a common fluid, termed *endolymph*. The complicated system which they constitute is closed, and communicates neither with the subdural nor the subarachnoid space. On the other hand, the perilymph drains into the subarachnoid space through the *aqueduct of the cochlea*, which is a minute bony canal, leading from the scala tympani to the surface of the petrous part of the temporal bone at the upper border of the jugular foramen.

The membranous labyrinth is developed from the ectoderm on the side of the head opposite the hindbrain. At first a thickened plate, or *placode*, it becomes depressed from the surface and closed off to form the otic or auditory vesicle.

THE EYE

The **Eyeball** consists of three concentric tunics, which enclose three refracting media. The outermost tunic is fibrous in character and is formed by the sclera and the cornea; the middle is vascular and includes the choroid, the ciliary body and the iris; the innermost is nervous in character and is termed the retina.

The **Sclera** covers the posterior five-sixths of the eyeball. Anteriorly it is continuous with the cornea at the corneoscleral junction or *limbus*, and beyond the margin of the cornea the sclera can be seen through the conjunctiva as "the white of the eye." Composed of dense white fibrous tissue, the sclera contains few blood vessels, but it is pierced by the vessels which ramify in the choroid tunic. A little below and medial to the posterior pole of the eyeball the sclera is pierced by the optic nerve and, around the point of entry of the nerve, by the posterior ciliary arteries. The large *venæ vorticosæ*, which return the blood distributed by the ciliary arteries, are usually four in number. They are symmetrically disposed and their points of emergence are situated further away from the optic nerve. The anterior ciliary arteries pierce the sclera near the corneoscleral junction.

The **Cornea** consists of fibrous tissue which, although transparent, is directly continuous with the substance of the sclera. Its superficial aspect is covered by a layer of stratified epithelium, the *bulbar conjunctiva.* Posteriorly it is limited by a *posterior elastic membrane*, covered in its turn by a layer of endothelium which is in contact with the aqueous humour. At its peripheral margin the fibres of the posterior elastic membrane divide into three groups. The innermost fibres turn medially into the iris and constitute the *ligamentum pectinatum* of the (iridocorneal) angle; the middle fibres give origin to the ciliary muscle; and the outermost fibres become continuous with fibres of the sclera. Owing to the need for transparency, the cornea contains no blood vessels, but derives its nourishment from the lymph which circulates in its numerous lymph spaces. Note that pain is the only sensation that is ordinarily aroused from the cornea. Its nerve supply is derived from the ophthalmic division of the trigeminal through the short ciliary nerves and the fibres form both a subepithelial and an intra-epithelial plexus which send free nerve endings between the cells of the epithelium covering its free surface.

At the corneoscleral junction a circular *scleral venous sinus* (Canal of Schlemm) is situated in the deeper part of the coat. It communicates, on the one hand, with the scleral veins, and, on the other, with the aqueous humour, the latter communication being possible owing to the presence of the *spaces of the iridocorneal angle* on the posterior aspect of the cornea, near its periphery. These spaces lie between the bundles of ligamentum pectinatum at their corneal ends, and permit the endothelium which covers the posterior aspect of the cornea to be brought close to the scleræ.

The **Choroid Tunic** consists of an outer pigmented layer adherent to the sclera, and an inner, higher vascular, layer, in which the short posterior ciliary arteries ramify (p. 276). Anteriorly the choroid expands into the **Ciliary Body**, which lies behind the peripheral part of the iris. It consists of a number of *ciliary processes* separated from one another by radial furrows and having free, rounded, central extremities. The *ciliary muscle* lies in the substance of the ciliary body. Its fibres arise at the corneoscleral junction and radiate backwards and inwards to the ciliary processes. In addition there are a certain number of circular fibres, placed medial to the rest of the muscle. (For Action and Nerve Supply, *see* p. 378.)

The **Iris,** which forms part of the intermediate coat of the eyeball, is a contractile diaphragm with a central aperture. Peripherally it is continuous with the ciliary body, while its central free margin bounds the pupil. The anterior aspect of the iris is covered by a layer of endothelium which is continuous with the endothelium on the posterior surface of the cornea. Its posterior aspect is covered by a double layer of columnar epithelium, containing pigment, which is continuous with the *pars ciliaris retinæ* (see below).

The iris contains a well-marked *sphincter* muscle, which consists of circular fibres, and a less clearly defined *dilator* muscle, consisting of a thin sheet of radial fibres, which lies near its posterior surface.

The **Retina** consists of an outer pigmented layer and an inner nervous layer, the latter being in contact with the vitreous body. The nervous layer lines the posterior three-fourths of the eyeball, and its anterior limit forms a wavy ring, termed the *ora serrata* (*i.e.*, the nervous layer does not cover that part of the interior of the eyeball on which no light rays can fall). It is, however, continued onwards, as a single layer of columnar epithelium, over the ciliary processes (pars ciliaris retinæ) and the posterior aspect of the iris (pars iridica retinæ) in company with the outer pigmented layer.

A little below and to the medial side of the posterior pole of the eyeball, the optic nerve reaches the retina and its fibres spread out over its surface. The point of entrance is termed the **Optic Disc** and, as it is not covered by rods or cones, it constitutes the physiological "blind spot." Above and to the lateral side of the optic disc, *i.e.*, at the posterior pole of the eye, there is a small area, somewhat yellowish in colour and devoid of blood vessels. This is termed the *macula lutea* and over its depressed central portion (*fovea centralis*) the rods are absent and only cones are present. *It is the part of the retina which is most sensitive to light stimuli.* In the peripheral retina, on the other hand, the rods predominate, and in nocturnal animals the cones are almost entirely absent from the retina. The *arteria centralis retinæ* (p. 276) appears at the optic disc, and its retinal branches can easily be seen in the living eye by ophthalmoscopic examination.

The three *Refracting Media* which are enclosed by the coats of the eyeball are (1) the aqueous humour, (2) the lens, and (3) the vitreous body.

The **Aqueous Humour** is a clear fluid which occupies the space between the cornea in front and the lens behind (anterior segment). This space includes both the *anterior and posterior chambers of the eye.* The former is limited posteriorly by the anterior aspect of the iris and the central part of the lens; the unfortunately named posterior chamber lies between the posterior aspect of the iris and the lens. The two chambers, therefore, communicate freely with each other through the aperture of the iris. The aqueous humour is secreted into the posterior chamber from the ciliary body and circulates into the anterior chamber through the pupil. From the anterior chamber, it drains away into the scleral venous sinus (p. 376). (Following inflammation of the iris, adhesions may form between the iris and the front of the lens, obstructing the outflow of the aqueous humour from the posterior to the anterior chamber. When this happens, secretion of the aqueous humour continues and the intra-ocular pressure may rise to a dangerous degree).

The **Vitreous Body** fills the whole of the eyeball behind the lens ('posterior segment'). It is a transparent, jelly-like substance, enclosed by the *hyaloid membrane.* Anteriorly the hyaloid membrane becomes somewhat thickened, and presents a number of radial furrows and elevations. The furrows receive the ciliary processes, and the elevations fit into the corresponding furrows in the ciliary body. Near the margin of the lens this part of the hyaloid membrane divides into a posterior layer, which lines the hollowed-out anterior aspect of the vitreous body, and an anterior layer, which is attached to the anterior aspect of the lens, constituting its *suspensory ligament.*

The **Lens** is a transparent, bi-convex body, which lies between the aqueous humour in front and the vitreous body behind (i.e., it separates the anterior and posterior segments of the eyeball). Circular in outline, it consists of concentric laminæ of elongated cells, which are termed the lens fibres, the whole being enclosed within an elastic capsule. When the eye is at rest the anterior surface of the lens is flattened by the tension of the suspensory ligament. Contraction of the ciliary muscle relaxes the ligament by drawing forwards the hyaloid membrane, and the anterior surface of the lens becomes more convex, owing to the elasticity of the lens substance.

Both muscles of the iris and the ciliary muscle are supplied by the *short ciliary nerves* from the ciliary ganglion, but the fibres which supply the sphincter of the iris and the ciliary muscle are parasympathetic, and travel in the oculomotor nerve from their origin in the accessory (Edinger-Westphal) nucleus (p. 330), whereas those which supply the dilator muscle are sympathetic in origin (p. 239).

The eye begins to develop before the cerebral hemispheres make their appearance. The *optic vesicle*, which grows out from the fore-brain and remains connected to it by the *optic stalk*, becomes invaginated to form the *optic cup*, and the two layers of the cup give origin to the pigmented and nervous layers of the retina. In addition, the periphery of the cup gives rise to the ciliary body and a part of the iris (*pars iridica retinæ*), including its unstriped muscle. All these structures therefore are derived from the ectoderm.

The invagination which forms the optic cup is eccentric and affects the optic stalk as well as the optic vesicle. The groove on the stalk and the notch on the margin of the cup, with which it is continuous, constitute the *choroidal fissure* of the developing eye. It is invaded by the hyaloid artery and surrounding mesoderm; and, when its two edges unite, the distal part of the artery becomes enclosed in the stalk and passes through the floor of the cup to reach and supply the mesoderm which surrounds the developing lens. Occasionally the lips of the choroidal fissure fail to fuse and the condition is marked by a congenital deficiency in the iris and choroid, termed *coloboma of the choroid.*

The ectoderm of the head, which overlies the optic vesicle, becomes thickened, depressed from the surface, and finally closed off to form the *lens vesicle*, which soon loses its connexion with the ectoderm and sinks into the hollow of the optic cup. Mesoderm grows into the interval between the ectoderm and the vesicle and a cleft, which represents the anterior chamber of the eye, appears in its substance. The posterior wall of the cleft forms a vascular layer over the margin of the optic cup and the front of the lens, forming the stroma of the iris and the pupillary membrane in these situations. The cells of the posterior wall of the lens vesicle lengthen to form the lens fibres, encroaching on and obliterating the cavity of the vesicle. The cells of the anterior wall, on the other hand, undergo little change and constitute a single layer of epithelium over the front of the lens.

In the seventh month of intra-uterine life the pupillary membrane breaks down centrally, and, later, the hyaloid artery, which has already given origin to retinal branches, becomes obliterated from the optic disc to the back of the lens. In rare cases, the pupillary membrane fails to break down—the condition known as Congenital Atresia of the Iris—and the resulting opacity, which is normally complicated by Congenital Cataract (opacity of the lens), renders the eye useless. The conjunctiva also is ectodermal in origin, but the cornea, sclera and choroid are derived from the mesoderm.

Section VII

OSTEOLOGY

The student cannot effectively revise his knowledge of the skeleton, unless he has access to it and *unless he is prepared to refer frequently to those bones in his own body which he can examine conveniently*. It cannot be repeated too often that it is essential for the medical student to be really familiar with all the bony points which can be felt through the skin, for, except on rare occasions, it is only through the skin that he will be able subsequently to examine the bones of his patients, although he will often have the aid of X-ray photographs.

The **Skeleton** includes all bones and cartilages; it is divisible into axial and appendicular parts on the basis of its evolution. The *axial* skeleton includes the vertebral column, the skull, the sternum, the ribs and the hyoid bone; the *appendicular* skeleton comprises the bones of the upper and lower limbs, including the girdles which connect them to the axial skeleton.

THE VERTEBRAL COLUMN

The vertebral column constitutes the central axis of the body. It comprises twenty-four movable vertebræ, which can be examined individually in the disarticulated skeleton, and eight or nine fixed vertebræ, of which the upper five are fused to form the sacrum and the remainder are fused to form the coccyx.

Cervical Vertebræ. The atlas, axis and the seventh cervical vertebræ are atypical, but the others conform fairly closely to a common type.

A **Typical Cervical Vertebra** shows the following noteworthy features. The *body* is wide in proportion to its antero-posterior depth and is small relative to the size of the vertebral foramen, which is large and triangular. The lateral edge of the upper surface of the body project upwards, and the corresponding edges of the lower surface are bevelled. The line of the neuro-central joint in the child is antero-posterior and lies just medial to these edges. The *spine* is bifid.

The *transverse process* exhibits a foramen for the passage of the vertebral vessels, and this—being present in all cervical, but in no other vertebrae—is their most distinctive feature. The anterior and lateral boundaries of the foramen are derived from the costal element; the posterior boundary is the morphological transverse process. The lateral boundary is grooved by the emerging anterior primary ramus, which passes behind the vertebral artery and emerges behind the muscles attached to the anterior tubercle of the transverse process (longus cervicis, longus capitis and scalenus anterior), and in front of those attached to the posterior tubercle (levator scapulæ, scalenus medius). The anterior tubercles lie behind the common carotid artery, and that on the sixth vertebra (level of cricoid cartilage) is termed the *carotid tubercle*, because it is large enough to enable the artery to be obliterated by digital pressure in this situation. The *articular processes* form a cervical articular pillar. The superior articular facets are directed upwards, backwards and slightly medially, while the inferior facets face downwards, forwards and slightly laterally.

The **Atlas** is a ring of bone (Plate XXVII, p. 386). The obliquely set *lateral masses* are connected to each other by an anterior arch and a longer posterior arch. The upper articular surface of each lateral mass is concave in its long axis, while the lower articular surface is nearly flat and more nearly circular. The medial aspect of the lateral mass shows a prominent tubercle for the attachment of the transverse ligament. *The transverse processes project further laterally than those of the other cervical vertebræ, and act as the levers to enable the inferior oblique muscles to rotate the skull and the atlas around the odontoid process.* After passing through the foramen in the transverse process of the atlas the vertebral artery turns medially, grooving the upper surface of the posterior arch behind the projecting posterior part of the lateral mass. The first cervical nerve lies between the artery and the groove.

The atlas lacks its centrum, which has become fused to the centrum of the axis and forms the odontoid process. Its neural arch forms the posterior arch and the bulk of the lateral masses. The anterior arch and the anterior extremity of each lateral mass are formed from the *hypochordal bar.*

The spine of the atlas is reduced to a small tubercle; if large, it would interfere with extension in nodding movements.

The **Axis** is atypical in the following respects. From the upper aspect of the body the *odontoid process* projects upwards to articulate with the posterior surface of the anterior arch of the atlas (p. 284). It is held in place by the transverse ligament. Somewhat conical in shape, the odontoid process is firmly attached to the occipital bone by the alar ligaments, which pass from its flattened shoulders, and limit both nodding and rotatory movements. The superior articular facets are on the lateral parts of the upper surface of the body and the adjoining parts of the pedicles. They are directed upwards and slightly laterally. The transverse processes are diminutive and the anterior tubercle is feebly developed. *The spine is stout and strong,* and gives attachment to numerous muscles and to the ligamentum nuchæ.

The **Seventh Cervical Vertebra** is characterised by its long, non-bifid spine, which can be felt through the skin at the lower end of the nuchal furrow. The foramen in the transverse process transmits only an accessory vertebral vein. The costal element ossifies from a separate centre, but fuses with the body and the transverse process. Occasionally it remains separate and forms a cervical rib.

The **Thoracic Vertebræ** all conform to one type, but there are distinguishing features which enable an individual vertebra either to be identified or to be assigned to some particular region of the column. T. 1 and T. 2 have bodies which resemble those of the cervical vertebræ. T. 1 bears (as a rule) a whole facet for the head of the first rib and a half facet for the upper part of the head of the second rib. Its superior vertebral notch is recognisable, and its nearly horizontal spine is long and can be felt through the skin without difficulty. T. 2 bears demi-facets for the heads of the second and third ribs, and its superior vertebral notch is usually unrecognisable as such.

The bodies of T. 3–T. 12 show a gradual increase in size proportionate to the increased weight they have to support in the erect or sitting posture. The bodies of T. 5–T. 8 are asymmetrical, being flattened on the left side by the pressure of the descending thoracic aorta.

The *spines* become increasingly oblique from T. 3–T. 8, which has the longest and most nearly vertical spine of any of the vertebræ. From T. 1 to T. 6 (as a rule) the articular facets on the transverse processes are appreciably concave and are directed forwards and laterally. From T. 7–T. 10 they are flattened and face upwards, laterally and forwards. The shapes of these facets indicate the character of the movement which occurs at the costotransverse joints. Above, the ribs tend to rotate, whereas, below, the movement is a gliding one.

The body of T. 10 bears only one demi-facet on each side, as a rule. The bodies of T. 11 and T. 12 have a single facet for the head of the corresponding rib; the facet tends to be slightly lower down on T. 12 and encroaches on the side of the pedicle. The transverse process of T. 11 is short, but can *easily be gripped between the finger and thumb. It has no articular facet.* This is also true of the transverse process of T. 12, which is very insignificant and rarely big enough to grip. The inferior articular facets of T. 12 are out-turned and therefore lumbar in type.

The **Lumbar Vertebræ** are characterised by the size of their bodies and by small triangular vertebral foramina, they are, however, more surely identified by absence of costal facets and transverse foramina. Their transverse processes increase in length from L. 1 to L. 3 (Plate XX, p. 172), and then show a slight diminution. L. 5 is characterised by three features. (Morphologically they are *costal* elements.) The fifth lumbar vertebra has particularly massive transverse processes, and its inferior articular facets face more anteriorly to meet the backwardly direct sacral facets. (This vertebra may be wholly or partly fused to the sacrum—*sacralization.* Conversely, the first sacral vertebra may fail to fuse with the second—*lumbarization.*) The depth of its body is usually greater in front than it is behind; the distance between the inferior articular processes is equal to that between the superior articular processes; *and the transverse process encroaches along the pedicle until it reaches the body.*

The adult **Sacrum** is formed by the fusion of five sacral vertebræ, which diminish in size from above downwards. The *lateral mass* represents the fused costal and transverse process elements, and forms a substantial mass of bone in the region of S. 1–S. 3. It bears the *auricular surface* for articulation with the ilium, and the bulk of this part of the bone is explained by the need of a strong bearing surface for the transmission of the body weight from the vertebral column to the hip girdle. The auricular surface is formed by the costal elements and the roughened tuberosity behind it, to which the posterior sacro-iliac ligaments are attached, is formed by the fused transverse processes. The lateral parts of S. 4 and S. 5 have no weight to transmit and are thin and sharp. They give attachment to the sacrotuberous and sacrospinous ligaments. The laminæ of S. 5 always (and of S. 4 frequently) fail to meet in the median plane. On this account the sacral canal opens on the dorsal surface through the sacral hiatus.

The sacral canal contains part of the cauda equina, filum terminale and meninges *down to the lower border of the second sacral vertebra. There the meninges terminate as such,* and the lower part of the canal contains only the nerve roots of the lower sacral and the coccygeal nerves and the filum terminale, together with the coverings they separately acquire from the meninges.

The male sacrum is long in proportion to its width. The female sacrum is broad in proportion to its length. This difference is associated with corresponding differences in the male and female pelves (p. 412). The typical male sacrum shows a gradual curve, affecting all the segments of the bone. The typical female sacrum looks as if it had been bent sharply at the third sacral vertebra and is flat above and below the bend. On the upper, or basal, surface of the bone the upper surface of the body of the first sacral vertebra forms a disproportionately small area in the female as compared with the male, for in the latter the body of the fifth lumbar vertebra is much larger and the lateral mass of the sacrum is relatively narrower.

The **Coccygeal Vertebræ** are all rudimentary. The first has a body and rudimentary transverse and superior articular processes. The others are represented only by their centra.

The Vertebral Column as a Whole. The intervertebral discs make up one quarter of the length of the whole column. They are thicker in the cervical and lumbar parts than they are in the thoracic part of the column and thus provide for the wider range of movement possible in the neck and loins. The spinal curves are primary and secondary. In the fœtus the cervical, thoracic and lumbar vertebræ form originally one continuous curve, concave ventrally. This feature is to be associated with the attitude of full flexion which accommodates the fœtus to the shape of the uterine cavity. The thoracic curve is a persistent part of this fœtal curve and is therefore primary. The sacrum and coccyx also form a slight forward concavity in the fœtus, and this primary curve becomes accentuated later. The cervical convexity, associated with the power to elevate the head and keep it poised on the vertebral column, and the lumbar convexity, associated with the adoption of the erect attitude by the child, are both secondary curves.

THE STERNUM AND RIBS

The *suprasternal notch* can easily be felt through the skin. It lies on the same horizontal plane as the disc between the second and third thoracic vertebræ. The manubrium is widest opposite the first costal cartilages. The *sternal angle* is in the same horizontal plane as the disc between the fourth and fifth thoracic vertebræ (Plate XVII, p. 124). The body of the sternum is widest below, at the junction of its third and fourth segments, *i.e.*, opposite the fifth costal cartilage. Its anterior surface, like the front of the manubrium, gives origin to the pectoralis major muscle, whilst its posterior surface is smooth and related to the pleuræ and pericardium.

The xiphoid process is rarely completely ossified, and it may be perforated. Its posterior surface gives attachment to the short anterior fibres of the diaphragm.

In early fœtal life the sternum is represented by right and left cartilaginous sternal plates or bars, with which the rib cartilages are continuous. Later these two plates unite, but union may be incomplete and foramina may be present in the adult bone. The sternum becomes ossified in late fœtal life, but the constituent parts of the body (sternebræ) do not begin to fuse until puberty.

The ribs increase in length from the first to the seventh and below that are successively shorter. With the exception of the first, which is obscured by the clavicle, and occasionally the twelfth, which may be absent or may be so short that it fails to project beyond the lateral edge of the sacrospinalis, all the ribs can be felt through the skin and overlying muscles. *The second rib can always be identified with certainty, for its cartilage reaches the sternum at the sternal angle.* When it is necessary to identify a given rib in the living body, the second should be identified and the succeeding ribs counted from above downwards, following a line which commences on the second 2.5 cm. from the sternum and runs downwards and laterally.

The articular surface on the *head* of a typical rib is divided into upper and lower parts by the transverse *crest.* It is the lower area which articulates with the body of the numerically corresponding vertebra. The crest gives attachment to the intra-articular ligament. The posterior surface of the *neck* is rough for the attachment of the inferior costotransverse ligament. The articular part of the *tubercle* articulates with the transverse process of the numerically corresponding vertebra. It forms a convex surface directed backwards and medially on the upper six ribs; on the seventh to tenth, however, it is flattened and directed downwards and backwards and slightly medially. The vertical ridge which marks the *angle* on the outer surface is caused by the adjoining attachments of the iliocostocervicalis part of the sacrospinalis. The *costal groove*, on the lower part of the inner surface, lodges the intercostal vessels and nerve.

The *first rib* is the broadest of all the ribs, and its *angle coincides with its tubercle*. The neck, like the shaft, has upper and lower surfaces. The lower surface of the shaft is smooth and featureless as a rule, but the upper surface presents several recognisable features. Posteriorly, it is roughened for the insertion of scalenus medius and, along the outer border, for the origin of the first digitation of serratus anterior. In front of this rough area, the rib is crossed by a wide shallow groove, which lodges the subclavian artery. Occasionally, this groove is sub-divided into two, corresponding to the lower trunk of the brachial plexus behind, and the subclavian artery in front. On the inner border of the rib, the arterial groove is limited anteriorly by the *scalene tubercle*, which, together with a small part of the upper surface, gives insertion to the scalenus anterior. In some cases the tubercle forms a prominent spicule, but in others it may be difficult to recognise. In front of the scalene tubercle the upper surface shows a second wide shallow groove, and this lodges the subclavian vein.

The surfaces of the *second rib* are oblique. The outer surface looks upwards as well as outwards and the inner surface downwards as well as inwards. In addition the shaft is not twisted and the lower border can rest evenly on a plane surface. A prominent roughened area marks the outer surface about its middle. It gives origin to the lower part of the first and the whole of the second digitation of serratus anterior.

The *eleventh* and *twelfth ribs* are degenerate. On each the head bears a single articular facet for the numerically corresponding vertebra; the neck is merely a slight constriction adjoining the head; and the tubercle is absent. The eleventh has a suspicion of an angle and a trace of a costal groove. Both these features are absent in the twelfth. *Note that in both cases the inner surfaces look definitely upwards as well as inwards.*

THE SKULL

The student is advised not to devote too much time to the study of the individual bones of the skull. It is with the articulated skull that he should be familiar, considered (1) as a whole, (2) with the vault removed, and (3) on median sagittal section.

The upper part of the skull, frequently termed the *calvaria*, contains and protects the brain (a skull minus its mandible is a *cranium*). The lower and anterior part of the skull forms the skeleton of the face. It provides the orbits, to lodge and protect the eyeballs; the skeleton of the nose, to provide permanently patent air passages; and the bony framework of the mouth. The skeleton of the face is therefore especially associated with the respiratory and alimentary systems and special senses.

Norma Verticalis

When the skull is viewed from above, the sagittal, coronal and lambdoid sutures can all be identified. The meeting place of the sagittal and coronal sutures is marked in the fœtal skull by a diamond-shaped, membrane-filled gap, termed the *anterior fontanelle.* Its anterior angle extends forwards between the two frontal bones and its posterior angle backwards between the two parietal bones. *When ossification has proceeded normally, the anterior fontanelle has disappeared by the end of the second year.* The meeting place of the sagittal and lambdoid sutures marks the site of the

PLATE XXVII. LATERAL RADIOGRAPH OF THE SKULL OF A YOUNG ADULT.

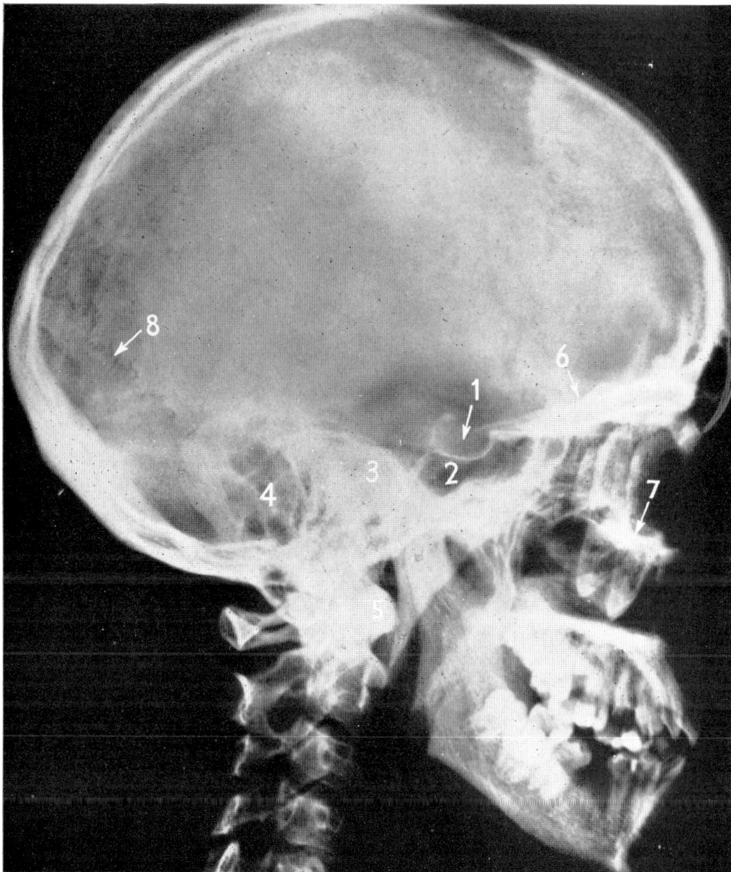

1. Hypophyseal fossa.
2. Sphenoid sinus.
3. Petrous part of temporal bone.
4. Mastoid air cells.
5. Anterior arch of atlas.
6. Roof of orbit.
7. Floor of orbit.
8. Lambdoid suture.

The broad dark band, which crosses the ramus of the mandible obliquely a short distance in front of 5, is due to air in the nasal and oral parts of the pharynx.

by the lesser wing, below by the greater wing and medially by the body of the sphenoid. Its long axis passes downwards and medially from its narrow lateral extremity to its wider medial end. *The lacrimal, frontal and trochlear nerves traverse the narrow part of the fissure, i.e.*, outside the annular tendon (p. 373). They are usually accompanied by the superior ophthalmic vein, which passes backwards to join the cavernous sinus. *The nasociliary, both divisions of the oculomotor nerve and the abducent nerve*, together with the inferior ophthalmic vein as a rule, *traverse the wider, medial, part of the fissure* within the tendinous ring.

The side of the body of the sphenoid is *directly related to the cavernous sinus*, and is grooved by the internal carotid artery, which lies within the sinus in this situation. Three foramina pierce the greater wing and open out of the fossa. The *foramen rotundum*, placed anteriorly and separated from the superior orbital fissure by a narrow bar of bone, *transmits the maxillary nerve*. The *foramen ovale* pierces the posterior part of the greater wing, close to its junction with the body of the sphenoid. *It transmits the mandibular nerve, which carries off the whole of the motor root of V for distribution to the muscles of mastication.* Close to the lateral corner of the foramen ovale, the *foramen spinosum* perforates the greater wing at the root of the sphenoidal spine, and *gives passage to the middle meningeal artery*. The groove formed by the trunk of this vessel runs forwards and laterally, marking the greater wing, and divides into two, one for the anterior division, which ascends over the deep surface of the pterion (p. 390), and one for the posterior division, which runs backwards on to the squamous part of the temporal bone.

The *foramen lacerum* pierces the floor of the fossa between the apex of the petrous part of the temporal bone and the angle of union of the greater wing with the body of the sphenoid. It is occluded in life by cartilage—a remnant of the embryonic chondrocranium—and in its upper part transmits the internal carotid artery from its canal in the petrous part of the temporal bone.

The anterior surface of the petrous part of the temporal bone forms a large and important part of the floor of the fossa. Its lateral part, which immediately adjoins the squamous portion of the bone, forms the *tegmen tympani. This is a thin plate of bone, which successively roofs in the tympanic antrum, the tympanic cavity and the auditory tube*, from behind, forwards and medially. A slight elevation to its medial side, the *arcuate eminence* is formed by the superior semicircular canal. The upper aspect of the apex of the petrous temporal shows a slightly hollowed rea, in which is the trigeminal

PLATE XXVII. LATERAL RADIOGRAPH OF THE SKULL OF A YOUNG ADULT.

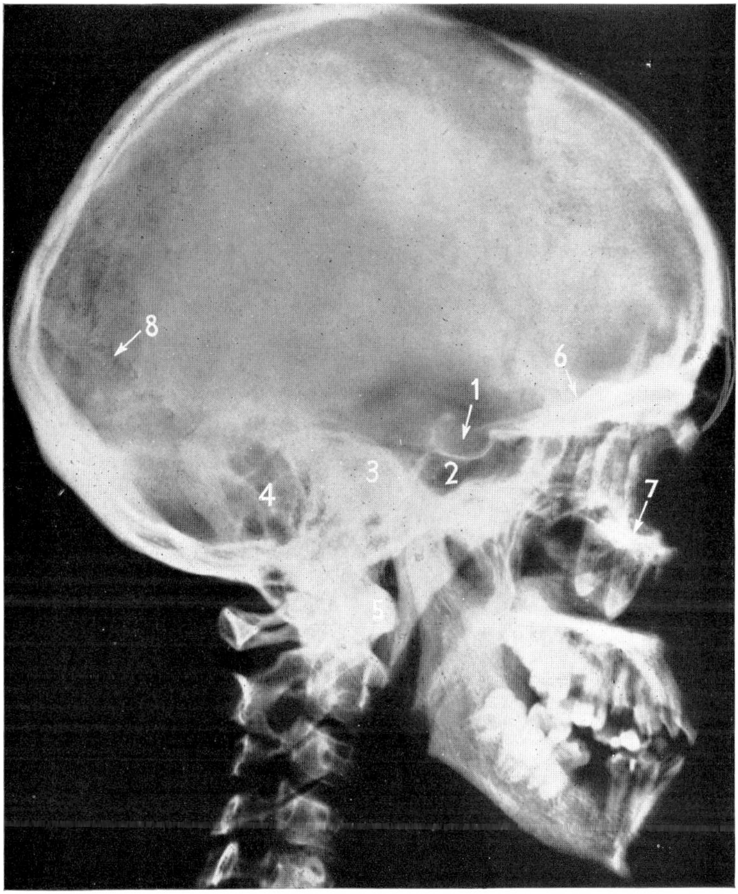

1. Hypophyseal fossa.
2. Sphenoid sinus.
3. Petrous part of temporal bone.
4. Mastoid air cells.
5. Anterior arch of atlas
6. Roof of orbit.
7. Floor of orbit.
8. Lambdoid suture.

The broad dark band, which crosses the ramus of the mandible obliquely a short distance in front of 5, is due to air in the nasal and oral parts of the pharynx.

triangular *posterior fontanelle*, which becomes closed within two or three months after birth.

The Interior of the Skull

The inner surface of the vault is marked by vascular grooves for the superior sagittal sinus and the branches of the meningeal vessels. On each side of the groove for the sinus the bone is pitted by arachnoid granulations (p. 361).

The inner surface of the base of the skull shows a natural subdivision into the anterior, middle and posterior cranial fossæ.

The Cranial Fossæ

The **Anterior Cranial Fossa** is limited posteriorly by the sharp posterior edges of the lesser wings and, in the median part, by the anterior edge of the optic groove of the sphenoid. It supports the frontal lobes and the olfactory bulbs and tracts. Its floor is depressed in its median part, which is part of the roof of the nasal cavity. It is formed by the *cribriform plate of the ethmoid* with its projecting *crista galli*, which gives attachment to the anterior end of the falx cerebri. The foramina which pierce the cribriform plate transmit the fila of the olfactory nerves from the olfactory cells in the nasal mucosa. A narrow slit-like foramen transmits the anterior ethmoidal nerve and vessels. Antero-lateral to this median area, the floor forms the roof of the frontal sinus, and behind that the roof of the orbit.

The **Middle Cranial Fossa** consists of a small median and expanded lateral portions. The *median part* is formed by the upper surface of the body of the sphenoid, from the optic groove in front to the dorsum sellæ behind. The optic groove leads on each side to the *optic foramen, which transmits the optic nerve and the ophthalmic artery*, a branch of the internal carotid artery. This foramen is bounded laterally by the lesser wing, in front and behind by the roots of the lesser wing and medially by the body of the sphenoid. Behind the optic groove the body of the sphenoid is hollowed out to form the *sella turcica, which contains the hypophyis cerebri* (Plate XXVII, p. 386).

The *lateral part* of the floor of the middle cranial fossa is formed by the greater wing of the sphenoid, the front aspect of the petrous part of the temporal bone and a portion of the squamous part of the same bone. It contains the temporal pole and the adjoining part of the temporal lobe of the brain.

The *superior orbital fissure* lies in its anterior part, bounded above by the lesser wing, below by the greater wing and medially by the body of the sphenoid. Its long axis passes downwards and medially from its narrow lateral extremity to its wider medial end. *The lacrimal, frontal and trochlear nerves traverse the narrow part of the fissure, i.e.*, outside the annular tendon (p. 373). They are usually accompanied by the superior ophthalmic vein, which passes backwards to join the cavernous sinus. *The nasociliary, both divisions of the oculomotor nerve and the abducent nerve*, together with the inferior ophthalmic vein as a rule, *traverse the wider, medial, part of the fissure* within the tendinous ring.

The side of the body of the sphenoid is *directly related to the cavernous sinus*, and is grooved by the internal carotid artery, which lies within the sinus in this situation. Three foramina pierce the greater wing and open out of the fossa. The *foramen rotundum*, placed anteriorly and separated from the superior orbital fissure by a narrow bar of bone, *transmits the maxillary nerve.* The *foramen ovale* pierces the posterior part of the greater wing, close to its junction with the body of the sphenoid. *It transmits the mandibular nerve, which carries off the whole of the motor root of V for distribution to the muscles of mastication.* Close to the lateral corner of the foramen ovale, the *foramen spinosum* perforates the greater wing at the root of the sphenoidal spine, and *gives passage to the middle meningeal artery.* The groove formed by the trunk of this vessel runs forwards and laterally, marking the greater wing, and divides into two, one for the anterior division, which ascends over the deep surface of the pterion (p. 390), and one for the posterior division, which runs backwards on to the squamous part of the temporal bone.

The *foramen lacerum* pierces the floor of the fossa between the apex of the petrous part of the temporal bone and the angle of union of the greater wing with the body of the sphenoid. It is occluded in life by cartilage—a remnant of the embryonic chondrocranium—and in its upper part transmits the internal carotid artery from its canal in the petrous part of the temporal bone.

The anterior surface of the petrous part of the temporal bone forms a large and important part of the floor of the fossa. Its lateral part, which immediately adjoins the squamous portion of the bone, forms the *tegmen tympani. This is a thin plate of bone, which successively roofs in the tympanic antrum, the tympanic cavity and the auditory tube*, from behind, forwards and medially. A slight elevation to its medial side, the *arcuate eminence* is formed by the superior semicircular canal. The upper aspect of the apex of the petrous temporal shows a slightly hollowed rea, in which is the trigeminal ganglion in its *cavum trigeminale*. The ganglion usually extends forwards over the upper and lateral part of the foramen lacerum. *The intimate relation of the tympanic cavity to the inferior surface of the temporal lobe of the brain, the tegmen tympani intervening, is probably the most important feature of this region, from the clinical point of view.*

The **Posterior Cranial Fossa** is somewhat rounded and is the deepest of the three fossæ. Its floor is formed by the basilar, condylar and squamous parts of the occipital bone; its lateral wall chiefly by the posterior surface of the petrous and the medial surface of the mastoid part of the temporal bone. The *foramen magnum* transmits a number of structures, including (1) the medulla oblongata, (2) the meninges, (3) the vertebral arteries and (4) the ascending spinal parts of the accessory nerves. *The hypoglossal nerve passes through the anterior condylar canal,* which lies above the antero-lateral boundary of the foramen magnum. The nerve arises by several rootlets, which represent the roots of origin of three or four pre-cervical anterior primary rami and the occasional division of the anterior condylar canal into two parts by a small bar of bone may be associated with this fact.

The *internal auditory meatus* is a deep depression in the posterior surface of the petrous temporal and runs in a lateral direction. *The auditory nerve and the motor and sensory roots of the facial nerve pass into it.*

The *jugular foramen* lies between the lower border of the petrous temporal and the condylar part of the occipital bone. *Its posterior part transmits the sigmoid sinus, which becomes the internal jugular vein* on emerging from the skull. *In front of the sinus, the eleventh, tenth and ninth cranial nerves pass through the foramen,* the tenth and eleventh sharing a common tube of dura mater, a fact in keeping with their evolutionary history. The *inferior petrosal sinus,* which emerges from the posterior end of the cavernous sinus and grooves the lower border of the petrous temporal, *passes through the anterior part of the jugular foramen* to join the internal jugular vein immediately outside the skull.

Where the mastoid part of the temporal bone adjoins the petrous temporal, it is deeply grooved by the *sigmoid sinus. This vessel, in its upper part, lies immediately posterior to the tympanic antrum* (p. 370). It receives the superior petrosal sinus, which runs backwards and laterally from the cavernous sinus along the upper border of the petrous temporal bone. This groove is interrupted by the trigeminal impression.

Just lateral to the foramen magnum, the occipital bone may be pierced by the *posterior condylar canal* for the passage of an emissary vein.

Norma Lateralis

The *superior temporal line*, which commences at the zygomatic process of the frontal bone and curves upwards and backwards from it, is easily felt in the living subject in its anterior and upper parts. Posteriorly, it curves downwards and forwards into the *supramastoid crest*. It marks the attachment of the temporal fascia, and the area which it encloses, as low down as the infratemporal crest on the greater wing of the sphenoid, constitutes the temporal fossa and serves as the origin for the temporalis muscle. The *pterion* is a point in the anterior part of the fossa, where the greater wing of the sphenoid meets the anterior inferior angle of the parietal bone. In this situation a small circular area can be drawn which includes, in addition to the two bones named, portions of the frontal and the squamous temporal. A point near the pterion, nearly 4 cm. above the zygoma and 2.7 cm. behind the frontal process of the zygomatic bone, overlies *the anterior division of the middle meningeal artery*.

The mastoid part of the temporal bone is a backward extension from the petrous part of the temporal bone. The *mastoid process*, which can be palpated medial to the lobule of the auricle, is *not recognisable as a bony projection until the end of the second year*. The *suprameatal triangle* lies immediately behind the upper part of the external auditory meatus. Its floor is often marked by a small depression, on the margin of which the suprameatal spine forms a tiny projection. In this situation the bone forms *the lateral wall of the tympanic antrum*. In the adult this wall is nearly 1.25 cm. thick, but it is considerably less in the young child.

The bony *external auditory meatus* is formed by the trough-like tympanic and the squamous parts of the temporal bone. The former constitutes the floor, the anterior and the lower part of the posterior wall, but the roof and the upper part of the posterior wall are formed by the squamous temporal. The limits of the tympanic part can easily be seen at the orifice of the external auditory meatus. In the newly born child the tympanic part of the temporal bone is represented by the *incomplete tympanic ring*, which surrounds the margin of the tympanic membrane, in front, below and behind but not above. As the meatus grows and deepens, the incomplete ring forms a gutter-like trough, which is roofed in above by the squamous part of the temporal bone.

The *zygomatic arch*, which gives origin to the posterior fibres of the masseter, can be examined in the living subject. Immediately in front of the tragus it is crossed by the superficial temporal artery. Anteriorly, it is completed by the zygomatic bone. The posterior root of the zygomatic process of the temporal bone is continued backwards above the meatus as the supramastoid crest.

The *infratemporal fossa* lies below the infratemporal crest on the greater wing. It is bounded medially by the lateral pterygoid plate and in front by the posterior surface of the maxilla. Above, it is partly roofed in by the infratemporal surface of the greater wing and the adjoining part of the squamous temporal, and communicates with the temporal fossa through the wide gap between the zygoma and the rest of the skull. This gap is traversed by the converging fibres of the temporalis muscle as they descend to their insertion. The fossa contains the lateral and medial pterygoid muscles, the maxillary artery and its middle meningeal branch, the pterygoid venous plexus, the mandibular nerve and its branches and the chorda tympani nerve.

Two fissures are present in the depths of the fossa: (1) The *pterygomaxillary fissure*, placed vertically, intervenes between the medial and anterior walls of the fossa and leads medially into the pterygopalatine fossa. It contains the terminal part of the maxillary artery.

(2) The *inferior orbital fissure* lies horizontally and is situated between the anterior wall and the roof of the fossa, leading into the orbit. It transmits the *maxillary nerve* from the pterygopalatine fossa to the orbit, and a *communicating branch from the inferior ophthalmic veins to the pterygoid venous plexus.*

The *pterygopalatine fossa* contains the *terminal part of the maxillary artery, and is crossed, in its upper part, by the maxillary nerve*, as it runs forwards and laterally from the foramen rotundum to gain the orbit. The *pterygopalatine ganglion* lies in the fossa below the maxillary nerve, and its various branches (p. 281) traverse the fossa. Through the upper part of its medial wall the fossa communicates with the nasal cavity through the *sphenopalatine foramen*, which transmits the nasopalatine nerve and the sphenopalatine vessels.

The Norma Frontalis

The depression at the root of the nose is termed the *nasion*. The *glabella* forms a rounded elevation immediately above the nasion; it connects the medial ends of the two *superciliary arches*. The *supra-orbital foramen* (or notch) lies immediately above the upper border of the orbital opening at the junction of its medial third with its lateral two-thirds. It transmits the vessels and nerve of the same name.

The margins of the *orbital opening* are easily felt through the skin, with the exception of the medial margin, which is flattened above and masked below by the fascia which covers the lacrimal sac.

The *infra-orbital foramen* lies a little less than 1 cm. below the orbital opening. It lies on the anterior surface of the maxilla, *vertically below the supra-orbital foramen*, and transmits the infra-orbital vessels and nerve.

The dorsum of the nose is formed by the nasal bones, which articulate with each other medially, and with the frontal process of the maxilla laterally. The *piriform* (anterior nasal) *aperture* is bounded by the nasal bones and maxillæ. Its lower margin projects forwards in the median plane, forming the *anterior nasal spine*, which can be felt on upward pressure over the posterior part of the lower border of the free part of the nasal septum (Plate XXVIII).

The Orbit

The orbit is a pyramidal cavity, narrow behind and wide in front. The *roof* of the orbit separates it from the frontal sinus antero-medially and from the anterior cranial fossa and the frontal lobe of the brain elsewhere. The lacrimal gland lies in a fossa in the antero-lateral part of the roof. A deep groove on the anterior part of the *medial wall* contains the lacrimal sac and is traversed by the vertical suture between the lacrimal bone and the frontal process of the maxilla. Laterally, it is bridged over by the lacrimal fascia. Inferiorly, it communicates with the inferior meatus of the nose through the nasolacrimal canal. Behind the lacrimal bone the medial wall of the orbit is formed by the orbital plate of the ethmoid, which separates the orbit from the ethmoidal sinuses. The anterior and posterior ethmoidal foramina, which transmit the corresponding nerves and vessels, lie in the fronto-ethmoidal suture at the junction of the roof and the medial wall. The *optic foramen* lies in line with but behind these foramina, and conducts the optic nerve and the ophthalmic artery forwards, downwards and laterally. The *floor* lies above the maxillary sinus, and is limited postero-laterally by the inferior orbital fissure. The *infra-orbital groove* leads forwards on the floor for a short distance from the fissure and then tunnels through the floor to reach the infra-orbital foramen. It transmits the infra-orbital nerve and vessels. The *lateral wall* of the orbit is devoid of any special feature. Posteriorly, it is separated from the roof by the *superior orbital fissure* (p. 387). The medial walls of the two

PLATE XXVIII. ANTERO-POSTERIOR RADIOGRAPH OF THE SKULL OF A YOUNG ADULT.

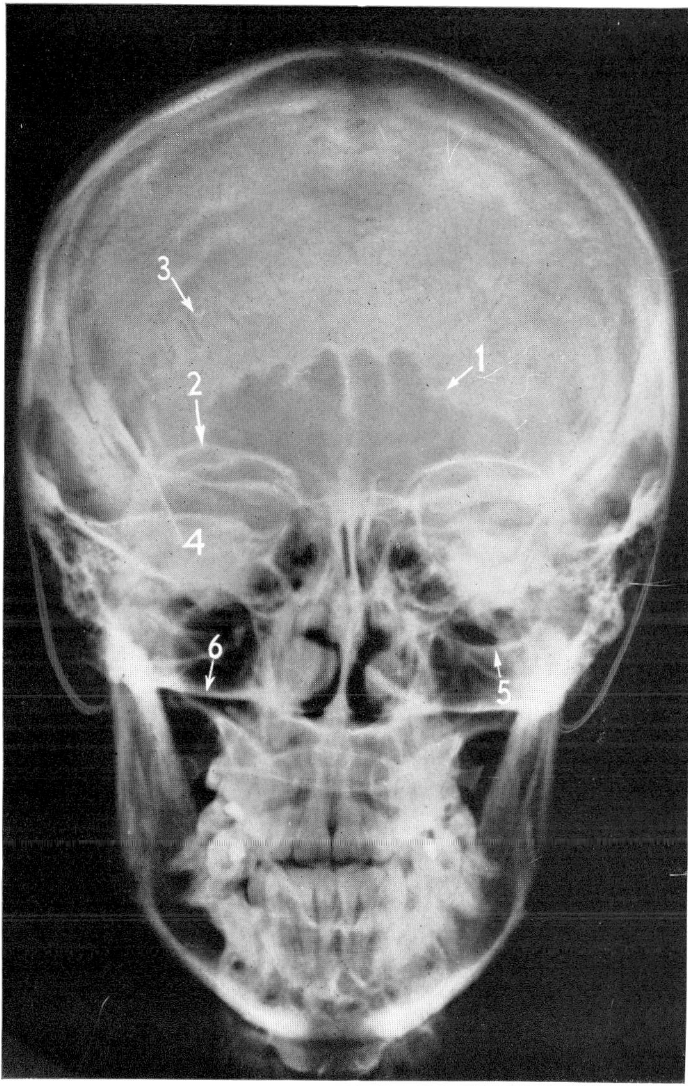

1. Frontal sinus.
2. Roof of orbit.
3. Lambdoidal suture.
4. Petrous part of temporal bone seen through orbit.
5. Floor of orbit.
6. Floor of posterior cranial fossa.

To face p. 392

orbits are parallel, but their lateral walls are set at right angles to each other (Plate XXVII).

The Norma Basalis

The anterior part of this aspect of the skull is occupied by the *bony palate*, which is formed by the palatine processes of the maxillæ and the horizontal plates of the palatine bones. The *greater palatine foramen* opens at its postero-lateral corner and transmits the greater palatine vessels and nerve. The lesser palatine foramina lie immediately behind it. In the median plane anteriorly the *incisive fossa* receives the openings of the lateral incisive canals; they transmit the terminal parts of the greater palatine vessels to the nose and the descending terminal branches of the nasopalatine nerves. Anterior and posterior median incisive canals are sometimes present; they serve for the transmission of the nasopalatine nerves, which otherwise traverse the lateral incisive canals.

The *choanae* (*posterior nasal apertures*) lie above the back of the bony palate, separated from each other by the vomer and bounded laterally by the medial pterygoid plates. The *pterygoid hamulus* curves downwards and laterally at the lower end of the medial pterygoid plate. It gives attachment at its tip to the pterygomandibular ligament, and by its posterior border to the upper fibres of the superior constrictor muscle of the pharynx. The tensor veli palatini tendon twists round its lateral and anterior aspects. A small spicule on the posterior border of the medial pterygoid plate marks the lower limit of the expanded pharyngeal end of the pharyngotympanic tube. Superiorly, this border widens to enclose the *scaphoid fossa*, which gives origin to the anterior fibres of the tensor palati.

The medial pterygoid plate has a separate centre of ossification, which appears in mesenchyme, but the lateral pterygoid plate is ossified in cartilage as a downward extension from the root of the greater wing. The medial plate fuses with the lateral and with the greater wing before birth. The lateral pterygoid plate gives origin to the deep head of the medial pterygoid muscle on its medial aspect, and to the lower head of the lateral pterygoid on its lateral aspect.

Postero-lateral to the root of the lateral pterygoid plate, the posterior part of the greater wing of the sphenoid is pierced by the *foramen ovale* and the *foramen spinosum* (p. 388). The *spine of the sphenoid* lies postero-lateral to the latter foramen, medial to the articular fossa of the temporal bone, and is intimately related to the upper and medial part of the tympanic part of the temporal bone.

Attached to it is the sphenomandibular ligament, which represents the perichondrium around the upper end of Meckel's cartilage.

The upper end of the medial border of the scaphoid fossa is marked by a small tubercle, above which the sphenoid is pierced by the *pterygoid canal*, with its contained nerve and vessels. It is along the line of this canal that the lateral part of the sphenoid, consisting of the pterygoid process and the greater wing, joins the body of the bone in the first year.

The interval between the posterior border of the greater wing and the inferior surface of the petrous temporal forms a groove, which is occupied by the cartilaginous part of the auditory tube. Just above and postero-medial to the spine of the sphenoid the tube emerges from the temporal bone, and runs forwards and medially to the posterior border of the medial pterygoid plate.

The *articular fossa* of the temporal bone lodges the condylar process of the mandible, when the mouth is closed. Its anterior wall is formed by the convex *articular eminence*, on to which the condylar process passes when the mouth is opened. Both these surfaces are covered with articular cartilage, *which is white fibrocartilage in this situation.* The articular fossa is limited behind by the squamotympanic fissure, at the medial end of which a thin edge of bone can be detected as a rule. This is the lower border of the down-turned lateral part of the tegmen tympani (petrous temporal), and it divides the squamotympanic fissure into a petrosquamous fissure anteriorly and a petrotympanic fissure posteriorly. Through the medial end of the latter the *chorda tympani* makes its exit from the tympanic cavity.

The medial portion of the tympanic part of the temporal bone adjoins the orifice of the *carotid canal* on the inferior surface of the petrous part. This canal transmits the internal carotid artery (p. 279) and the carotid sympathetic plexus. A bony ridge separates the opening from the *jugular foramen* behind (p. 389).

The lower margin of the tympanic part of the temporal bone grips and forms a sheath for the root of the *styloid process.* This process juts downwards and forwards immediately lateral to, but on a lower level than, the jugular foramen. It represents the dorsal or cephalic end of the skeletal element of the second visceral arch, and the stylomastoid foramen, which transmits the facial nerve (second arch), lies immediately behind its root. The process gives attachment to a number of structures. The stylohyoid ligament springs from its tip; the styloglossus from the anterior aspect of its tip; the stylohyoid from its posterior aspect, and the stylopharyngeus from the medial side of its base.

Behind the posterior bony apertures of the nose the inferior surface of the sphenoid joins the basilar part of the occipital bone. *Up to the twenty-fifth year a plate of cartilage separates the two bones.* The *pharyngeal tubercle* forms a small elevation in the median plane on the basilar part of the occipital bone. It gives attachment to the uppermost fibres of the superior constrictor muscles. Postero-lateral to this tubercle the longus capitis is attached to a roughened impression on the bone.

The basilar part of the occipital includes the anterior margin of the foramen magnum, the anterior ends of the occipital condyles and the anterior walls of the anterior condylar canals. The *anterior condylar canal,* therefore, lies in the line of union between the basilar and the condylar portion of the occipital bone, which fuse with each other about the sixth year. The hypoglossal nerve runs laterally and slightly forwards as it passes through the anterior condylar canal, and so comes into close relationship with the ninth, tenth and eleventh cranial nerves as they leave the skull.

The *occipital condyle* articulates with the upper aspect of the lateral mass of the atlas. Its long axis passes forwards and medially. Posterior to the condyle the occipital bone shows a distinct depression, which may or may not be perforated by a *posterior condylar canal* for the passage of an emissary vein.

Medial to the mastoid process, the mastoid part of the temporal bone is marked by the *mastoid notch* for the origin of the posterior belly of the digastric muscle, and to the medial side of this notch the bone may be grooved by the occipital artery.

Behind the foramen magnum in the median plane the *external occipital crest* runs backwards and upwards to the *external occipital protuberance*, marking the attachment of the ligamentum nuchal. About the middle of the crest, the *inferior nuchal line* curves laterally, limiting the insertions of the rectus capitis posterior minor and major muscles. Opposite the protuberance, the *superior nuchal lines* curve laterally on each side with an upward convexity. Medially they are sharp and prominent, but laterally they tend to fade away. The semispinalis capitis is inserted into the depression between the nuchal lines lateral to the external occipital crest. The *highest nuchal line*, the attachment of the occipital bellies of the occipito-frontalis and the epicranial aponeurosis, lies about 1 cm. above the superior nuchal line.

Norma Occipitalis

The chief features on this aspect of the skull have already been included under the norma verticalis and the norma basalis.

The Nasal Cavity

The lateral wall of the nasal cavity is marked by the presence of the inferior, middle and superior nasal conchæ and meatuses and the spheno-ethmoidal recess.

The *inferior nasal concha* is a separate bone, which helps to cover in the lower part of the large gap on the nasal surface of the maxilla and so forms a part of the medial wall of the maxillary sinus. It roofs in the inferior meatus and hides the orifice of the *nasolacrimal canal*, which opens at the highest part of the meatus, *i.e.*, at the junction of its anterior third with the posterior two-thirds.

The *superior and middle nasal conchæ* are elevations on the medial aspect of the ethmoidal labyrinth. Anteriorly a small part of the wall of the middle meatus is formed by the lacrimal bone, but behind that it is constituted by the lower part of the labyrinth and its *uncinate process*, which curves downwards and backwards to articulate with the inferior concha. This articulation is often imperfect, and a varying number of small gaps are left which lead into the maxillary sinus. As a rule, these are closed in life by mucous membrane. When the middle concha is removed, the curved upper and posterior border of the uncinate process can be seen. Clothed by mucous membrane, it forms the medial edge of the *hiatus semilunaris* (p. 295). Above and behind the uncinate process the *ethmoidal bulla* forms a projection on the lateral wall of the middle meatus. Between the bulla and the uncinate process anteriorly the *infundibulum of the frontal sinus* opens. Above the bulla the middle ethmoidal sinuses communicate with the nasal cavity. The *maxillary sinus* opens, in an upward direction, through the floor of the hiatus semilunaris. *The orifice is difficult to see, as it is hidden by the uncinate process when viewed from the medial side.*

The *superior meatus* is short and receives the opening of the posterior ethmoidal sinuses.

The *spheno-ethmoidal recess* lies between the superior concha and the front of the sphenoid, which forms its posterior wall. It is through this aspect of the sphenoid that the sphenoidal sinus communicates with the nasal cavity.

Posteriorly, the lateral wall of the nasal cavity is formed by the perpendicular plate of the palatine bone, which forms the posterior part of the medial wall of the maxillary sinus. Just behind the superior meatus the lateral wall of the nasal cavity is pierced by the *sphenopalatine foramen* (p. 391), which communicates with the pterygopalatine fossa. This foramen is bounded in front by the orbital process and behind by the sphenoidal process of the palatine bone, and above by the body of the sphenoid.

The *floor* of the nasal cavity is formed by the upper surface of the bony palate. It slopes backwards and slightly upwards.

The *roof* is highest at its central part, where it is formed by the cribriform plate of the ethmoid. In front and behind it slopes downwards, and is formed, anteriorly, by the frontal and nasal bones, and, posteriorly, by the body of the sphenoid bone.

The *nasal septum* is partly bony and partly cartilaginous. The perpendicular plate of the ethmoid and the vomer play the largest part in its formation, but below and in front the septal cartilage occupies an extensive area. The septum is often deflected along the line of the vomero-ethmoidal articulation.

Development of the Skull

In the early embryo the skull is represented by a capsule of condensed mesenchyme which surrounds the developing brain. During the second and third months, portions of this mesenchyme are replaced by cartilage, and these are sooner or later replaced by bone. The remainder of the mesenchymatous capsule of the brain ossifies without passing through a cartilaginous stage.

The bones of the base of the skull are, for the most part, preformed in cartilage. These include the whole of the occipital bone (except the upper portion of the squamous part, which ossifies directly in membrane), the petrous part of the temporal bone, the body, lesser wings and roots of the greater wings of the sphenoid and the ethmoid bone. All the other bones of the skull, including all the bones of the cranial vault but excluding the styloid process, the inferior concha and the auditory ossicles, ossify in membrane.

The basilar parts of the occipital and the sphenoid, collectively called the clivus and closely related to the cephalic end of the notochord, together with the condylar parts of the occipital, may be regarded as representing greatly modified precervical vertebræ. The petrous temporal is developed in connexion with the membranous labyrinth, and represents the ossified auditory capsule, while the ethmoid is an ossified part of the nasal capsule. *The bones of the cranial vault*—parietals, frontals, squamous temporals and the upper portion of the squamous occipital—*all ossify in mesenchyme* and are to be regarded as *dermal* bones, *i.e.*, as originally derived from the skin.

In the skull of the newly-born child the fontanelles form membrane-filled gaps which permit of rapid enlargement of the skull. The anterior fontanelle (p. 386) is placed at the middle of the coronal suture, the posterior fontanelle at the lambda, the sphenoidal (antero-lateral) at the pterion, and the mastoid (postero-lateral) at the junction of the mastoid part of the temporal bone with the parietal and the occipital bones. *During the first year of life the size of the brain is trebled, and the skull grows very rapidly.* Increase in length occurs chiefly at the fontanelles, at the coronal and lambdoid sutures and at the spheno-occipital joint, in height at the lateral fontanelles and at the temporoparietal suture, in breadth at the fontanelles and at the sagittal suture. After the first year the rate of growth becomes much slower, and *after the closure of the anterior fontanelle at the end of the second year* most of the growth occurs at the sutures.

The growth of the face is associated to a very large extent with the growth of the jaws, and is therefore particularly active during the period of the eruption of the deciduous teeth (sixth month—second year), and again during the eruption of the permanent teeth (sixth year—fourteenth year).

The Mandible

The mandible ossifies in two halves, each from a single centre, which appears in the sixth or seventh week in a sheet of connective tissue lateral to Meckel's cartilage. At birth the two halves are united in front by fibrous tissue, but bony union occurs during the first year. As the mandible enlarges its alveolar arch lengthens to provide the necessary accommodation for the additional teeth of the permanent set. The ramus, relatively, moves backwards by a combined process of absorption along the front of the ramus and deposition along its posterior border. At the same time the condyle goes through a continuous process of remodelling until the adult stage is reached.

The *mental foramen*, which transmits the cutaneous branch of the inferior alveolar (dental) nerve and vessels, lies below the interval between the first and second premolar teeth, and in the adult it is placed about midway between the lower border and the alveolar part. In the young child it lies close to the lower border; in the edentulous jaw the alveolar part becomes absorbed to a large extent and the foramen lies near the upper border.

When teeth are extracted, the alveoli become absorbed but the process affects the thinner of the two alveolar walls to a greater degree. In the mandible the labial wall is the thinner in the incisor and canine regions, but in the molar region it is the lingual wall which is the thinner. The alveolar ridge which is found on edentulous mandibles after absorption has taken place lies within the line of the incisor and canine teeth, but lies outside the line of the molar teeth. It may be noted that in the maxilla, on the other hand, the labial walls of the alveoli are everywhere the thinner, so that the maxillary alveolar ridge lies within the line of the teeth in all regions. These facts are of considerable practical importance in connexion with the planning of complete upper and lower dentures.

The inner surface of the body of the mandible is marked in the median plane by the *genial tubercules*, which give origin to the genio-hyoid muscles below, and the genioglossi above. On each side the *mylohyoid line* is an outstanding feature. It begins just behind the last molar tooth and runs downwards and forwards to reach the median plane immediately *below the genial tubercles.* In its posterior part it is sharp and salient and overhangs the *submandibular fossa*, which lodges the submandibular salivary gland. Anteriorly, the line is faint and not always easy to trace. Throughout its extent it gives origin to the mylohyoid muscle. The area above the mylohyoid line is narrow behind, *where it is closely related to the lingual nerve* (p. 270), but wider in front, where it is covered with mucous membrane above, and in contact with the sublingual gland below.

The *angle of the mandible* is subcutaneous and can be palpated without difficulty. Its deep surface shows a triangular roughened area, which extends as far forwards as the mylohyoid groove and is the attachment of the medial pterygoid muscle.

The lateral surface of the ramus gives attachment to the masseter muscle. The medial surface is marked by the *mandibular foramen*, into which the inferior alveolar vessels and nerve enter. Its medial edge may project and constitutes the *lingula*, which gives attachment to the sphenomandibular ligament. Behind and below the lingula the *mylohyoid groove*, containing the corresponding branches of the inferior alveolar vessels and nerve, runs downwards and forwards, below and behind the posterior end of the mylohyoid line.

The thin, sharp *coronoid process* gives attachment along its edges and on its deep surface to the temporalis. The anterior fibres of the muscle descend beyond the process and are inserted into the anterior border of the ramus. If the finger is pressed into the angle between the zygomatic bone and the anterior border of the masseter, the anterior edge of the coronoid process will impinge on it when the mouth is opened.

The *condylar process* articulates with the articular fossa on the infratemporal surface of the squamous temporal. Articular cartilage covers its superior and anterior but not its posterior aspect, which is separated from the tympanic part of the temporal bone by an upward extension of the parotid gland. *The lateral aspect of the condylar process is covered by the parotid gland* and lies immediately in front of the lower part of the tragus of the auricle. When a finger is placed in this position and the mouth is alternately opened and closed, the movements of the process can be appreciated. The condylar process is connected to the ramus by a short neck, which bears on its anterior aspect a depression, sometimes roughened, for attachment of the lateral pterygoid muscle.

The mandibular notch transmits the nerve and vessels of supply to the masseter.

The Hyoid Bone

The hyoid bone lies at the root of the tongue. The body is difficult to feel, but the tips of the greater cornua can be gripped between the finger and thumb a little above the level of the thyroid cartilage. The body of the hyoid overhangs the thyrohyoid membrane, which is attached to the upper part of its posterior surface, the subhyoid bursa, when present, intervening. *The upper part of the posterior surface is related to the epiglottis, to which it is attached by its hyo-epiglottic ligament.*

The lesser cornu projects upwards and backwards, and the stylohyoid ligament is attached to its tip. Along its posterior border the middle constrictor muscle is attached. The elongated greater cornu gives origin along its upper border to the hyoglossus and, under cover of that muscle, to the middle constrictor. Its lower border is the attachment to the thyrohyoid membrane.

The body of the hyoid bone represents the fused ventral ends of the skeletal elements of the second and third visceral arches. The lesser cornu represents the adjoining part of the second and the greater cornu that of the third arch.

THE BONES OF THE UPPER LIMB

The *shoulder girdle* consists of two independent bones, viz., the clavicle and the scapula, which are able to move on each other at the acromioclavicular point. It must be noted that the girdle articulates with the axial skeleton only through the medium of the sternoclavicular joint, a fact which permits the wide range of movement possible at the shoulder. Further, the two girdles are not connected to each other. Compare the shoulder girdle with the girdle of the lower limb and observe how the rigidity of the latter is enhanced and its mobility proportionately diminished by (1) the fusion of its three elements into a single bone, (2) the presence of the pubic symphysis, and (3) the size and character of the sacro-iliac joints.

The Clavicle

The clavicle is subcutaneous throughout its whole length. Its sternal end is expanded, and is triangular or quadrilateral on transverse section. Its acromial end is flattened, and articulates with the medial side of the acromion. The clavicle is convex forwards in its medial half, and concave forwards in its lateral half. Its inferior surface is marked in its intermediate third by a longitudinal groove for the attachment of the subclavius. To the medial third of its upper border, or surface, the clavicular head of the sternomastoid is attached, and to its anterior surface the clavicular head of the pectoralis major. To the lateral third of its anterior border the deltoid and to the posterior border the trapezius are attached. The intermediate third forms the base of the posterior triangle of the neck and the upper boundary of the infraclavicular fossa.

The articular facet at its sternal end is continued round on to the inferior surface of the bone, and there articulates with the upper aspect of the medial end of the first costal cartilage. Lateral to this area the inferior surface of the bone shows a prominent marking, either a depression or a roughened area, for the attachment of the strong *costoclavicular ligament* (p. 245).

A short distance from the acromial end, the posterior margin of the inferior surface is marked by the *conoid tubercle*, to which the conoid part of the coracoclavicular ligament (p. 14) is attached. From this tubercle the *trapezoid line*—a linear marking of variable breadth—runs forwards and laterally, providing attachment for the trapezoid part of the same ligament.

The clavicle acts as a strut to the shoulder and enables the upper limb to work clear of the body. In addition, it helps to transmit the weight of the limb to the axial skeleton (p. 14).

The clavicle is the *first bone in the body to ossify* and the process of ossification starts in mesenchyme. The bone usually possesses one epiphysis only, viz., for the sternal end. This epiphysis is usually late (eighteenth to twentieth year) in appearing, and it fuses with the shaft about the twenty-fifth year.

The Scapula

When the arm is by the side, the glenoid cavity faces forwards and laterally and the coracoid process points almost directly forwards.

Most of the *costal surface*, including the grooved strip along the lateral border, but excluding the area adjoining the neck of the bone, has attached to it the subscapularis muscle.

The medial two-thirds of the *supraspinous fossa* provides origin for the supraspinatus, which runs below the acromion as it passes to its insertion into the greater tuberosity of the humerus. The medial three-fourths of the *infraspinous fossa* gives origin to the infraspinatus. In neither case does the origin of the muscle extend on to the neck of the bone. Lateral to the origin of the infraspinatus, and immediately adjoining the lateral border, the bone is flattened and forms a striplike area above for teres minor and an oval area below for teres major. The teres minor area is crossed by a vascular groove, produced by the circumflex scapular vessels.

The bone adjoining the *lateral border* is markedly thickened to provide a strong lever for those fibres of the serratus anterior which are inserted on the costal surface of the inferior angle of the bone. The border itself is a linear ridge and its upper part is marked by the *infraglenoid tubercle* for the origin of the long head of triceps. The lateral border is thickly covered by muscle and cannot be felt satisfactorily through the skin.

The *medial border* is thin and to it are attached the upper fibres of the serratus anterior on its costal aspect and to the levator scapulæ and the rhomboid muscles.

The *inferior angle* of the scapula and the lower part of the medial border can easily be felt through the skin. *With the arm by the side, the inferior angle lies over the seventh intercostal space.*

The *superior angle* is covered by the trapezius and is difficult to feel, and this applies to the whole of the superior border. At the lateral end of the superior border the *suprascapular notch* is bridged by the suprascapular ligament and converted into a foramen, which transmits the suprascapular nerve. The corresponding vessels lie above the ligament.

The lateral angle is truncated to form the shallow *glenoid cavity*, which is deepened by the labrum glenoidale. In the fresh specimen the cartilage is thinner over the central area and thicker at the periphery. Immediately above the cavity the *supraglenoid tubercle* gives origin to the intracapsular tendon of the long head of the biceps, and it is only in this situation that the capsular ligament of the shoulder joint is attached directly to the bone.

The *coracoid process* springs by a stout root from the lateral part of the superior border of the bone and almost at once bends forwards and slightly laterally at a right angle. A flattened impression marks the posterior aspect of the bend and gives attachment to the conoid part of the coracoclavicular ligament. The trapezoid part is attached to the upper surface of the process, and in front of the ligament the pectoralis minor is inserted into the bone. The lateral border gives attachment to the coraco-acromial ligament, which helps the acromion to form an arch above the head of the humerus. The tip of the coracoid process, to which are attached coracobrachialis and the short head of biceps, is covered by the anterior fibres of deltoid, *but can be felt on deep pressure through the lateral boundary of the infraclavicular fossa, about 2.5 cm. below the clavicle.*

The crest of the *spine of the scapula* is subcutaneous. Its flattened medial end lies opposite the spine of the third thoracic vertebra with the arm by the side. The lateral part of the spine forms the *acromion.* It projects laterally, and then bends forwards sharply at the *acromial angle.* The upper surface and borders of the *acromion* can be felt through the skin. Its medial border bears the small, oval, sloping clavicular facet, and to the bone immediately in front of the joint is attached to the narrow lateral extremity of the coraco-acromial ligament.

The mobility of the bone is its outstanding characteristic, for it greatly increases the range of movement at the shoulder and renders it possible to raise the arm above the head (p. 13).

At birth the body and spine of the scapula are ossified, but the acromion and the coracoid process are cartilaginous as well as the glenoid cavity, the inferior angle and the medial border of the bone. A centre of ossification appears in the coracoid in the first year. Its early appearance may be correlated with the fact that the *coracoid* process corresponds to the ischium in the lower limb girdle and is, therefore, morphologically a distinct element. It joins the rest of the bone at the fifteenth year. Other centres appear between the tenth and twentieth years. Of these the most important are two which appear in the acromion about the fifteenth year. They soon unite with each other forming an epiphysis which later joins the spine. It sometimes fails to unite, and in this event the condition is always bilateral.

The Humerus

The cartilage over the *head* of the humerus is thickest in its central part and thins off towards the circumference. The anatomical neck is the faint constriction which *immediately adjoins the head.* The capsular ligament of the shoulder joint is attached to it except on the medial side, where the ligament descends on to the shaft. The *greater tuberosity* is the *most lateral bony point of the shoulder* (Plate V, p. 32) and, although covered by the deltoid, can be felt in the living subject on deep pressure. The *lesser tuberosity* is placed on the front of the shaft immediately below the anatomical neck. Like the greater tuberosity it is obscured by the deltoid, but can be felt on deep pressure, especially during rotation of the humerus. The two tuberosities are separated by the *bicipital groove,* in which lies the long head of the biceps and its synovial sheath.

The *upper epiphyseal line* is almost horizontal. It coincides with the lower margin of the head on the medial side, but passes through the lowest part of the bulge caused by the greater tuberosity on the lateral side. The upper epiphysis comprises the head, the anatomical neck and all but the lowest parts of the tuberosities. Its lower surface is slightly hollowed out, to conform to the convex upper end of the diaphysis, which is a conspicuous feature in X-ray photographs of the young bone (Plate VI, p. 28). The two unite between twenty and twenty-two.

The *deltoid tuberosity* forms a roughened area, somewhat V-shaped, with the apex downwards. It is placed on the lateral aspect of the shaft about half-way down the bone. The shallow *radial groove* lies immediately behind the tuberosity. It contains the radial nerve and profunda artery, and gives origin to some of the fibres of the upper and lateral part of the brachialis.

The *lateral supracondylar ridge* is salient and roughened by the attachments of brachioradialis and extensor carpi radialis longus. The *medial supracondylar ridge* is inconspicuous; the medial intermuscular septum is attached to it.

The *medial epicondyle*, easily felt through the skin, has a muscular impression on its medial and anterior aspects, for the superficial flexors of the forearm. This area forms a scale-like epiphysis, which joins the rest of the bone about the eighteenth year. *The rest of the epicondyle ossifies as a downward extension of the shaft.*

The *lateral epicondyle* is much less conspicuous. Its lateral and anterior aspects show a muscular impression for the common extensor origin. *It can be felt easily both on the lateral and on the posterior aspects of the elbow.* When the arm is at rest by the side, a line drawn through the lower end of the humerus from the lateral to the medial epicondyle passes backwards and medially. This does not mean that the humerus is rotated medially, for in the resting position the anterior surface of the bone faces in the same direction as the costal surface of the scapula. The lateral epicondyle has a separate centre of ossification, but it joins the epiphysis for the trochlea and capitulum (*vide infra*).

The medial edge of the trochlea descends to a lower level than the lateral edge, and consequently the line of the elbow-joint is not horizontal (Plate VII, p. 28). When the forearm is supine, the long axis of the arm meets the long axis of the forearm at an angle of about 170 degrees, open to the lateral side. This is the "carrying angle," and it enables the long axis of the forearm to be brought into line with the long axis of the arm, when the forearm and hand are in the mid-prone position. N.B. *The hand is most frequently used in the mid-prone position.* However, the elbow is very commonly flexed to bring the fully supinated forearm and hand towards the face, in which position the axes of the two segments of the limb do not and must not coincide.

The capsular ligament of the elbow-joint extends above the level of the articular surfaces both in front and behind, *but it skirts the epicondyles and leaves their muscular impressions extracapsular.* Anteriorly its line of attachment follows the upper borders of the coronoid and radial fossæ; posteriorly it follows, roughly, the upper border of the olecranon fossa; medially it is attached to the root of the epicondyle, and laterally it runs close to the edge of the capitulum.

The *lower epiphysis of the humerus* includes the lateral epicondyle, the capitulum and the trochlea. The epiphyseal line is practically horizontal at the level of the upper border of the trochlea. On the medial side, it descends across the root of the medial epicondyle, corresponding to the capsular attachment in this situation, and an interval intervenes between it and the epiphyseal line of the medial epicondyle. The lower epiphysis joins the shaft at the seventeenth year or earlier.

The Radius

The circumference of the disc-like *head* of the radius can be felt easily from the posterior aspect of the limb. When the elbow is extended passively, *a depression is visible on the posterior aspect of the elbow on the lateral side*, placed immediately medial to the curved fleshy projection formed by the superficial extensor muscles of the forearm (Plate IB, p. 16). *The head of the radius can be felt in the lower part of this depression*, and it can be felt rotating within the annular ligament when the hand is alternately pronated and supinated. In the upper part of the depression, the back of the lateral epicondyle and the adjoining part of the humerus can be felt. Between these two bones, the finger sinks into the line of the radio-humeral joint. The *upper epiphyseal line* runs round the lower border of the flattened circumference of the head. This epiphysis does not begin to ossify until the fifth year and it joins the shaft at puberty. N.B. *The annular ligament is not attached to the radius.*

The biceps is attached to the posterior part of the *radial tuberosity*, and insertion enables the muscle to act to good mechanical advantage as a supinator, especially when the forearm is flexed. A roughened area marks the lateral aspect of the shaft at the region of its maximum curvature. It marks the insertion of the pronator teres. The interosseous membrane is attached to the interosseous border of the shaft, but it does not extend so high as the radial tuberosity. Below, it follows the posterior of the two lines into which the interosseous border divides.

The lower end of the radius is the widest and bulkiest part of the bone. The *lateral aspect* is prolonged downwards as the *styloid process*, which is partially obscured in the living subject by the tendons of abductor pollicis longus and extensor pollicis brevis. These tendons must be kept relaxed when the bone is being examined. Just above the styloid process, the lateral aspect of the bone receives the insertion of the brachioradialis. *The anterior margin of this area is sharp and easily felt through the skin.* It gives attachment to the extensor retinaculum. The *anterior border* of the lower end is projected forwards and can be felt on deep pressure about 1.5 to 2 cm. *above* the base of the thenar eminence. It is obscured by the flexor tendons, which must be kept relaxed during its examination. The *dorsal aspect* of the lower end presents the prominent *dorsal tubercle*, grooved obliquely on its medial aspect by the tendon of the extensor pollicis longus. It intervenes between the grooves for the radial extensors of the wrist, on its lateral side, and the wide groove for the extensor digitorum and extensor indicis, on its medial side. This tubercle lies in line with the radial border of the middle finger. The *medial aspect* of the lower end articulates with the side of the head of the ulna. *The sharp ridge which separates this surface from the carpal articular surface gives attachment to the lateral border of the articular disc of the inferior radio-ulnar joint* (*vide infra*).

The *lower epiphyseal line* of the radius passes round the bone on a level with the upper margin of the ulnar notch (Plate VIII, p. 33), and, on the lateral side, includes the area for the insertion of brachioradialis. It does not join the shaft until about the twentieth year.

The Ulna

The upper end of the ulna is the bulkiest part of the bone. The posterior aspect of the *olecranon* and the edge which separates it from the superior aspect are subcutaneous and easily palpable. In extension of the forearm, this edge is on the same level as the epicondyles of the humerus. The superior aspect of the olecranon gives insertion to the tendon of triceps, and, *in most cases, the upper epiphysis of the ulna is scale-like and restricted to this area.* It is a traction epiphysis, the centre for which appears at about eight or nine. It joins the shaft at about sixteen. The lateral aspect of the olecranon gives insertion to the upper part of anconeus, and its medial aspect gives origin to the ulnar head of the flexor carpi ulnaris.

The *coronoid process ossifies with the shaft.* Its anterior aspect is covered by, and gives insertion to, the brachialis. Its medial edge is prominent: to the rounded tubercle at its upper end the anterior band of the medial ligament of the elbow joint is attached. This band gives origin to part of the humero-ulnar head of the flexor digitorum sublimis, which extends downwards to share the tubercle with the ligament. The deep head of pronator teres arises from the same edge at a lower level, and a small additional head for flexor pollicis longus may arise below it.

The *lateral aspect* of the coronoid process is marked by the *radial notch* for articulation with the head of the radius. *Its anterior and posterior borders give attachment to the annular ligament.* Below the notch the bone is slightly hollowed out to give clearance for the radial tuberosity during the movements of pronation and supination. The posterior part of this area gives origin to the supinator. Below this area the interosseous membrane is attached to the interosseous border of the bone.

The posterior border of the shaft of the ulna is subcutaneous in its whole length (Plate IB, p. 16), from the posterior aspect of the olecranon down to the styloid process.

The posterior surface of the shaft is marked by two ridges of variable prominence. An upper oblique ridge can usually be traced from just below the radial notch downwards and medially to the posterior border; it marks the lower limit of the insertion of anconeus. A vertical ridge commences near the upper end of this oblique ridge and runs downwards for about three-fourths of the length of the bone; it separates a narrow lateral strip, which adjoins the interosseous border and gives origin to some of the deep extensors, from a broader medial strip, *which is covered by the extensor carpi ulnaris but is free from muscular attachments.*

The small rounded *head* of the ulna has the *styloid process* projecting from its postero-medial aspect. A small non-articular area intervenes between the root of the process and the inferior articular surface of the head; *it gives attachment to the apex of the articular disc of the inferior radio-ulnar joint.* The inferior articular surface is separated from the triquetral bone by the disc. The articular circumference forms a somewhat semilunar area on the lateral and anterior aspects of the head for articulation with the ulnar notch of the radius. Posteriorly a groove, which lodges the extensor carpi ulnaris tendon, separates the styloid process from the rest of the head.

The head of the ulna can be gripped between the finger and thumb, when both the flexor and the extensor carpi ulnaris are relaxed.

In full pronation it forms a prominence, conspicuous in some individuals, on the medial part of the dorsal aspect of the wrist.

The Carpus

The *scaphoid*, *lunate* and *triquetral bones* form the carpal articular surface in the radiocarpal joint. The *tubercle of the scaphoid* can be felt through the skin at the base of the thenar eminence, in line with the radial side of the middle finger. Occasionally it forms a visible elevation, but it is usually concealed by the tendon of the flexor carpi radialis, and can be felt only when that muscle is relaxed. The *pisiform bone* lies at the base of the hypothenar eminence on the medial side of the front of the wrist. When the flexor carpi ulnaris, in the tendon of which it lies, is relaxed, it can be moved about on the palmar surface of the triquetral bone.

Of the bones of the distal row of the carpus, only the *trapezium* and the *hook of the hamate bone* can be identified with certainty through the skin. The ridge on the trapezium lies immediately below the tubercle of the scaphoid, but it is rarely easy to feel. The hook of the hamate can be felt through the medial part of the hypothenar eminence. *It lies 2.5 cm. below the level of the pisiform and in line with the ulnar border of the ring finger. The superficial terminal branch of the ulnar nerve can be rolled across the tip of the hook.*

As a whole the carpus forms a surface which is concave from side to side on its palmar aspect, and the extremities of the concavity form the palpable bony points which have just been mentioned. To them is attached the flexor retinaculum (p. 30), forming an osteofascial tunnel for the flexor tendons of the fingers.

The carpus is cartilaginous at birth. The capitate, which is the largest of the carpal bones, begins to ossify in the first year and, with the exception of the pisiform, which does not undergo ossification until the twelfth year, all the carpal bones are in process of ossification by the eighth year.

The Metacarpus and Phalanges

The *first metacarpal bone* is the *shortest* and *most movable* of all the metacarpals. It lies in a plane anterior to the other metacarpal bones, and has been rotated medially through a right angle so that the thumbnail faces *laterally* in the resting position. Its dorsal surface is the same breadth throughout and shows no trace of the flattened elongated triangular areas which mark the dorsal aspects of the distal halves of the shafts of the other metacarpals. This aspect can easily be examined through the skin, and *in the living hand it is directed laterally. On this account flexion of the thumb carries it medially across the front of the palm and opposition of the thumb to the other digits is rendered possible.* The saddle-shaped base of the first metacarpal articulates with the trapezium. The importance of this articulation has already been emphasised (p. 47). The first metacarpal bone always has an epiphysis at its proximal end, *i.e.*, it ossifies like a phalanx; but it is by no means uncommon to find an epiphysis present for the distal end as well, which, when present, unites between the ages of 12 and 14.

The remaining four metacarpal bones exhibit flattened triangular areas on the dorsal aspect of the shaft, towards the distal end. These areas are covered by the extensor tendons of the fingers and are devoid of muscular attachments. *Each of these bones has an epiphysis at the distal end only, whereas the phalanges have their single epiphyses at their proximal ends.* At the metacarpophalangeal joints of the fingers, the epiphyseal ends of the metacarpals articulate with the epiphyseal ends of the phalanges, and this circumstance may be associated with the fact that the metacarpophalangeal joints enjoy a wider range of movement than any other digital joint.

The prominence of the knuckles is formed by the distal aspects of the heads of the metacarpal bones.

It should be noted that the tuberosity which marks the distal phalanx of each of the five digits is placed on the *palmar* aspect and has nothing to do with the attachment of the nail.

THE BONES OF THE LOWER LIMB

The Hip Bone

The three constituent parts of the hip bone meet one another in the acetabulum, and, up to the age of twelve, the connecting medium is a *triradiate* piece of *cartilage*, which begins to ossify at that period (Plate IX, p. 64). *By the age of sixteen, the ossification of the acetabulum is complete.* The whole of the floor of the acetabular fossa, including the acetabular notch, belongs to the ischium, as well as the lower two-fifths of the articular surface. The upper and anterior one-fifth of the articular surface belongs to the pubis, and the remainder to the ilium. Apart from the acetabular region, the ilium does not come into contact with the pubis or the ischium, but the inferior pubic ramus meets the ischial ramus and *fuses with it about the eighth year.*

The *bodies* of the two pubic bones articulate with each other at the pubic symphysis. The posterior surface of the body is directed upwards and backwards, and is related to the retropubic fat and the infero-lateral surfaces of the urinary bladder. It gives attachment to the anterior fibres of the levator ani and to the puboprostatic ligaments. The anterior surface faces downwards and laterally towards the adductor region of the thigh. In the angle between the pubic crest and the symphysis it gives origin to the adductor longus and along its medial edge to the gracilis.

The *pubic crest* forms the upper border of the body of the pubis and terminates laterally in the *pubic tubercle*, to which the medial end of the inguinal ligament is attached. The upper border of the superior pubic ramus (*pectineal line*) is sharp and gives attachment at its medial end to the conjoint tendon and to the inguinal and lacunar ligament. The inferior or obturator surface of the superior ramus presents the *obturator groove* for the passage of the obturator vessels and nerve.

The *crest of the ilium* can be felt through the skin over its whole length. The *anterior superior spine* lies at the upper end of the fold of the groin. The *posterior superior spine* can be identified easily, for it lies on a level with the second sacral spine *at the bottom of a small dimple*, which is usually plainly visible in the upper and medial part of the buttock (Plate III, p. 16). *It lies opposite the centre of the sacro-iliac joint*. The *tubercle of the crest* lies 5 cm. behind the anterior superior spine and one hand's breadth above the greater trochanter. The crest possesses outer and inner lips and an intervening intermediate area; to the *outer lip* is attached the fascia lata of the thigh throughout its whole extent. In its anterior half it gives insertion to the external oblique; behind that it gives origin to part of the latissimus dorsi. Between the two it forms the base of the lumbar triangle. The *intermediate area* in its anterior two-thirds gives origin to the internal oblique, and more posteriorly to the lumbar fascia and the sacrospinalis. The *inner lip* in its anterior two-thirds gives origin to the transversus and, just behind that muscle, to the lateral fibres of the quadratus lumborum and the anterior layer of the lumbar fascia. The *anterior inferior spine* is situated too deeply to be palpable through the skin. Its upper part gives attachment to the straight head of the rectus femoris and its lower part, which lies immediately above the hip-joint, to the upper end of the strong iliofemoral ligament.

The *iliac fossa* in its upper two-thirds gives origin to the iliacus muscle. Inferiorly, it is occupied by the iliacus, laterally, and by the psoas major tendon, medially, and these two structures traverse the wide shallow groove which lies between the anterior inferior spine and the iliopubic eminence. The psoas bursa is situated between the tendon and the groove.

The *gluteal surface* is divided into four areas by the three gluteal lines. The *posterior gluteal line* runs upwards and slightly forwards from the neighbourhood of the posterior inferior spine to the crest. The upper part of the area behind it gives origin to the highest fibres of the gluteus maximus; the lower part is smooth and gives attachment to the longest fibres of the sacrotuberous ligament. The *middle gluteal line* begins near the middle of the upper border of the greater sciatic notch and runs forwards and upwards to reach the crest just in front of its tubercle. The area between the middle and posterior gluteal lines and the crest gives origin to the gluteus medius. The *inferior gluteal line* is very indistinct. It runs from the apex of the greater sciatic notch to the notch between the anterior superior and the anterior inferior spines. The area above it gives origin to the gluteus minimus, which covers the bone below it and the groove for the origin of the reflected head of the rectus femoris. Behind the acetabulum the gluteal surface of the ilium becomes continuous with the posterior surface of the body of the ischium, and the site of union is marked by a low rounded elevation, covered in the recent state by the piriformis muscle.

The *sacropelvic surface* of the ilium is divided into three areas. The uppermost is very rough and forms the *iliac tuberosity*, which gives attachment to the posterior sacro-iliac ligaments. The middle area bears the *auricular surface* for articulation with the lateral mass of the sacrum. The lowest area is smooth and featureless and gives partial origin to the obturator internus.

The *ischial spine* is placed on the posterior border of the ischium and intervenes between the greater and the lesser sciatic notches. Its apex and margins give attachment to the sacrospinous ligament and its pelvic surface to the posterior fibres of levator ani and coccygeus. The *ischial tuberosity* caps the posterior aspect of the lower part of the body of the bone. *Its sharp medial edge gives attachment to the sacrotuberous ligament.* Its surface is subdivided into an upper and a lower portion by a transverse ridge. The upper portion is further subdivided by an oblique ridge into an upper and lateral part for the origin of semimembranosus, and a lower and medial part for the semitendinosus and the long head of biceps femoris. (Note that the area for the latter adjoins the attachment of the sacrotuberous ligament, and the fibres of the ligament can often be traced down into the tendon of the biceps femoris). The lower portion of the tuberosity is divided into a lateral area for the origin of the adductor magnus and a medial area, covered by fatty connective tissue containing a bursa, on which the body rests in the sitting posture. The floor of the lesser sciatic notch is smooth and its cartilage-covered surface is grooved by the tendon of obturator internus.

The ramus of the ischium ascends from the lower part of the body to join the ramus of the pubis.

In the erect posture the weight of the body is transmitted through the auricular surface to the ilium and along the region of the iliac part of the arcuate line, which separates the iliac fossa from the sacropelvic surface to the iliac, *i.e.*, the upper part of the acetabulum. *The compact bone of the ilium is thickest along the line of weight transmission.*

The cartilage-covered articular surface of the *acetabulum* forms a horse-shoe shaped strip, deficient below at the acetabular notch. It is deepest in its upper part, where the weight of the trunk is transmitted to the head of the femur in the erect attitude. The acetabular fossa is occupied by a pad of fat covered with synovial membrane. The margins of the acetabulum give attachment to the acetabular labrum, which is continued across the acetabular notch as the transverse ligament. Through the gap between the ligament and the floor of the notch the fat in the fossa becomes continuous with the extra-articular fibro-fatty tissue, and arteries of supply enter the joint from the obturator and the medial circumflex femoral arteries.

Sexual characters are usually strongly marked in the hip bone and *they depend on the necessity for a wider and shorter pelvis in the female.* Some of them (*e.g.*, the size of the subpubic angle) are not easy to gauge in the single hip bone as compared with the articulated pelvis; but the following facts may be found helpful in dealing with a single bone. (1) The male bone is heavier and stronger and the muscular markings are more pronounced. (2) The subpubic angle and the greater sciatic notch are wider (almost 90 degrees) in the female; in the male they are more acute. (3) The acetabulum is smaller in the female, conforming to the size of the femoral head. The breadth of the acetabulum in the female is definitely less than the distance from its anterior margin to the pubic symphyseal surface. In the male the two measurements are nearly equal. (4) The body of the pubis is wide in the female and, consequently, the crest is long, but the depth of the symphysis is less. (5) The anterior superior iliac spines are in-turned in the male, so that the crest, viewed from above, shows a more accentuated curve anteriorly. (6) The presence of a pre-auricular sulcus for the iliac attachment of the lower fibres of the anterior sacro-iliac ligament is much commoner in the female bone. It lies close to the lateral side of the lower part of the auricular surface, between it and the upper border of the greater sciatic notch. (7) The ischiopubic ramus is far more ruggedly marked by the attachment of the crus penis than by the crus clitoridis.

It must be remembered that these features show a wide range of individual variation. Points (3) and (7) are regarded generally as the most reliable basis for identification of sex.

THE PELVIS

In the living body the pelvis is tilted forwards, so that the anterior superior iliac spines lie on or near the same coronal plane as the upper border of the pubic symphysis. As a result the plane of the pelvic inlet makes an angle of from 50 to 60 degrees with the horizontal plane drawn through the pubic crests. On this account, the posterior surfaces of the bodies of the pubic bones look upwards as well as backwards and so help to sustain the downward pressure of the abdominal viscera.

The *pelvic inlet* is bounded behind by the sacral promontory and on each side by the arcuate line. Its transverse diameter is considerably greater than its median antero-posterior measurement. The *pelvic cavity* is a short, curved canal, with a shallow anterior and a much deeper posterior wall. The curve of the cavity reflects the curvature of the sacrum (p. 383). The *pelvic outlet* is of little importance unless the position of the sacrotuberous ligaments is taken into consideration. Together with the ischial and pubic rami, they give the outlet a diamond-shaped outline.

In order that space may be provided for the fœtal head and that its passage through the pelvis may be expedited, *the female pelvis is roomier than the male, and the distance from the inlet to the outlet is appreciably shorter*. When viewed from above and in front, the lateral walls of the female pelvis are seen to be almost parallel to each other, whereas in the male pelvis they converge towards the outlet. *The female pelvic cavity can be likened to a short segment of a long cone, the male to a long segment of a short cone.*

The Femur

The rounded *head* of the femur is securely gripped by the acetabular labrum *beyond its maximum diameter*. In the erect posture its upper aspect is pressed against the iliac part of the acetabular articular surface. *The head forms a separate epiphysis and the epiphyseal cartilage separates it from the neck of the bone* (Plate IX, p. 64). This *epiphysis* ossifies at the end of the first year and joins the shaft about eighteen or nineteen. *It is entirely intracapsular.*

The *neck*, which ossifies as an upward extension of the shaft, passes downward, backwards and laterally and makes an angle of about 125 degrees (rather less in the female) with the long axis of the shaft. *The anterior surface of the neck lies entirely within the capsular ligament of the hip-joint,* which is attached laterally to the trochanteric line. On the posterior aspect, the capsular ligament and the synovial membrane cover the neck in its medial part but never extend so far as the intertrochanteric crest. *This aspect is therefore partly intra- and partly extra-capsular.*

The *greater trochanter* can be felt through the skin, a hand's breadth below the iliac crest. It has a separate centre of ossification, and its epiphysis includes the attachments of the gluteus minimus in front, gluteus medius on the lateral side, piriformis and obturator internus on its free upper border, and obturator externus in the trochanteric fossa.

The *lesser trochanter* cannot be palpated in the living subject. It gives attachment to the tendon of psoas major and forms a scale-like epiphysis between the fourteenth and eighteenth years.

The *intertrochanteric line* crosses the front of the upper end of the shaft. *It gives attachment to the capsular ligament, and the upper and lower parts of the iliofemoral ligament of the hip-joint.* Below and medially it runs into the *spiral line,* which passes below the lesser trochanter and reaches the medial lip of the linea aspera. The origin of the vastus medialis follows the lower part of the intertrochanteric line and the spiral line to the linea aspera. The *intertrochanteric crest* crosses the posterior aspect of the bone and runs into the lesser trochanter below. A small rounded tubercle about its middle gives insertion to quadratus femoris.

To the *linea aspera* are attached the vasti, the adductors and the short head of biceps femoris. *In this situation the compact bone shows a marked thickening,* to compensate for the forward curve of the shaft. The lateral lip is continued upwards into the roughened *gluteal tuberosity,* which gives attachment to the lower and deeper fibres of the gluteus maximus. The upper end of the tuberosity sometimes forms a distinct roughened elevation, termed the *third trochanter.* The medial edge of the tuberosity gives insertion to the upper, horizontal fibres of the adductor magnus, and its lateral edge gives origin to the vastus lateralis. The interval between the spiral line and the gluteal tuberosity gives insertion to the pectineus medially, and the adductor brevis laterally.

The medial aspect of the shaft is devoid of muscular attachments. Inferiorly, the linea aspera divides into the *lateral* and *medial supracondylar lines,* which enclose the *popliteal surface* of the femur. A roughened area marks the lower and medial part of the popliteal surface; it gives origin to the medial head of gastrocnemius. The medial supracondylar line can be traced down to the *adductor tubercle* (Plate XI, p. 60), which is the highest point on the medial epicondyle. *This bony point is subcutaneous* and can be identified most easily in the living subject when it is approached from above. It gives attachment to the tendon of the adductor magnus.

The lower end of the femur ossifies from a singe centre which appears during the *ninth month of intrauterine life* and joins the shaft about the twenty-first year. On the medial side, the epiphyseal line passes through the adductor tubercle. Immediately below the tubercle, the medial epicondyle, which is subcutaneous, gives attachment to the upper end of the medial ligament of the knee joint. The lateral ligament of the knee-joint is attached to the lateral epicondyle, and below it the lateral condyle is marked by the groove for the popliteus tendon, which lies within the capsule of the knee-joint (p. 75). This muscle arises from the anterior end of the groove and occupies its posterior part in full flexion only. Above the lateral epicondyle the lateral aspect of the condyle is marked by a muscular impression, which gives origin to the lateral head of gastrocnemius.

The articular surfaces of the condyles are crossed anteriorly by faintly marked curved grooves which correspond to the semilunar cartilages. The periphery of the cartilage fits into the groove only in full extension. These grooves therefore separate the patellar from the tibial surfaces. The lateral tibial surface is wider and straighter than the medial tibial surface, which curves medially as it passes backwards. The *intercondylar line* gives attachment to the posterior part of the capsular ligament and laterally to the oblique posterior ligament of the knee-joint. The *intercondylar fossa* is occupied by the cruciate ligaments. The anterior cruciate ligament is attached to the medial aspect of the lateral condyle, while the posterior is attached to the lateral aspect of the medial condyle.

The Patella

This little bone functions as a sesamoid bone in the tendon of the quadriceps femoris, and its anterior surface is easily felt through the skin, from which it is separated partly by the subcutaneous prepatellar bursa. X-ray photographs show that the line of the knee-joint lies below the patella and intersects the line of the ligamentum patellæ at or a little above its middle. The femoral articular surface covers all but the projecting lower part of the deep surface. It is subdivided by a vertical ridge into a *larger lateral and a smaller medial area.* A small strip at the medial side of the medial area comes into contact with the medial femoral condyle in full flexion of the knee. Below the articular surface the bone is roughened and non-articular. The lower half of this area covers the posterior aspect of the apex and gives attachment to the ligamentum (tendo) patellæ. The upper, lateral and medial margins of the bone give insertion to the rectus femoris and the vasti.

The Tibia

The *upper end* of the tibia is greatly expanded to provide a good bearing surface for the lower end of the femur, and its lateral and medial condyles can be felt through the skin. The anterior margin of the lateral condyle can be felt in the depression which lies to the lateral side of the upper end of the ligamentum patellæ when the knee is passively flexed, and the border of the medial condyle can be felt in the corresponding depression on the medial side, but not so distinctly. *These edges indicate the level of the knee-joint.*

The superior articular surface is divided into two by a non-articular *intercondylar area*, which is narrow in the centre and widens out in front and behind. The central part of this area is marked by the lateral and medial intercondylar tubercles, which are formed by the raised adjoining margins of the two articular surfaces. The intercondylar area gives attachment to the horns of the semilunar cartilages and the cruciate ligaments.

The posterior margin of the lateral condyle shows a faint groove due to the pressure of the popliteus tendon and, lateral to this groove, its projecting part bears on its under surface a circular articular facet for the head of the fibula.

The *tibial tuberosity*, which is rough and subcutaneous in its inferior part, gives attachment on its smooth upper part to the ligamentum patellæ (which is in reality the *tendon* of the quadriceps).

The postero-medial aspect of the medial condyle shows a transverse groove, to which the semimembranosus is attached.

The centre of ossification for the upper end of the tibia appears very early, *just before or very soon after birth.* The upper epiphysis includes both condyles and extends downwards in front to include the tibial tubercle, which may occasionally possess a separate centre of ossification. This epiphysis does not join the shaft until the twentieth year.

The medial, subcutaneous, surface of the shaft of the tibia is smooth everywhere except at the most posterior part of its upper end. In this situation a slightly roughened strip extends downwards for 5 or 6 cm. from the lower border of the medial condyle. It gives attachment to the medial ligament of the knee-joint. The sartorius, gracilis and semitendinosus are inserted a little in front of this area.

The *soleal line* crosses the upper part of the posterior surface obliquely downwards and medially; it gives origin to soleus and attachment to the fascia covering the popliteus. The vertical line which descends from it separates the origin of flexor digitorum longus, on the medial side, from the tibial origin of tibialis posterior, on the lateral side. The interosseous border is scarcely discernible at its upper end, where there is a wide gap in the interosseous membrane for the passage of the anterior tibial vessels.

The *medial malleolus* can be palpated without difficulty. It lies somewhat anterior to the lateral malleolus and does not extend so far downwards. Its pitted apex gives attachment to the deltoid ligament of the ankle-joint, and its posterior aspect is grooved by the tendon of tibialis posterior. The lateral aspect of the lower end of the tibia is roughened for the attachment of the interosseous tibiofibular ligament. The posterior aspect may show a shallow groove at its lateral part for the tendon of flexor hallucis longus, but the flexor digitorum longus tendon does not mark the bone.

The lower end forms a substantial epiphysis, which includes the medial malleolus. Its centre of ossification appears early (second year) and it fuses with the shaft about the eighteenth year.

The Fibula

The *head* of the fibula possesses an articular surface which is directed *upwards and slightly forwards and medially* to articulate with the under aspect of the posterior part of the lateral condyle of the tibia. It can be felt through the skin on the *postero-lateral aspect of the knee, below the level of the joint*. At the same time the student should identify the lateral popliteal nerve, which can be rolled against the postero-lateral aspect of the bone immediately below the head. The styloid process projects upwards from the postero-lateral aspect of the head. It is usually a rounded elevation, showing an impression on its anterior aspect for the tendon of biceps femoris and the attachment of the lateral ligament of the knee-joint (p. 87).

The student often experiences difficulty in assigning a fibula to its correct side and in identifying the various surfaces of the shaft. The ends can always be differentiated by examination of their articular surfaces, which face in different directions. The articular surface of the head, as already stated, is directed upwards, and slightly forwards and medially; *that on the lower end faces medially*, is somewhat triangular in outline and is slightly convex from above downwards; further, a non-articular depression marks the bone behind it (*vide infra*). The subcutaneous lateral surface of the lateral malleolus is continuous above with an *elongated triangular area on the shaft, which is also subcutaneous.* From the apex of this triangle the anterior border of the bone passes upwards, separating the peroneal surface on the lateral side from the extensor surface on the medial side.

The shaft of the fibula shows considerable variation. It may be flattened from side to side, or it may be compressed from before backwards. The former variety is the commoner. *The extensor surface*, which gives origin to extensor digitorum longus, extensor hallucis longus and peroneus tertius, *is exceedingly narrow in its upper part* where its boundaries—the anterior and the interosseous borders of the bone—may run into each other. It is wider below.

The lateral (peroneal) surface is grooved and gives origin to the peroneus longus and brevis. Inferiorly, this surface curves so as to pass behind the lateral malleolus. The posterior (flexor) surface is very extensive, and is subdivided into two areas by the *medial crest*. The slightly hollowed-out area in front of the medial crest extends forwards as far as the interosseous border and gives origin to the tibialis posterior muscle. *The medial crest is closely related to the peroneal artery.*

The *lateral malleolus* can be palpated without difficulty and traced upwards into the triangular area, referred to above. The anterior margin of this triangular area gives attachment, below, to the upper extensor retinaculum. The triangular articular facet of the malleolus articulates with the lateral aspect of the body of the talus. The roughened area above it gives attachment to the interosseous tibiofibular ligament. The depression behind and below the articular facet, termed the *malleolar fossa*, gives attachment above to the transverse inferior tibiofibular ligament, and below to the posterior talofibular ligament. The anterior margin of the lateral malleolus gives attachment to the anterior talofibular ligament, and the depression just in front of the apex of the malleolus to the calcaneofibular ligament.

Although, as a general rule in long bones, the epiphysis which begins to ossify first is the last to join the shaft, the lower epiphysis of the fibula, which begins to ossify in the second year, joins the shaft about the eighteenth year, whereas the upper epiphysis, which does not begin to ossify until the fifth year, does not unite with the shaft until some time between the twentieth and twenty-fifth years.

The Tarsus

The student has already revised the arches of the foot (p. 94), and he would be well advised to study the articulated foot and observe how the arches are built up. The position of the talus relative to the calcaneum and the shapes of the cuneiform bones and of the bases of the metatarsals are important points to observe.

The **calcaneus** is the largest bone of the tarsus. *Its long axis is directed forwards and laterally* (Plate XIV, p. 92), and its small anterior aspect is covered by an obliquely set concavoconvex articular facet for the cuboid. The medial surface is hollowed out and *is overhung by the projecting sustentaculum tali* (Plate XIII, p. 92). The superior surface presents, about its middle, a large, oval, convex facet for the body of the talus.

In the upright posture it is only the tuberculated posterior part of the *plantar surface* that rests on the ground. To the tubercles, of which the medial is the larger, the superficial layer of muscles in the sole of the foot and the plantar aponeurosis are attached. In front of the tubercles an elongated rough area gives attachment to the long plantar ligament; this area is limited in front by the anterior tubercle, to which the short plantar ligament is attached.

The *medial surface* is concave from above downwards and backwards, and the *sustentaculum tali projects from its upper border.* Its upper aspect is covered by an elongated oval articular facet for the inferior surface of the head of the talus. Anteriorly, it gives attachment to the plantar calcaneonavicular ligament, which passes forwards below the infero-medial part of the head of the talus to reach the navicular bone. Its medial aspect receives fibres of the deltoid ligament above, and, below, the bone is in contact with the tendon of the flexor digitorum longus. Occasionally this tendon lies in a shallow groove. The medial aspect of the sustentaculum tali lies a little more than 1 cm. below the tip of the medial malleolus, and it can be felt indistinctly in this situation in the living subject. The inferior surface of the sustentaculum tali is marked by a groove for the tendon of the flexor hallucis longus, which is directly continuous with the groove on the posterior aspect of the talus.

The *lateral surface* of the calcaneus is flattened and non-articular, and may show two small elevations. The *peroneal tubercle* lies on the anterior part of this surface, almost directly below the lateral tubercle of the talus. It varies considerably in size. When well developed, it shows a groove on its upper surface for the peroneus brevis, and a groove on its lower surface for the peroneus longus tendon. The second elevation, low and rounded, is situated more posteriorly and gives attachment to the calcaneofibular ligament.

The *posterior surface* is divided into three areas. The uppermost area is covered by a bursa, which separates it from the tendo calcaneus; the middle area gives insertion to that tendon, and, on its medial side, to the plantaris; the lowest area is covered with a pad of fat in which a second bursa may be present.

The *superior surface* is covered about its middle by a convex oval facet for articulation with the body of the talus. Behind that the bone supports a mass of fibro-fatty tissue which intervenes between the tendo calcaneus and the back of the ankle-joint. In front, the superior surface is partly articular and partly rough. The articular facet is borne almost entirely by the sustentaculum tali. Between it and the facet for the body of the talus the interosseous talocalcaneal ligament is attached. In front and laterally, the inferior extensor retinaculum and the extensor digitorum brevis are attached to the bone.

The **talus** has a somewhat rounded *head,* directed forwards, medially and downwards to articulate with the navicular. The *upper surface* of the body is covered with a large trochlear facet for the tibia, continuous on the *lateral surface* with a large, triangular articular facet for the lateral malleolus.

The articular surface of the *head* is carried round on to its inferior surface, *where it rests on the plantar calcaneonavicular ligament in front and on the sustentaculum tali behind.* The upper aspect of the *neck* lies within the capsular ligament of the ankle-joint; its lower aspect is deeply grooved and gives attachment to the interosseous talocalcanea ligament. In the articulated foot this groove forms part of a bony tunnel, termed the *sinus tarsi.*

The trochlear facet for the tibia on the *superior surface* is wider in front than behind, a point of considerable importance from a practical point of view. The *lateral surface* is covered by the facet mentioned above. It is slightly concave from above downwards, and its lower part forms the *lateral tubercle,* which gives attachment to the lateral talocalcanean ligament. Its anterior border gives attachment above to the anterior talofibular ligament. The *medial surface* presents, above, a comma-shaped articular facet for the medial malleolus, which is deeper in front than behind. Below the facet the bone is rough for the attachment of the deeper fibres of the deltoid ligament.

The *posterior aspect* of the talus is marked by a groove which runs obliquely downwards and medially, curving forwards below, to become continuous with a groove on the under aspect of the sustentaculum tali. This groove lodges the tendon of the flexor hallucis longus. On the talus it lies between the posterior tubercle on the lateral side, and the medial tubercle on the medial side. The *posterior tubercle* is the larger and may ossify from a separate centre. When that happens, the tubercle may remain throughout life as a separate ossicle, termed the *os trigonum,* which is connected to the rest of the bone by a thin plate of cartilage. It gives attachment to the posterior talofibular ligament.

The *inferior surface* is covered by a concave facet, oval in outline, which articulates with the corresponding facet on the superior surface of the calcaneus.

The remaining bones of the tarsus need less detailed description.

The *tuberosity of the navicular bone* projects downwards immediately in front of the head of the talus; it gives insertion to a part of the tibialis posterior. The tuberosity can be felt through the skin on the medial border of the foot, about 2.5 cm. in front of the medial malleolus, on a slightly lower level. A flattened impression marks the antero-inferior part of the medial aspect of the *medial cuneiform bone*. Together with the adjoining part of the base of the first metatarsal, it gives insertion to the tibialis anterior tendon.

The tuberosity of the navicular bone overhangs a shallow groove on the medial part of the inferior surface of the bone. This groove contains slips of the tibialis posterior tendon which run forwards to be attached to the cuneiform and cuboid bones and the bases of the middle three metatarsal bones. The posterior border of the plantar surface of the navicular gives attachment to the anterior extremity of the plantar calcaneonavicular or "spring" ligament, which contains little or no elastic tissue.

The inferior surface of the *cuboid bone* is marked by an oblique ridge, which may be faceted at its lateral end, where it is in contact with the sesamoid bone in the peroneus longus tendon. The tendon itself occupies the medial part of the groove which lies in front of the ridge, crosses the plantar aspects of the lateral and intermediate cuneiform bones and is inserted into a roughened area on the antero-inferior part of the lateral aspect of the medial cuneiform and the adjoining part of the base of the first metatarsal.

The tarsus, unlike the carpus, is partly ossified at birth. Large ossific nuclei are present in the calcaneus and the talus, and the centre of ossification for the cuboid bone, if not present at birth, appears very soon after. By the end of the fourth year ossification is in progress in all the tarsal bones. *Only one*, viz., *the calcaneus, normally possesses an epiphysis.* It forms the posterior surface below the bursal area, and the adjoining part of the plantar surface. The centre of ossification appears about the sixth or seventh year and joins the rest of the bone at puberty.

The Metatarsus

The metatarsal bones resemble the metacarpals in a general way, and their mode of ossification is similar (p. 409). With the exception of the first, the metatarsals are more slender and taper towards their heads. *The first metatarsal plays a very important part in supporting the weight of the body, in standing, walking and running, and it is proportionately large and strong.* At its base it articulates with the medial cuneiform bone by means of a large kidney-shaped facet, the notch of which is placed on the lateral side. The bases of the first and second metatarsals do not articulate with each other, although a pressure facet may indicate where they come into contact. *The head of the first metatarsal shows two grooves on its plantar aspect, produced by the sesamoid bones incorporated in the tendons of the flexor hallucis brevis.* (Though doubtless of considerable functional importance, the role of sesamoids in general is still uncertain.)

The *second metatarsal* is the longest of the metatarsal bones and its base projects backwards further than any of the others so that it interrupts the line of the tarsometatarsal joints (p. 94).

The *fifth metatarsal* is flattened from above downwards. The *tubercle* on its base projects backwards and laterally and can be palpated without difficulty. To it is attached the peroneus brevis tendon. The plantar surface of the base presents a grooved area medial to the tubercle for the flexor digiti minimi brevis.

INDEX